The Changing World of Inflammatory Bowel Disease

IMPACT OF GENERATION, GENDER, AND GLOBAL TRENDS

The Changing World of Inflammatory Bowel Disease

IMPACT OF GENERATION, GENDER, AND GLOBAL TRENDS

ELLEN J. SCHERL, MD, FACP, AGAF

Director,
Inflammatory Bowel Disease Center

Associate Professor of
Clinical Medicine

Weill Medical College of
Cornell University

New York Presbyterian Hospital

Adjunct Associate Professor

Columbia University Medical School

New York, New York

MARLA C. DUBINSKY, MD

Associate Professor of Pediatrics

David Geffen School of Medicine, UCLA

Director,
Pediatric IBD Center

Cedars-Sinai Medical Center

Los Angeles, California

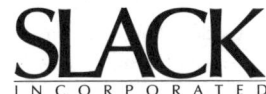

SLACK
INCORPORATED

www.slackbooks.com

ISBN: 978-1-55642-841-8

Copyright © 2009 by SLACK Incorporated

The procedures and practices described in this book should be implemented in a manner consistent with the professional standards set for the circumstances that apply in each specific situation. Every effort has been made to confirm the accuracy of the information presented and to correctly relate generally accepted practices. The authors, editor, and publisher cannot accept responsibility for errors or exclusions or for the outcome of the material presented herein. There is no expressed or implied warranty of this book or information imparted by it. Care has been taken to ensure that drug selection and dosages are in accordance with currently accepted/recommended practice. Due to continuing research, changes in government policy and regulations, and various effects of drug reactions and interactions, it is recommended that the reader carefully review all materials and literature provided for each drug, especially those that are new or not frequently used. Any review or mention of specific companies or products is not intended as an endorsement by the author or publisher.

SLACK Incorporated uses a review process to evaluate submitted material. Prior to publication, educators or clinicians provide important feedback on the content that we publish. We welcome feedback on this work.

Published by: SLACK Incorporated
                 6900 Grove Road
                 Thorofare, NJ 08086 USA
                 Telephone: 856-848-1000
                 Fax: 856-853-5991
                 www.slackbooks.com

Contact SLACK Incorporated for more information about other books in this field or about the availability of our books from distributors outside the United States.

Library of Congress Cataloging-in-Publication Data

The changing world of inflammatory bowel disease : impact of generation, gender, and global trends / edited by Ellen J. Scherl, Marla C. Dubinsky.
       p. ; cm.
    Includes bibliographical references and index.
    ISBN 978-1-55642-841-8 (alk. paper)
    1. Inflammatory bowel diseases--Epidemiology. I. Scherl, Ellen J. II. Dubinsky, Marla.
    [DNLM: 1. Inflammatory Bowel Diseases--epidemiology. 2. Age Factors. 3. Sex Factors. WI 420 C456 2009]
    RA645.I53C43 2009
    362.196'344--dc22
                                          2009019079

Last digit is print number: 10   9   8   7   6   5   4   3   2   1

Dedication

I dedicate this book to my husband, Fredric Harbus, and children, Michael and Carolyn Harbus, who continue to be my guiding light, best friends, and secret weapons in the fight against inflammatory bowel disease. I would also like to dedicate this book to my mother, Lila Scherl, and in memory of my father, Siegfried Scherl, MD.

Ellen J. Scherl, MD, FACP, AGAF

I would like to dedicate this book to my family and mentors who continue to guide and support me in my career and help shape my vision of managing the life cycle of IBD.

Marla C. Dubinsky, MD

Contents

Acknowledgments

We would like to acknowledge those committed to our patients and families living with inflammatory bowel disease, including the following associations and individuals:

* Crohn's and Colitis Foundation of America and their founders, Henry D. Janowitz, MD; Irwin M. and Suzanne Rosenthal; and William D. and Shelby Modell

* WE CARE and its officers, including Judith F. Collins, MD; Sunanda V. Kane, MD, MSPH,; Sonia Friedman, MD; Uma Mahadevan, MD; Maria T. Abreu, MD; Kim L. Isaacs, MD, PhD; and Jane Elizabeth Onken, MD

* New York Crohn's Foundation, including the Litwin and Kerr families

* Jill Roberts and her family

* The contributing authors who made this book a reality

* The staff at SLACK Incorporated, including Carrie Kotlar, Acquisitions Editor; April Billick, Senior Project Editor; and Debra Toulson, Managing Editor, as well as Kristin Della Volpe, Freelance Editor. Without their tireless work and dedication, this book would not be possible

About the Editors

Ellen J. Scherl, MD, FACP, AGAF, is the Jill Roberts Associate Professor of Clinical Medicine and Director of The Roberts Center for Inflammatory Bowel Disease at Weill Medical College of Cornell University/New York-Presbyterian Hospital. She holds a Bachelor's degree in English from Barnard College, Columbia University, and a medical degree from New York Medical College. She is a fellow of the American College of Physicians and the American Gastroenterological Association (AGA), a member of the American Society of Gastrointestinal Endoscopy, and a past president of the New York Society for Gastrointestinal Endoscopy (NYSGE). She is currently Vice President of the New York Academy of Gastroenterology.

Dr. Scherl is Chairperson of the New York Chapter of the Crohn's and Colitis Foundation of America and is involved in the New York Crohn's Foundation. She received the 2008 AGA Outstanding Women in Science award, 2006 NYSGE Florence Lefcourt Distinguished Service Award, and has been awarded by the Crohn's and Colitis Foundation of America. She is an American Society of Gastrointestinal Endoscopy Circle of Life Member and a member of the AGA Legacy Society. She is board certified in medicine and gastroenterology.

Dr. Scherl is an editorial reviewer for *IBD Journal, Journal of Clinical Gastroenterology, Gastrointestinal Endoscopy, Digestive Diseases and Sciences*, and *Journal of Gastroenterology and Hepatology*. She is coauthor of the chapter "Crohn's Disease of the Small Intestine" in *Gastroenterology and Hepatology: The Comprehensive Visual Reference*, associate editor of *Inflammatory Bowel Disease: The Complete Guide to Medical Management*, and coauthor of *An Interactive Dialogue on IBD*.

Dr. Scherl established the first IBD tissue bank in New York City at Weill Medical College of Cornell University/New York-Presbyterian Hospital. She has extensive experience as an investigator in clinical trials and is currently participating in national multicenter trials and in investigator-initiated trials focusing on ulcerative colitis and Crohn's disease.

Marla C. Dubinsky, MD received a medical degree from Queen's University in Canada and completed her clinical pediatric gastroenterology training at Sainte-Justine Hospital, University of Montreal in Quebec, Canada. Currently, Dr. Dubinsky is Director of the Pediatric Inflammatory Bowel Disease Center at Cedars-Sinai Medical Center in Los Angeles, CA. In addition, Dr. Dubinsky is Associate Professor of Pediatrics at the University of California, Los Angeles, David Geffen School of Medicine.

Board certified in pediatrics and pediatric gastroenterology, Dr. Dubinsky holds positions of prominence with several advisory bodies, including Chair of the Western Regional Pediatric IBD Research Alliance. She is a member of several professional societies, including the American Gastroenterology Association, the American College of Gastroenterology, and the American Academy of Pediatrics. Among her many awards, Dr. Dubinsky was a Crohn's and Colitis Foundation of America Medical Honoree in 2004 and recently received the Lenny and Corinne Sands Clinical Investigator Award.

Dr. Dubinsky's main research interests are health outcomes and the epidemiology and genetic influences of inflammatory bowel disease (IBD) in children. Her objective is to study the influence of genetics and immune responses on the variability in clinical presentations of early-onset IBD. Additional interests include the study of pharmacogenetics to evaluate how heredity influences drug responses and optimizing and individualizing the management of IBD. Dr. Dubinsky's work has been published in numerous peer-reviewed journals, including *Gastroenterology, The Journal of Pediatric Gastroenterology and Nutrition, Inflammatory Bowel Diseases*, and the *American Journal of Gastroenterology*. In addition, she has authored book chapters for *Trends in Inflammatory Bowel Disease Therapy* and *Inflammatory Bowel Disease: Diagnosis and Therapeutics*. Dr. Dubinsky has lectured widely both nationally and internationally.

Contributing Authors

Maria T. Abreu, MD (Chapter 14)
Professor of Medicine
Chief, Division of Gastroenterology
University of Miami Miller School of
Medicine
Miami, Florida

Devendra K. Amre (Chapter 4)
Research Center, Sainte Justine Hospital
Department of Pediatrics
University of Montreal
Montreal, Quebec, Canada

Daisy Batista, MD (Chapter 2)
Senior Resident
Massachusetts General Hospital
Harvard Medical School
Boston, Massachusetts

Wallace V. Crandall, MD (Chapter 10)
Director, The Center for Pediatric and
Adolescent Inflammatory Bowel Disease
Associate Director, Pediatric Gastroenterology
Fellowship Training Program
Nationwide Children's Hospital
Associate Professor of Clinical Pediatrics
The Ohio State University College of
Medicine
Columbus, Ohio

Lee A. Denson, MD (Chapter 3)
Associate Professor, Pediatrics
Cincinnati Children's Hospital Medical Center
University of Cincinnati College of Medicine
Cincinnati, Ohio

William Faubion, MD (Chapter 6)
Department of Internal Medicine
Division of Gastroenterology
Mayo Clinic
Rochester, Minnesota

Sonia Friedman, MD (Chapter 13)
Assistant Professor of Medicine
Harvard Medical School
Boston, Massachusetts

Kim L. Isaacs, MD, PhD (Chapter 12)
Professor of Medicine
University of North Carolina at Chapel Hill
Division of Gastroenterology and Hepatology
Chapel Hill, North Carolina

Tine Jess, MD, DrMedSci (Chapter 1)
Associate Professor
Institute of Preventive Medicine
Copenhagen University Hospital
Copenhagen, Denmark

Sunanda Kane, MD, MSPH, FACG, FACP, AGAF
(Chapter 15)
Mayo Clinic
Rochester, Minnesota

Joshua Korzenik, MD (Chapter 2)
Co-Director, MGH Crohn's and Colitis
Center
Massachusetts General Hospital
Harvard Medical School
Boston, Massachusetts

Oren L. Koslowe, MD (Chapter 9)
Department of Pediatrics
Division of Pediatric Gastroenterology and
Nutrition
New York-Presbyterian Hospital-Weill Cornell
Medical College
New York, New York

Subra Kugathasan, MD (Chapter 5)
Division of Pediatric Gastroenterology
Department of Pediatrics
Medical College of Wisconsin &
Children's Research Institute
Milwaukee, Wisconsin

Fabrizio Michelassi, MD (Chapter 18)
Lewis Atterbury Stimson Professor
Chairman, Department of Surgery
Surgeon-in-Chief
New York-Presbyterian Hospital-Weill Cornell
Medical College
New York, NY

Darrell S. Pardi, MD (Chapter 16)
Inflammatory Bowel Disease Clinic
Miles and Shirley Fiterman Center for Digestive
Diseases
Mayo Clinic College of Medicine
Rochester, Minnesota

Robert James Pattison (Chapter 5)
Division of Pediatric Gastroenterology
Department of Pediatrics
Medical College of Wisconsin &
Children's Research Institute
Milwaukee, Wisconsin

David T. Rubin, MD, FACG, AGAF (Chapter 17)
Associate Professor of Medicine
Co-Director, Inflammatory Bowel Disease
Center
University of Chicago Medical Center
Chicago, Illinois

John M. Russo, MD (Chapter 10)
Nationwide Children's Hospital
Assistant Professor of Clinical Pediatrics
The Ohio State University College of
Medicine
Columbus, Ohio

Ernest G. Seidman, MD (Chapter 4)
Division of Gastroenterology
Montreal Children's Hospital
Departments of Medicine and Pediatrics
McGill University
Montreal, Quebec, Canada

Corey A. Siegel, MD (Chapter 19)
Assistant Professor of Medicine
Dartmouth Medical School
Director, Dartmouth-Hitchcock IBD Center
Section of Gastroenterology and Hepatology
Dartmouth-Hitchcock Medical Center
Lebanon, New Hampshire

Robbyn E. Sockolow, MD (Chapter 9)
Department of Pediatrics
Division of Pediatric Gastroenterology and
Nutrition
New York Presbyterian Hospital-Weill Cornell
Medical College
New York, New York

Aliza B. Solomon, DO (Chapter 9)
Department of Pediatrics
Division of Pediatric Gastroenterology and
Nutrition
New York Presbyterian Hospital-Weill Cornell
Medical College
New York, New York

Sharon L. Stein, MD (Chapter 18)
Assistant Professor of Surgery
Case Western Reserve University
Division of Colorectal Surgery
University Hospitals, Case Medical Center
Cleveland, Ohio

Michael C. Stephens, MD, FAAP (Chapter 7)
Medical Director, Pediatric Inflammatory
Bowel Disease Program
Children's Hospital of Wisconsin
Assistant Professor of Pediatrics
Medical College of Wisconsin & Children's
Research Institute
Milwaukee, Wisconsin

Francisco A. Sylvester, MD (Chapter 8)
Associate Professor of Pediatrics
University of Connecticut School of Medicine
Pediatric Gastroenterologist
Connecticut Children's Medical Center
Hartford, Connecticut

Amy B. Trachter, PsyD, PhD (Chapter 11)
Private Practice
New City, NY

Yuki Young, MD (Chapter 14)
Clinical Instructor
Division of Gastroenterology
Mount Sinai School of Medicine
New York, New York

Foreword

Inflammatory bowel disease (IBD), specifically Crohn's disease and ulcerative colitis, represent chronic idiopathic inflammatory intestinal disorders marked by cyclical periods of symptomatic intestinal inflammation and remittance. Since Drs. Burrill Crohn, Leon Ginzburg, and Gordon Oppenheimer's initial description of Crohn's disease in 1932 and Sir Samuel Wilks and W. Moxon's original description of ulcerative colitis in 1875, much has been learned about these two disorders. Both occur worldwide and spare no socioeconomic group. These diseases have been estimated to afflict nearly 1.4 million people in the United States and 2.2 million Europeans.[1] There is no known cure for these chronic and potentially debilitating diseases, although patients with ulcerative colitis can undergo a total colectomy to remove the affected organ. Colectomy is not curative in patients with Crohn's disease since inflammation can recur anywhere throughout the gastrointestinal tract, and most often recurs postsurgically at the site of the anastomosis. Current medical therapy for IBD is aimed at alleviating symptoms and inducing a state of remission. Recent scientific and technological advances have not only promoted a greater understanding of the pathogenesis underlying these disorders, but have also led to the discovery and use of new medications for the treatment of inflammatory bowel disease.

In this book East coast meets West coast; Dr. Ellen J. Scherl and Dr. Marla C. Dubinsky join together and compile an enormously successful comprehensive textbook. This unique textbook focuses on the patient life cycle as it relates to IBD. Dr. Scherl and Dr. Dubinsky cover the continuum of inflammatory bowel disease from the pediatrics to the elderly. An overview of the epidemiology and immunology of IBD is initially reviewed. Then, they highlight areas of intense interest to the reader—sex, fertility, pregnancy, and even menopause. Additionally, pediatric and adolescent patients are focused upon as related to the natural history of disease, medical therapy, genetics, and bone disease.

A vast amount of clinical trial literature in IBD is evidence based. The use of an evidence-based approach to objectively evaluate the quality of clinical research by critically assessing techniques reported by researchers in their publications has been the primary approach. To exclusively rely upon this approach is near sighted. Dr. Scherl and Dr. Dubinsky astutely recognized this. They have ventured into arenas where controlled trial data are sparse yet clinical experience is rich; they rely on the experience and the ability of their nationally recognized expert authors to recount personal experiences and in this manner they offer clinical guidance to the readership for management of specific clinical scenarios.

The authors and editors should be congratulated for their accomplishment. They have assimilated a textbook that is likely to be in press for a long time and with many forthcoming editions. This book is a "must have" for people who desire a book focused on these specific aspects of IBD.

Reference

1. Loftus E. Clinical epidemiology of inflammatory bowel disease: incidence, prevalence, and environmental influences. *Gastroenterology.* 2004;126:1504-1517.

Gary R. Lichtenstein, MD, FACP, FACG, AGAF
Professor of Medicine
University of Pennsylvania School of Medicine
Director, Center for Inflammatory Bowel Disease
Department of Medicine
Division of Gastroenterology
Philadelphia, Pennsylvania

Preface

With the changing diagnostic and therapeutic options for patients with inflammatory bowel disease (IBD), the greatest challenge for clinicians is to move from symptom-oriented step-up strategies toward proactive preventive-oriented (early intervention) approaches aimed at altering the natural history of IBD. Major progress has been made in both the diagnosis and treatment of IBD, resulting in a better quality of life for individuals affected by Crohn's disease and ulcerative colitis. Despite these advances, many questions remain unanswered regarding the developmental history, epidemiology, pathogenesis, genetic and immune mechanisms of these diseases, and disease-modifying potential of IBD therapies.

IBD does not discriminate based on age, gender, or socioeconomic class. *The Changing World of Inflammatory Bowel Disease: Impact of Generation, Gender, and Global Trends* will feature new information on how IBD progresses through the life cycle of patients with these diseases. Age of onset influences the phenotypic variability, and early onset, or childhood onset, IBD appears to be one of the fastest growing populations of interest. Similarly, novel populations, such as the rising incidence in the developing world, generate questions as to the influence of the environment on diverse genetic backgrounds and the life cycle of the disease.

A female patient's journey from menarche to menopause will be highlighted in this book. The authors address issues ranging from those pertinent to female adolescents with IBD to those of women with IBD inquiring about conception and pregnancy. The purpose of *The Changing World of Inflammatory Bowel Disease* is to describe the exciting advances in our understanding of disease pathogenesis, epidemiology, natural history, the life cycle of disease, and the population it impacts in the context of rapidly changing diagnostic and therapeutic approaches.

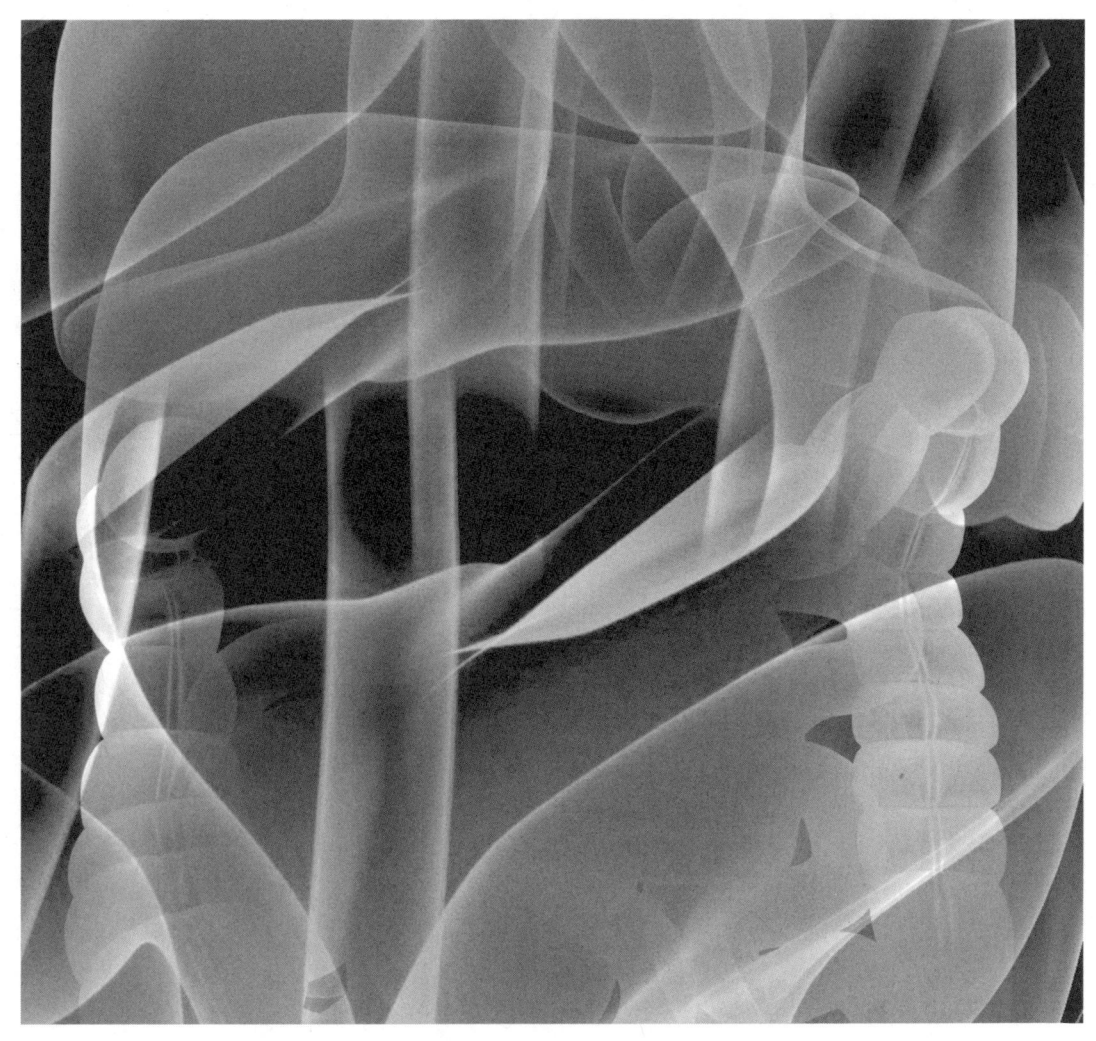

SECTION I

INTRODUCTION TO THE LIFE CYCLE OF INFLAMMATORY BOWEL DISEASE

CHAPTER 1

EPIDEMIOLOGY OF THE LIFE CYCLE OF INFLAMMATORY BOWEL DISEASE

Tine Jess, MD, DrMedSci

Epidemiology is the study of diseases in human populations and describes features such as occurrence, course, and prognosis of disease. Although ulcerative colitis (UC) and Crohn's disease have been recognized as disease entities since the 19th and early 20th centuries, respectively,[1] it was not until the 1960s that epidemiological methods were properly implemented in research on inflammatory bowel disease (IBD). It was Truelove and colleagues who recognized the importance of using diagnostically well-defined and unselected patient cohorts for studies on the course and prognosis of IBD.[2,3] The reaching of an international consensus on diagnostic criteria for the 2 diseases[4] has made comparison and generalization of epidemiological data on patients with IBD from different countries possible.

Most epidemiological studies derive from Western countries, where the incidence of IBD is highest and identification of populations of adequate size for such studies is therefore easiest. The countries with free or partly free access to health care have further epidemiological advantages, since access to health care increases the likelihood of identifying all variants of disease, including patients with only mild symptoms, and thereby helps guarantee that patients under investigation are representative of the general IBD population.

In this chapter, epidemiological features of the life cycle of IBD will be presented, beginning with incidence, prevalence, patient characteristics, disease course, and risk of surgery. A description of the long-term risk of cancer and death will follow.

The focus will be on patients with IBD diagnosed in childhood or adolescence (these subgroups are often presented as one group in the literature) and to a lesser extent—and primarily for comparison—on patients diagnosed with Crohn's disease or UC in adulthood.

Incidence of Inflammatory Bowel Disease

The incidence of IBD varies within populations and throughout the world, with the highest incidences observed among adults in Western countries. In the United States and northern

Scherl EJ, Dubinsky MC.
*The Changing World of Inflammatory Bowel Disease:
Impact of Generation, Gender, and Global Trends (pp 3-16)*
© 2009 SLACK Incorporated.

Europe, the annual incidence of IBD has reached levels of 7.9 to 8.6/100,000 for Crohn's disease and 8.8 to 13.4/100,000 for UC, with a steeper increase in incidence of Crohn's disease than of UC occurring during the last decades.[5,6]

It has been estimated that approximately 25% to 30% of patients with Crohn's disease and 20% of patients with UC are younger than 20 years old at diagnosis.[7] However, annual incidence rates for pediatric IBD vary from 0.1 to 8.5/100,000 for Crohn's disease and 0.5 to 5.0/100,000 for UC, even when focusing exclusively on studies of unselected patient cohorts (Table 1-1).[6,8-20] There are several reasons for these. First, the quoted studies cover several decades (from 1962 to 2004) and the incidence of pediatric IBD may have changed during this period along with the overall incidence of IBD and especially Crohn's disease. In fact, based on the middle year in the inclusion period of each individual study, it can be estimated that the annual incidence of pediatric UC has remained fairly stable—around 2.0/100,000—during the last 4 decades, whereas the annual incidence of pediatric Crohn's disease has increased from a mean of 1.2/100,000 to 3.9/100,000 during the same period. Secondly, the before-mentioned studies are fairly heterogeneous in the definition of childhood, some including patients up to 16 to 19 years of age, thereby potentially increasing the number of pediatric cases and the associated incidence estimates. Thirdly, the size of the study populations varies from 27 to 739; the smaller the study, the greater the risk that estimates may not reflect the true incidence. Fourthly, despite internationally implemented diagnostic criteria for IBD,[4] studies may still demonstrate inconsistency in exact definitions of and distinction between Crohn's disease, UC, and indeterminate colitis (IC). The annual incidence of IC has remained fairly stable during the last decades (0.5/100,000 [range, 0.2 to 0.6/100,000]).[13,15,16] Exclusion of IC cases may reduce overall estimates of IBD incidence, whereas categorizing IC as Crohn's disease or UC may provide falsely high incidence estimates for these subtypes. New diagnostic serologic assays may help discriminate between subtypes of IBD at an early stage.[21] Lastly, geographic variations may result in varying incidence estimates. As mentioned above, the risk of IBD is highest in Western countries, among which the Scandinavian countries have reported some of the highest incidence and prevalence rates.[22] Genetic predisposition and environmental influences may to some extent explain these differences, but easy access to public health care and thorough registration of citizens, as seen in Scandinavia, may also influence incidence estimates.

An increasing temporal trend in the *prevalence* of IBD and especially Crohn's disease has also been observed during the second half of the 19th century.[23] This increase may reflect changes in incidence of IBD, age distribution of the population, and survival of patients. The current overall prevalence of IBD (US estimates) is 174/100,00 for Crohn's disease, which is 31% higher than in 1991, and 214/100,000 for UC, which is similar to 1991 figures of UC.[5] In children under the age of 15 years (Scandinavian estimates), the current prevalence is 8.3/100,000 for UC, 6.7/100,000 for CD, and 0.8/100,000 for IC.[9] The steep increase in incidence of especially CD observed during the last decades points toward a significant role of environmental factors in the etiology of IBD. Among these, smoking is the most central factor yet identified.[24] At the same time, twin and family studies underscore the importance of genetics in development of IBD and especially Crohn's disease, with a proband concordance rate for Crohn's disease of approximately 64% among monozygotic twins.[25,26] Family studies have shown that IBD also occurs with high frequency among other relatives[22] and that the prevalence of affected first-degree relatives is greater in pediatric cases than in adult cases.[27] Up to 31% of pediatric cases have a family member with IBD,[27,28] with an even higher number of affected first-degree relatives (44% to 56%) of children younger than age 3 to 5 years at onset of IBD.[7,28] In comparison, up to 15% of the general IBD population has first-degree relatives with IBD.[6,7] Both in children and adults, a family history of IBD is more common among patients with Crohn's disease than patients with UC.[6,29] The role of genetics in IBD is supported by the identification of a number of gene polymorphisms related to development of both subtypes but especially Crohn's disease.[30]

Table 1-1

POPULATION-BASED STUDIES ON INCIDENCE OF PEDIATRIC CROHN'S DISEASE AND ULCERATIVE COLITIS

Author	Geographic Area	Time Period	Age Group (at Onset or Diagnosis)	Number of Cases	Incidence of CD/100,000/year	Incidence of UC/100,000/year
Scandinavia						
Langholz et al[8]	Denmark	1962 to 1987	<15 yrs	103	0.2	2.0
Vind et al[6]	Denmark	2003 to 2004	<15 yrs <18 yrs		2.7 4.4	2.4 5.0
Urne et al[9]	Denmark	1998 to 2000	<15 yrs	98	2.3	1.8
Olafsdottir et al[10]	Norway	1984 to 1985		27	2.5	4.3
Bentsen et al[11]	Norway	1990 to 1993		29	2.0	2.1
Lindberg et al[12]	Sweden	1984 to 1986 1993 to 1995	<16 yrs	639	1.2 1.3	1.4 3.2
Hildebrand et al[13]	Sweden	1990 to 2001	<16 yrs	152	1.7 (1990 to 1992) 8.4 (1999 to 2001)	3.3 (1990 to 1992) 1.8 (1999 to 2001)
Bjornsson et al[14]	Iceland	1990 to 1994	10 to 19 yrs	287	8.5	
Europe						
Sawczenko et al[15]	British Isles	1998 to 1999	<16 yrs	739	3.1	1.4
Hassan et al[16]	Wales, UK	1995 to 1997	<17 yrs	38	1.4	0.8
Tourlelier et al[17]	France	1994 to 1997	<17 yrs	88	1.6	0.6
Gottrand et al[18]	France	1984 to 1989	<17 yrs	47	2.1	0.5

CD = Crohn's disease, UC = ulcerative colitis

Table 1-1 (continued)

POPULATION-BASED STUDIES ON INCIDENCE OF PEDIATRIC CROHN'S DISEASE AND ULCERATIVE COLITIS

Author	Geographic Area	Time Period	Age Group (at Onset or Diagnosis)	Number of Cases	Incidence of CD/100,000/year	Incidence of UC/100,000/year
	United States					
Kugathasan et al[19]	Wisconsin, US	2000 to 2001	<18 yrs	199	4.6	2.1
	Australia					
Phavichitr et al[20]*	Victoria, Australia	1971 to 2001	<17 yrs	351	0.1 (1971 to 1976) 2.0 (1996 to 2001)	

*May not represent all cases in area.

CD = Crohn's disease, UC = ulcerative colitis

Patient Demographics

The incidence of disease peaks between 15 to 30 years of age in both Crohn's disease and UC.[22] An increase in median age at diagnosis of Crohn's disease was observed between the 1960s (25 years) and the 1980s (32 years) due to an increase in the proportion of patients diagnosed late in life[22] and has remained fairly stable since then.[5,31] A more recent increase in median age at diagnosis has been observed (from early 30s to middle/late 30s) in UC.[5,31] The median age at diagnosis of IBD in children is approximately 12 years,[15,16,20] both in Crohn's disease and UC.[12,13]

According to population-based studies, 4% to 8% of pediatric cases have onset of disease before the age of 5 years, 17% to 20% at age 5 to 10 years, the majority (58%) at age 10 to 14 years, and approximately 10% at age 15 to 16 years.[12,15,20] In addition, a recent North American tertiary center study of 1370 pediatric IBD cases (The Pediatric IBD Consortium Registry; PediIBDC) reported that 3% of children were less than 12 months old at the onset of the disease.[28] In children with onset of IBD before age 6 to 8 years, Crohn's disease (mainly colonic) and UC are either equally distributed or UC and IC are the most common subtypes.[12,28] After this age, Crohn's disease becomes more frequent[9] and the predominant form of IBD[28] as UC remains equally distributed throughout childhood and adolescence.[9]

The median time from onset to diagnosis of IBD has decreased in adults during the last 5 decades—from 2.2 to 0.7 years in Crohn's disease and from 1.0 to 0.4 years in UC.[31] This delay has apparently always been shorter in children (ie, 7 to 11 months for Crohn's disease and 5 to 8 months for UC)[27] with recent evidence suggesting that this delay has decreased to only 5 months for Crohn's disease and 4 months for UC.[9,11]

Cohort studies of IBD patients (of all ages) have shown a female-to-male ratio of close to 1 for UC, whereas the ratio in Crohn's disease varies from 1.1:1 to 1.8:1.[22] Although some pediatric studies, including the PediIBDC study,[28] suggest that there is no gender predisposition for IBD among children, unselected population-based cohort studies tend to report a pattern opposite to that observed among adults (ie, a slightly increased preponderance of Crohn's disease in boys and no difference between genders in frequency of UC). The female-to-male ratio in pediatric cases with Crohn's disease varies from 1:1.6 to 1:4.0.[12,16,17,19]

Initial Disease Extent and Severity

CROHN'S DISEASE

Crohn's disease may affect one or more parts of the gastrointestinal tract. However, classification of disease extent as well as the ability to discover upper gastrointestinal inflammation has changed over time. Before the era of the Vienna and Montreal Classifications of Crohn's disease and the introduction of capsule endoscopy, population-based inception cohort studies tended to simply focus on prevalence of pure ileal disease (22% to 36%), ileocolonic disease (33% to 45%), and pure colonic disease (18% to 32%) at the time of diagnosis[32-34] and focused less systematically on frequency of upper gastrointestinal involvement.

A comparison of population-based inception cohorts from Denmark showed that cohorts including both adult and pediatric cases had a higher prevalence of pure ileal disease and a lower prevalence of pure colonic disease than cohorts including patients aged 15 years or above.[31] However, in pure pediatric studies, disease distribution is apparently similar to that of adults, as 15% to 38% present with small bowel disease, 38% to 58% with ileocolonic disease, and 20% to 30% with pure colonic disease.[8,17,27] Among these pediatric cases, 17% to 40% also have upper gastrointestinal involvement.[6,13,27] However, when assessed specifically by upper endoscopy and histology, as many as 80% of pediatric cases have upper gastrointestinal inflammation.[27]

Similarly, the prevalence of fistulas and perianal involvement at the time of diagnosis of Crohn's disease is similar in pediatric and adult cases (15% to 26%), with a predominance occurring (at least among adults) in male patients.[13,27,32,34]

Within the first year of diagnosis, disease activity is similar in pediatric and adult cases with Crohn's disease, with approximately 20% having low (or no) activity after initial inflammation and 80% having moderate to high disease activity.[8]

ULCERATIVE COLITIS

Seventeen percent to 44% of adult patients with UC present with proctitis, 16% to 42% with left-sided colitis, and 14% to 47% with extensive colitis or pancolitis.[5,6,27,31] The frequency of proctitis is particularly high in patient cohorts excluding pediatric cases (up to 60%),[31] and children appear to have more extensive disease than adults at diagnosis. In a population-based Danish inception cohort study, Langholz et al observed that significantly more children (29%) than adults (16%) had pancolitis at diagnosis.[8] Similar percentages were reported in a French population-based pediatric study.[17] Other studies have reported even higher frequencies of pancolitis in children (43% to 90%), possibly reflecting selected patient materials or more systematic use of endoscopies in the diagnosis of pediatric IBD.[11,13,19,35] Patients aged <6 years at diagnosis may have an even lower prevalence of proctitis than older children.[28]

Forty-three percent of children present with mild initial disease, whereas 57% have moderate to severe UC at diagnosis.[35] Despite a higher prevalence of extensive disease at diagnosis among children, disease activity appears to be similar in children and adults within the first year after diagnosis.

Extraintestinal Manifestations

Extraintestinal manifestations (EIMs) are observed in up to 35% of patients with IBD and may occur concomitantly with intestinal inflammation or occur unrelated to disease activity.[7,36] Among the most common EIMs are rheumatologic disorders (peripheral and axial arthropathy), dermatologic disorders (erythema nodosum and pyoderma gangrenosum), ophthalmologic disorders (episcleritis and uveitis), primary sclerosing cholangitis, nephrolithiasis, and thromboembolic events. In children, EIMs occur with similar overall frequency as in adults, but they have a tendency to precede the onset of gastrointestinal symptoms, which is rarely the case in adults.[7,22,27] Up to 35% of pediatric patients have at least one EIM at the time of diagnosis of IBD.[27]

Arthritis is the most common EIM observed in children, with a prevalence of 7% to 25%—a prevalence that is similar to that found in adults.[27,37] Pauciarticular arthritis affects large joints at times of IBD activity, whereas polyarticular and axial arthritis may give rise to symptoms independent of IBD activity.[36] Nevertheless, peripheral arthritis is commonly observed years prior to onset of IBD in pediatric cases.[27] Up to 50% of adult patients show radiological signs of sacroiliitis but may be asymptomatic,[36] whereas approximately 7% of children have symptomatic sacroiliitis.[29]

Dermatological manifestations are not as common in pediatric IBD as in adult IBD, with a prevalence of 3% for erythema nodosum in pediatric Crohn's disease (and less in UC) and a prevalence of <1% for pyoderma gangrenosum.[7,27] Primary sclerosing cholangitis is also less common in children than in adults[38] and occurs with a frequency of 3.5% in pediatric UC and <1% in pediatric Crohn's disease.[27] Ophthalmologic manifestations are markedly less frequent in children (4%) than in adults (10% to 45%).[7,27,37] Nephrolithiasis, on the other hand, occurs with approximately the same frequency in children and adults (2% to 6%) and is more common in Crohn's disease than in UC.[27,37] Thromboembolic events occur in 1% to 6% of both pediatric and adult patients, although necropsy studies have shown rates of up to 39%.[27,37]

In addition to the previously mentioned disorders, growth failure, osteopenia, and osteoporosis are sometimes categorized as EIMs of IBD. It has been reported that as many as 85% of children and prepubertal adolescents with Crohn's disease and 65% with UC show signs of growth failure, as measured by weight loss, at the time of diagnosis of IBD. Impaired linear growth is observed in 10% to 40% of children with Crohn's disease and 4% to 10% with UC at the time of diagnosis.[8,39-41] In a recent population-based study of growth failure among children diagnosed with IBD before the age of 15, height-for-age and body mass index (BMI)-for-age z scores were similar in children with UC and children from the general population, whereas both measures were significantly lower in children with Crohn's disease.[42]

In the majority of children with growth failure, reduced height velocity is observed prior to diagnosis of IBD[43] and growth failure may also be an early indicator of exacerbation of disease. Growth failure is thought to result from insufficient intake of calories, increased losses, and ongoing inflammation.[36]

Reassuringly—in terms of risk of osteoporosis—a study of 73 adolescents with IBD (median age, 13.5 years) showed that despite a high prevalence of "small bone for age" due to growth retardation, the majority had adequate bone mass after adjusting for bone size when interpreting data from dual energy x-ray absorptiometry.[44]

Disease Course and Risk of Surgery

Both Crohn's disease and UC are typically characterized as chronic relapsing diseases that quite often lead to surgical interventions. It has been hypothesized that pediatric-onset IBD is linked to a more aggressive disease course than adult IBD due to a stronger genetic influence on disease,[27] but the available population-based literature does not unequivocally support this theory.

CROHN'S DISEASE

Except for the first 2 years following diagnosis, the disease course is relatively mild in the majority of adult patients with more than 50% being in clinical remission at any given point in time. Each year, 15% of patients experience low activity and 30% experience moderate to high disease activity.[32] The natural course is similar in pediatric Crohn's disease, with approximately 50% of children being in remission in each of the first 10 years following diagnosis[8] and 10% suffering from chronically active steroid-dependent or steroid-refractory disease. Overall, up to 80% of pediatric patients relapse during the first 5 years of follow-up.[29] Pure ileal disease may predict a milder course than ileocolonic disease in children with Crohn's disease,[27] whereas serum immune response may predict rapid disease progression.[45]

Progression of disease is more common in pediatric than in adult Crohn's disease.[8,32] Among children, involvement of both the ileum and colon is observed in 39% at diagnosis but in up to 65% during follow-up.[8]

Indications for surgery in patients with Crohn's disease include fistulas, abscesses, stenoses, obstruction, perforation, and cancer. The cumulative incidence of surgery among adult patients with Crohn's disease varies from 40% to 70% at 10 years,[46] seemingly reflecting both differences in phenotypic characteristics of patients under study and variations in treatment policies between countries and over time. Age may be an important phenotypic characteristic influencing the risk of surgery. In a case-control study from the Mayo Clinic, Tremaine and colleagues observed a significant decrease in risk of surgery for non-neoplastic Crohn's disease with increasing age, irrespective of disease distribution and history of cigarette smoking.[47] Smoking per se still influences the risk of surgery, especially early in the course of Crohn's disease.[48]

In children with Crohn's disease, early population-based studies have reported crude surgery rates of 28% to 80% (partly depending on length of follow-up) or cumulative probabilities of up to 95%[8,12,49] but no significant difference in probability of surgery between children and adults.[8] However, surgery rates may have changed because of better nutritional and medical treatments, especially following the introduction of immunomodulatory/biologic therapies serving as—at least initially—alternatives to surgery in patients not responding to conventional treatment with corticosteroids. During the period of 1984 to 1995, a significant decrease in risk of surgery before the age of 16 was observed in a population-based IBD study from Sweden.[12] In a recent study of 989 pediatric patients with Crohn's disease collected from 6 tertiary care referral centers in the United States, 13% required surgery during a median follow-up of 2.8 years, resulting in an estimated cumulative incidence of only 17% at 5 years and 28% at 10 years.[46] In the same study, the risk of surgery was related to poor growth at presentation, abscesses, fistulas, and strictures, whereas treatment with 5-aminosalicylic acid and infliximab was associated with decreased risk of surgery (seemingly reflecting either low disease activity or efficacy of treatment).[46] Mutations in the NOD2/CARD15 gene are also risk factors for early surgery in children with Crohn's disease.[50]

Surgical intervention may be beneficial in pediatric patients with severe disease not responding to medical therapy and/or with growth retardation, providing a disease-free interval of 2 to 3 years and thereby leaving time for both growth and sexual development.[36,51,52]

A second operation is required in 25% to 38% of patients with Crohn's disease (of all ages) at 5 years and 40% to 70% at 15 years. Of these patients, 37% will require a third operation.[22]

ULCERATIVE COLITIS

Among adults with UC who have not undergone surgery, 40% to 50% are in remission at any given point in time, at least after the initial 2 years following diagnosis. Some will undergo surgery and approximately 30% will have active disease in a given year of follow-up. Only a minority of patients have continuously active disease, and this proportion decreases with disease duration.[53]

Similarly, 50% to 70% of children with UC are in remission in each of the first 10 years following the year of diagnosis. Each year, the remaining 30% to 50% will experience symptoms, most as part of a chronic intermittent disease course and fewer due to continuous disease activity (5% to 10%).[8,35] Overall, relapse is observed in two-thirds of patients during the first 5 years following diagnosis with a resulting relatively high need for surgery.[29]

During the disease course, 65% of children with initial proctitis experience further spread of UC.[8] The cumulative risk of progression of proctitis or proctosigmoiditis during the first 15 years after diagnosis is 58% to 70% among children as compared with 48% among adults.[8,54] Among children presenting with substantial colitis, change of extent is observed in 50%, of whom 25% progress to pancolitis and 75% experience regression of disease, similar to frequencies observed in adult patients. Lastly, among children presenting with pancolitis, the cumulative probability of regression within the first 11 years is 80% versus 87% in adults. Still, the overall risk of developing extensive UC is greater in children than in adults.[8,54]

Indications for surgery in UC are both acute and elective and include severe bleeding, toxic megacolon, perforation, lack of response to medical treatment, severe growth retardation, and malignancy. Colectomy rates are similar in children and adults with UC (but varying between countries), with modest changes over time[31] and no difference among age groups.[47] Pediatric studies have reported crude colectomy rates of 21% at 5 years,[29] 26% at 15 years,[49] and approximately 30% after 20 years.[8,55] Apparently, female gender and systemic symptoms (weight loss and fever) at the time of diagnosis are more predictive of later need for colectomy than initial disease extent.[8]

Risk of Intestinal Cancer

The risk of intestinal cancer is increased in at least a subset of patients with long-standing active IBD.[56-58] Patients diagnosed in childhood may be expected to carry a higher risk of intestinal cancer later in life than patients diagnosed with IBD during adulthood because of a longer disease course. However, long-term risk of cancer among pediatric IBD patients in unselected cohorts is difficult to assess because of small sample sizes and limited follow-up time.

CROHN'S DISEASE

In a recent meta-analysis of 6 population-based cohort studies of pediatric and adult patients with Crohn's disease, a significantly increased risk of both colorectal cancer (standardized incidence ratio [SIR], 1.9; 95% CI, 1.4 to 2.5) and small bowel cancer (SIR, 27; 95% CI, 15 to 49) was observed.[56] However, these estimates were based on data from a past treatment era, and recent advances in medical treatment of Crohn's disease may potentially decrease the risk of intestinal cancer because of better disease control. On the other hand, these new treatments may increase the risk of other types of malignancies, such as lymphomas.[59]

The long-term risk of intestinal cancer specific to children with Crohn's disease is uncertain. In a population-based inception cohort study from Denmark involving 374 pediatric and adult patients with Crohn's disease followed for a median of 17 years, no intestinal cancers were observed among patients aged less than 20 years at diagnosis.[60] In a similar study from Olmsted County, Minnesota, a single patient diagnosed with Crohn's disease in childhood (age 13 years in 1962) developed metastasizing colorectal cancer at age 29 and died at age 30. The Olmsted County study also revealed that men aged less than 30 years at diagnosis had a significantly increased risk of colorectal cancer,[61] a finding also noted in population-based studies from Sweden[62] and Canada.[63] However, the data do not reveal how contemporary treatment of pediatric patients with Crohn's disease will influence the future risk of intestinal cancer.

ULCERATIVE COLITIS

The risk of colorectal cancer is also increased among adult patients with long-standing extensive and active UC but the magnitude of risk is debated, and reported estimates often reflect patient materials under study. In a meta-analysis by Eaden et al (based on referral center studies, surgical series, surveillance programs, histology series, inception cohorts, and private practice series), the overall cumulative probability of colorectal cancer among patients with UC increased from 3% at 10 years to 8.7% at 30 years.[57] However, population-based studies of unselected patient cohorts have shown an overall risk of colorectal cancer identical to that of the background population,[61,64] probably because unselected cohorts represent the whole spectrum of UC patients and the majority of these patients have well-controlled disease.

In one of the first systematic studies on colorectal cancer risk in pediatric UC (in a referral center population), Devroede et al observed a cumulative probability of developing colorectal cancer of 43% after 35 years duration of UC, with the greatest risk observed among children aged 5 to 9 years at diagnosis and/or with extensive disease.[65] In the above-mentioned meta-analysis by Eaden et al, 12 studies on the risk of colorectal cancer in children with UC were identified, yielding an overall cumulative probability of 5.5% at 10 years and 15.7% at 30 years.[57] In this respect, there is lack of accordance among population-based inception cohort studies. In the Olmsted County study, no cases of colorectal cancer were observed among patients with pediatric-onset of UC[61] and in the study from Denmark, only 1 of 80 patients with pediatric-onset UC developed colorectal cancer.[8] However, in the study from Sweden, the cumulative risk for colorectal cancer was 40% at 35 years among 266 patients diagnosed with UC before age 15.[66]

Mortality

As for cancer, there is a lack of population-based pediatric cohorts of sufficient sample size and follow-up time describing long-term mortality in childhood-onset IBD.

CROHN'S DISEASE

Population-based inception cohort studies, including both pediatric and adult cases, have revealed a slightly increased mortality rate in patients with Crohn's disease, especially in women with long disease duration.[67,68] In a meta-analysis of population-based, hospital-based, and referral center studies of patients with Crohn's disease, the overall pooled standardized mortality ratio (SMR) was 1.5 (95% CI, 1.3 to 1.7).[69]

In population-based studies stratifying for age at diagnosis, no increased mortality related to early-onset IBD has been identified.[67,68] In a study of 374 Danish patients followed for a median of 17 years, only one death was observed among a subgroup of patients diagnosed at age 0 to 19 years versus 0.9 expected deaths (NS). The patient died at age 33 of short bowel syndrome and hepatitis.[67]

ULCERATIVE COLITIS

Overall, mortality is not increased in patients with UC as shown in a meta-analysis of population-based inception cohort studies of both pediatric and adult patients (pooled SMR, 1.1; 95% CI, 0.9 to 1.2).[70] Nevertheless, 17% of all deaths in this study were related to UC and occurred early after diagnosis and in patients with extensive disease. The primary causes were postoperative complications, toxic megacolon, intestinal perforation, myocardial infarction secondary to anemia, colorectal cancer, and end-stage liver disease secondary to primary sclerosing cholangitis. Accordingly, analyses of cause-specific mortality show an increased risk of dying from nonalcoholic liver disease, pulmonary emboli, and respiratory diseases among patients with UC, which in turn is counterweighted by a reduced mortality from pulmonary cancer and a borderline reduced mortality from cardiovascular diseases.[70]

In the early study on prognosis in children with UC by Devroede et al, a high risk of dying was observed in patients with extensive colitis as compared to patients with less extensive disease, whereas comparison with the general population was not performed.[65] In a later population-based study from the Mayo Clinic, no deaths among pediatric-onset cases were observed.[68] In contrast, in the study from Denmark,[8] Langholz et al observed 4 deaths among pediatric patients (occurring 4 to 20 years after onset of disease) versus 0.76 expected deaths, yielding a significantly increased relative risk of 5.3. However, 2 of the 4 deaths had no relation to UC.[8] In the meta-analysis of mortality in UC, mortality was not increased among patients younger than 20 years of age at diagnosis (the highest SMR identified was 2.3, but this increase was only of borderline significance).[70]

Summary

Epidemiological data on patients with IBD have been collected since the middle of the last century. During this period, an increase in the incidence of IBD—and recently in particular in the incidence of Crohn's disease—has been observed among both children and adults. The etiology of IBD is multi-factorial, involving both environmental and genetic factors. According to twin studies, the genetic component is stronger in Crohn's disease than in UC, and genetics play a greater role in pediatric IBD than in adult IBD. Up to one-third of IBD patients are diagnosed during childhood and up to 8% of these are less than 5 years old at onset of disease. The female-to-male ratio is close to 1 for UC independent of age at diagnosis, whereas in Crohn's disease, male preponderance for disease is observed among children and female preponderance among adults.

Initial disease extent and severity of Crohn's disease is similar in different age groups, whereas UC tends to be most extensive in pediatric cases. Although progression of disease is common in pediatric Crohn's disease and UC, 50% of patients are in remission at any given point in time and surgery rates are similar to those observed in adults. Improved nutritional and medical treatment of IBD may lead to a decrease in surgery rates. EIMs occur with similar frequency in children and adults but are differently distributed and tend to be present at diagnosis among children with IBD. Intestinal cancer risk and mortality are slightly increased in adult patients with IBD (according to studies involving older treatment strategies), whereas data on long-term prognosis of patients with IBD diagnosed in childhood are sparse.

References

1. Baron JH. Inflammatory bowel disease up to 1932. *Mt Sinai J Med.* 2000;67:174-189.
2. Edwards FC, Truelove SC. The course and prognosis of ulcerative colitis. *Gut.* 1963;4:299-315.
3. Truelove SC, Pena AS. Course and prognosis of Crohn's disease. *Gut.* 1976;17:192-201.
4. Lennard-Jones JE. Classification of inflammatory bowel disease. *Scand J Gastroenterol Suppl.* 1989;170:2-6.
5. Loftus CG, Loftus EV Jr, Harmsen WS, et al. Update on the incidence and prevalence of Crohn's disease and ulcerative colitis in Olmsted County, Minnesota, 1940-2000. *Inflamm Bowel Dis.* 2007;13:254-261.
6. Vind I, Riis L, Jess T, et al. Increasing incidences of inflammatory bowel disease and decreasing surgery rates in Copenhagen City and County, 2003-2005: a population-based study from the Danish Crohn colitis database. *Am J Gastroenterol.* 2006;101:1274-1282.
7. Baldassano RN, Piccoli DA. Inflammatory bowel disease in pediatric and adolescent patients. *Gastroenterol Clin North Am.* 1999;28:445-458.
8. Langholz E, Munkholm P, Krasilnikoff PA, Binder V. Inflammatory bowel diseases with onset in childhood: clinical features, morbidity, and mortality in a regional cohort. *Scand J Gastroenterol.* 1997;32:139-147.
9. Urne FU, Paerregaard A. [Chronic inflammatory bowel disease in children: an epidemiological study from eastern Denmark 1998-2000]. *Ugeskr Laeger.* 2002;164:5810-5814.
10. Olafsdottir EJ, Fluge G, Haug K. Chronic inflammatory bowel disease in children in western Norway. *J Pediatr Gastroenterol Nutr.* 1989;8:454-458.
11. Bentsen BS, Moum B, Ekbom A. Incidence of inflammatory bowel disease in children in southeastern Norway: a prospective population-based study 1990-94. *Scand J Gastroenterol.* 2002;37:540-545.
12. Lindberg E, Lindquist B, Holmquist L, Hildebrand H. Inflammatory bowel disease in children and adolescents in Sweden, 1984-1995. *J Pediatr Gastroenterol Nutr.* 2000;30:259-264.
13. Hildebrand H, Brydolf M, Holmquist L, Krantz I, Kristiansson B. Incidence and prevalence of inflammatory bowel disease in children in south-western Sweden. *Acta Paediatr.* 1994;83:640-645.
14. Bjornsson S, Johannsson JH. Inflammatory bowel disease in Iceland, 1990-1994: a prospective, nationwide, epidemiological study. *Eur J Gastroenterol Hepatol.* 2000;12:31-38.
15. Sawczenko A, Sandhu BK, Logan RF, et al. Prospective survey of childhood inflammatory bowel disease in the British Isles. *Lancet.* 2001;357:1093-1094.
16. Hassan K, Cowan FJ, Jenkins HR. The incidence of childhood inflammatory bowel disease in Wales. *Eur J Pediatr.* 2000;159:261-263.
17. Tourtelier Y, Dabadie A, Tron I, et al. [Incidence of inflammatory bowel disease in children in Brittany (1994-1997). Breton association of study and research on digestive system diseases (Abermad)]. *Arch Pediatr.* 2000;7:377-384.
18. Gottrand F, Colombel JF, Moreno L, Salomez JL, Farriaux JP, Cortot A. [Incidence of inflammatory bowel diseases in children in the Nord-Pas-de-Calais region]. *Arch Fr Pediatr.* 1991;48:25-28.
19. Kugathasan S, Judd RH, Hoffmann RG, et al. Epidemiologic and clinical characteristics of children with newly diagnosed inflammatory bowel disease in Wisconsin: a statewide population-based study. *J Pediatr.* 2003;143:525-531.
20. Phavichitr N, Cameron DJ, Catto-Smith AG. Increasing incidence of Crohn's disease in Victorian children. *J Gastroenterol Hepatol.* 2003;18:329-332.
21. Seidman EG. Recent advances in the diagnosis and treatment of pediatric inflammatory bowel disease. *Curr Gastroenterol Rep.* 2000;2:248-252.
22. Andres PG, Friedman LS. Epidemiology and the natural course of inflammatory bowel disease. *Gastroenterol Clin North Am.* 1999;28:255-81, vii.
23. Ehlin AG, Montgomery SM, Ekbom A, Pounder RE, Wakefield AJ. Prevalence of gastrointestinal diseases in two British national birth cohorts. *Gut.* 2003;52:1117-1121.
24. Calkins BM. A meta-analysis of the role of smoking in inflammatory bowel disease. *Dig Dis Sci.* 1989;34:1841-1854.

25. Halfvarson J, Bodin L, Tysk C, Lindberg E, Jarnerot G. Inflammatory bowel disease in a Swedish twin cohort: a long-term follow-up of concordance and clinical characteristics. *Gastroenterology.* 2003;124:1767-1773.

26. Jess T, Riis L, Jespersgaard C, et al. Disease concordance, zygosity, and *NOD2/CARD15* status: follow-up of a population-based cohort of Danish twins with inflammatory bowel disease. *Am J Gastroenterol.* 2005;100:2486-2492.

27. Mamula P, Markowitz JE, Baldassano RN. Inflammatory bowel disease in early childhood and adolescence: special considerations. *Gastroenterol Clin North Am.* 2003;32:967-995, viii.

28. Heyman MB, Kirschner BS, Gold BD, et al. Children with early-onset inflammatory bowel disease (IBD): analysis of a pediatric IBD consortium registry. *J Pediatr.* 2005;146:35-40.

29. Stordal K, Jahnsen J, Bentsen BS, Moum B. Pediatric inflammatory bowel disease in southeastern Norway: a five-year follow-up study. *Digestion.* 2004;70:226-230.

30. Ahmed FE. Role of genes, the environment and their interactions in the etiology of inflammatory bowel diseases. *Expert Rev Mol Diagn.* 2006;6:345-363.

31. Jess T, Riis L, Vind I, et al. Changes in clinical characteristics, course, and prognosis of inflammatory bowel disease during the last 5 decades: a population-based study from Copenhagen, Denmark. *Inflamm Bowel Dis.* 2007;13(4):481-489.

32. Munkholm P. Crohn's disease: occurrence, course and prognosis: an epidemiologic cohort-study. *Dan Med Bull.* 1997;44:287-302.

33. Persson PG, Karlen P, Bernell O, et al. Crohn's disease and cancer: a population-based cohort study. *Gastroenterology.* 1994;107:1675-1679.

34. Loftus EV Jr, Silverstein MD, Sandborn WJ, Tremaine WJ, Harmsen WS, Zinsmeister AR. Crohn's disease in Olmsted County, Minnesota, 1940-1993: incidence, prevalence, and survival. *Gastroenterology.* 1998;114:1161-1168.

35. Hyams JS, Davis P, Grancher K, Lerer T, Justinich CJ, Markowitz J. Clinical outcome of ulcerative colitis in children. *J Pediatr.* 1996;129:81-88.

36. Caprilli R, Gassull MA, Escher JC, et al. European evidence based consensus on the diagnosis and management of Crohn's disease: special situations. *Gut.* 2006;55(Suppl 1):i36-i58.

37. Danese S, Semeraro S, Papa A, et al. Extraintestinal manifestations in inflammatory bowel disease. *World J Gastroenterol.* 2005;11:7227-7236.

38. Kaplan GG, Laupland KB, Butzner D, Urbanski SJ, Lee SS. The burden of large and small duct primary sclerosing cholangitis in adults and children: a population-based analysis. *Am J Gastroenterol.* 2007;102:1042-1049.

39. Motil KJ, Grand RJ, vis-Kraft L, Ferlic LL, Smith EO. Growth failure in children with inflammatory bowel disease: a prospective study. *Gastroenterology.* 1993;105:681-691.

40. Kim SC, Ferry GD. Inflammatory bowel diseases in pediatric and adolescent patients: clinical, therapeutic, and psychosocial considerations. *Gastroenterology.* 2004;126:1550-1560.

41. Seidman E, LeLeiko N, Ament M, et al. Nutritional issues in pediatric inflammatory bowel disease. *J Pediatr Gastroenterol Nutr.* 1991;12:424-438.

42. Paerregaard A, Uldall UF. Anthropometry at the time of diagnosis in Danish children with inflammatory bowel disease. *Acta Paediatr.* 2005;94:1682-1683.

43. Kanof ME, Lake AM, Bayless TM. Decreased height velocity in children and adolescents before the diagnosis of Crohn's disease. *Gastroenterology.* 1988;95:1523-1527.

44. Ahmed SF, Horrocks IA, Patterson T, et al. Bone mineral assessment by dual energy X-ray absorptiometry in children with inflammatory bowel disease: evaluation by age or bone area. *J Pediatr Gastroenterol Nutr.* 2004;38:276-280.

45. Dubinsky MC, Lin YC, Dutridge D, et al. Serum immune responses predict rapid disease progression among children with Crohn's disease: immune responses predict disease progression. *Am J Gastroenterol.* 2006;101:360-367.

46. Gupta N, Cohen SA, Bostrom AG, et al. Risk factors for initial surgery in pediatric patients with Crohn's disease. *Gastroenterology.* 2006;130:1069-1077.

47. Tremaine WJ, Timmons LJ, Loftus EV Jr, et al. Age at onset of inflammatory bowel disease and the risk of surgery for non-neoplastic bowel disease. *Aliment Pharmacol Ther.* 2007;25:1435-1441.

48. Sands BE, Arsenault JE, Rosen MJ, et al. Risk of early surgery for Crohn's disease: implications for early treatment strategies. *Am J Gastroenterol.* 2003;98:2712-2718.

49. Sedgwick DM, Barton JR, Hamer-Hodges DW, Nixon SJ, Ferguson A. Population-based study of surgery in juvenile onset Crohn's disease. *Br J Surg.* 1991;78:171-175.

50. Kugathasan S, Collins N, Maresso K, et al. *CARD15* gene mutations and risk for early surgery in pediatric-onset Crohn's disease. *Clin Gastroenterol Hepatol.* 2004;2:1003-1009.

51. Baldassano RN, Han PD, Jeshion WC, et al. Pediatric Crohn's disease: risk factors for postoperative recurrence. *Am J Gastroenterol.* 2001;96:2169-2176.

52. Diefenbach KA, Breuer CK. Pediatric inflammatory bowel disease. *World J Gastroenterol.* 2006;12:3204-3212.

53. Langholz E. Ulcerative colitis: an epidemiological study based on a regional inception cohort, with special reference to disease course and prognosis. *Dan Med Bull.* 1999;46:400-415.

54. Mir-Madjlessi SH, Michener WM, Farmer RG. Course and prognosis of idiopathic ulcerative proctosigmoiditis in young patients. *J Pediatr Gastroenterol Nutr.* 1986;5:571-575.

55. Barton JR, Ferguson A. Clinical features, morbidity and mortality of Scottish children with inflammatory bowel disease. *Q J Med.* 1990;75:423-439.
56. Jess T, Gamborg M, Matzen P, Munkholm P, Sorensen TI. Increased risk of intestinal cancer in Crohn's disease: a meta-analysis of population-based cohort studies. *Am J Gastroenterol.* 2005;100:2724-2729.
57. Eaden JA, Abrams KR, Mayberry JF. The risk of colorectal cancer in ulcerative colitis: a meta-analysis. *Gut.* 2001;48:526-535.
58. Jess T, Loftus EV Jr, Velayos FS, et al. Risk factors for colorectal neoplasia in inflammatory bowel disease: a nested case-control study from Copenhagen county, Denmark and Olmsted county, Minnesota. *Am J Gastroenterol.* 2007;102:829-836.
59. Ljung T, Karlen P, Schmidt D, et al. Infliximab in inflammatory bowel disease: clinical outcome in a population based cohort from Stockholm County. *Gut.* 2004;53:849-853.
60. Jess T, Winther KV, Munkholm P, Langholz E, Binder V. Intestinal and extra-intestinal cancer in Crohn's disease: follow-up of a population-based cohort in Copenhagen County, Denmark. *Aliment Pharmacol Ther.* 2004;19:287-293.
61. Jess T, Loftus EV Jr, Velayos FS, et al. Risk of intestinal cancer in inflammatory bowel disease: a population-based study from Olmsted County, Minnesota. *Gastroenterology.* 2006;130:1039-1046.
62. Ekbom A, Helmick C, Zack M, Adami HO. Increased risk of large-bowel cancer in Crohn's disease with colonic involvement. *Lancet.* 1990;336:357-359.
63. Bernstein CN, Blanchard JF, Kliewer E, Wajda A. Cancer risk in patients with inflammatory bowel disease: a population-based study. *Cancer.* 2001;91:854-862.
64. Winther KV, Jess T, Langholz E, Munkholm P, Binder V. Long-term risk of cancer in ulcerative colitis: a population-based cohort study from Copenhagen County. *Clin Gastroenterol Hepatol.* 2004;2:1088-1095.
65. Devroede GJ, Taylor WF, Sauer WG, Jackman RJ, Stickler GB. Cancer risk and life expectancy of children with ulcerative colitis. *N Engl J Med.* 1971;285:17-21.
66. Ekbom A, Helmick C, Zack M, Adami HO. Ulcerative colitis and colorectal cancer: a population-based study. *N Engl J Med.* 1990;323:1228-1233.
67. Jess T, Winther KV, Munkholm P, Langholz E, Binder V. Mortality and causes of death in Crohn's disease: follow-up of a population-based cohort in Copenhagen County, Denmark. *Gastroenterology.* 2002;122:1808-1814.
68. Jess T, Loftus EV Jr, Harmsen WS, et al. Survival and cause specific mortality in patients with inflammatory bowel disease: a long term outcome study in Olmsted County, Minnesota, 1940-2004. *Gut.* 2006;55:1248-1254.
69. Canavan C, Abrams KR, Mayberry JF. Meta-analysis: mortality in Crohn's disease. *Aliment Pharmacol Ther.* 2007;25:861-870.
70. Jess T, Gamborg M, Munkholm P, Sorensen TI. Overall and cause-specific mortality in ulcerative colitis: meta-analysis of population-based inception cohort studies. *Am J Gastroenterol.* 2007;102:609-617.

INFLAMMATORY BOWEL DISEASE IN THE DEVELOPING WORLD

A RAPID EVOLUTION OF GLOBAL EPIDEMIOLOGY

Daisy Batista, MD and Joshua Korzenik, MD

Inflammatory bowel disease (IBD) appears to be a recent medical phenomenon. Ulcerative colitis (UC) was first described in the latter half of the 19th century. Crohn's disease (CD) was first reported perhaps about 40 years later, a few decades prior to Burrill Crohn's initial report. Both diseases have increased significantly during the past century. A striking epidemiologic feature has been the geographic distribution of IBD, which has the highest prevalence in industrialized Western countries, particularly North America[1-9] and western Europe.[10-23] Until recently, CD and UC had been unusual diagnoses in the developing world. However, over the past few decades, this pattern appears to be shifting with increasing numbers of cases identified in the developing world.[24-28] The extent to which this reflects a detection bias rather than a genuine increase cannot be easily established, but the widespread nature of this phenomenon and its magnitude substantiate the likelihood of a real increase. Countries in which IBD had been previously an uncommon diagnosis, such as India,[25] Japan,[28] and Korea,[26] now report a frequent occurrence of both CD and UC. This possible environmental shift may offer vital clues with regard to a broader understanding of IBD and the factors that promote its development. This chapter focuses on the emergence of IBD in the developing world and its implications.

Epidemiology

The highest incidence and prevalence for IBD is found in North America[1-9] and northern/western Europe.[10-23] Geographic variation has previously suggested a higher prevalence and incidence in industrialized countries and a north-south gradient, with higher rates in northern climates.[13,29-31] These geographic distinctions may be eroding as reported by the European IBD Study Group.[11] Furthermore, epidemiologic studies from the last 2 decades demonstrate an increasing incidence of IBD around the world, but interpretation of these data is difficult due to marked differences in study methodology, case ascertainment, diagnostic tools available to make the diagnosis, and physician awareness of these diseases.

Scherl EJ, Dubinsky MC.
The Changing World of Inflammatory Bowel Disease:
Impact of Generation, Gender, and Global Trends (pp 17-32)
© 2009 SLACK Incorporated.

Table 2-1

INCIDENCE RATES FOR ULCERATIVE COLITIS AND CROHN'S DISEASE FROM NORTH AMERICAN STUDIES

Reference	Location	Case Ascertainment	Dates	Incidence of UC	Incidence of CD
Bernstein et al[6]	Manitoba	Population	1989 to 1994	14.3	14.6
Blanchard et al[8]	Manitoba	Population	1987 to 1996	15.6	15.6
Pinchbeck et al[1]	Northern Alberta	Population	1981	6	10
Loftus et al[5,7,9]	Olmsted County, MN	Population	1984 to 1993	8.3	6.9
			1990 to 2000	8.8	7.9
Stowe et al[3]	Monroe County, NY	Hospital	1980 to 1989	2.3	3.9
Hiatt et al[2]	Northern California	HMO	1980 to 1981	10.9	7.0
Kurata et al[4]	Southern California	HMO, outpatient HMO, hospital	1987 to 1988	NA	3.5
			1988	NA	5.4

NORTH AMERICA

As a background to understanding evolving patterns in the developing world, below is a brief review of the existing epidemiology of IBD in North America and western Europe. In North America, the incidence rate for UC and CD ranges from 2.2 to 14.3 per 10^5 and 3.1 to 14.6 per 10^5, respectively. Prevalence for UC is 37 to 246 cases per 10^5 and 26 to 199 cases per 10^5 for CD (Table 2-1). Few population-based estimates exist for the North American population and even the most rigorous studies vary considerably.

The highest incidence and prevalence rates for IBD have been identified in a study from the Canadian province of Manitoba.[6] Using computerized claims data from the universal insurance provider for the province, the incidence rates between 1984 and 1995 for UC were 14.3 per 10^5 and 14.6 per 10^5 for CD. The prevalence was estimated at 169.7 per 10^5 for UC and 198.5 per 10^5 for CD. Patients were identified as having CD or UC if they had at least 5 separate medical contacts with such diagnosis or at least 3 contacts if they had been registered for less than 2 years during the study period. Chart reviews and self-administered questionnaires were used to validate the accuracy of administrative health data. Of note, gastroenterologists were routinely providing care for only 60% of patients with IBD, which suggests that studies relying only on gastroenterologists' data underestimate the true incidence of these diseases.

A study by Pinchbeck et al[1] focused on the population of Edmonton in Northern Alberta from January 1977 to December 1981, the major city in this province with a population of 532,246 in the 1981 census. Possible IBD cases were identified by using ICD codes from the medical records of 5 teaching hospitals, 37 community hospitals, and 10 practicing gastroenterologists that service the city of Edmonton. The administrative database was validated through chart reviews

---

Table 2-2

DIAGNOSTIC CRITERIA FOR ULCERATIVE COLITIS AND CROHN'S DISEASE IN THE OLMSTED COUNTY STUDY

Diagnostic Criteria for CD (At least 2 out of 5, for at least 2 months)	Diagnostic Criteria for UC (On 2 studies separated by at least 6 months)*
Clinical history of abdominal pain, weight loss, malaise, diarrhea, and/or rectal bleeding	Diffusely granular or friable colonic mucosa on endoscopy
Endoscopic finding of mucosal cobblestoning, linear ulceration, skip areas, or perianal disease	Continuous involvement observed on endoscopy or barium x-ray
Radiologic findings of stricture, fistula, mucosal cobblestoning, or ulceration	
Macroscopic appearance of bowel wall induration, mesenteric lymphadenopathy, and creeping fat at laparotomy	
Pathologic findings of transmural inflammation and/or epithelioid granulomas	

* Probable UC if met only one diagnostic study or two diagnostic studies separated by less than 6 months.

---

confirming the diagnosis of UC or CD if the patient met clinical plus radiological and/or pathological criteria. The calculated incidence rates were 10 per 10^5 for CD and 6 per 10^5 for UC. The prevalence of CD was higher in urban than rural areas.

Loftus et al determined the epidemiology of UC and CD from Olmsted County, Minnesota between 1940 to 1993.[5,7] In 1990, the population of Olmsted County was approximately 106,000 people, with 76,000 living in the urban Rochester area and the remainder in rural areas. The majority (96%) of the population of Olmsted County was White with a high proportion from Northern European heritage. The investigators had complete access to both inpatient and outpatient medical records as the residents of Olmsted County received their care at one of two main organizations with their affiliates, the Mayo Medical Center and Olmsted Medical Center. Cases were identified through diagnostic index, and the diagnosis of CD or UC was made if a potential case met a rigorous set of criteria (Table 2-2).

The age and gender-adjusted incidence for CD was 5.8 per 10^5. In Rochester, the adjusted incidence was 6.4 per 10^5 compared to 4.6 per 10^5 in rural Olmsted County. The adjusted incidence rate for UC including probable cases was 7.6 per 10^5 and 6.8 per 10^5 when only definite cases were included. The adjusted incidence rate in Rochester was 9.6 per 10^5, which was significantly higher than 3.9 per 10^5 in rural Olmsted County.

The incidence of CD in Olmsted County peaked between the 1960s and 1970s and stabilized at a rate of approximately 7 cases per 100,000 person-years. For UC, the incidence peaked between 1984 to 1993 at a rate of 9.4 per 10^5 followed by a slight decline and stabilization thereafter. An update of the epidemiology of IBD in Olmsted County to the year 2000 showed that these rates remained stable. The incidence rate for UC was 8.8 cases per 10^5 and 7.9 per 10^5 for CD. At the end of 2000, the adjusted prevalence for UC and CD was 214 per 10^5 and 174 per 10^5, respectively.

While this study provided valuable epidemiologic information on IBD and case ascertainment approached nearly 100%, the population size was relatively small and homogenous.

Ninety-six percent of the population in Olmsted County was White compared to 77.1% of the US population based on the figures from the 2000 US Census. While the ethnic composition of Olmsted County is evolving, it may not account adequately for varying rates in different ethnic populations. Estimates of IBD prevalence for US Whites commonly use the epidemiologic data from Olmsted County. However, including only Whites to estimate the prevalence of IBD in the United States may underestimate the true prevalence of these diseases, especially after studies have shown that African Americans may have an incidence approaching that of US Whites.[32] At the same time, since it appears that Asian Americans and Hispanics have significantly lower rates of CD,[4] extrapolating the results from Olmsted County to the whole US population would over-estimate the true incidence and prevalence of CD.

A lower incidence rate has been suggested from data assessed through a review of medical records from a large health maintenance organization (HMO) in Southern California, revealing incidence rates of 3.6 to 5.4 per 10^5 for CD,[4] which is much lower than the rates found in the north. Although most epidemiologic studies in North America are consistent with the "north-south gradient" found in Europe, meaning a higher prevalence for IBD in northern latitudes, a study of African-American children in Georgia found incidence rates higher than previously reported.[32]

EUROPE

Significant variability in the incidence and prevalence of UC and CD is apparent throughout Europe, with much higher rates in the northern locales and western Europe.[10,11,13,15,17,18,21-23,29,33-40] The highest incidence rate for UC in Europe is found in Iceland (24.5 per 10^5), while the lowest was in Almada in southern Portugal (1.6 per 10^5). For CD, the highest incidence rate in Europe is found in Maastricht, The Netherlands, with 9.2 per 10^5, while Ioannina in northwest Greece reports an incidence of only 0.9 per 10^5.

To investigate this variation, the European Collaborative Study on Inflammatory Bowel Disease (EC-IBD)[11] enlisted 20 centers throughout Europe and used a standard protocol for case ascertainment for the 2-year period between 1991 and 1993. The study centers' requirements included a defined catchment area with up-to-date population data, high-quality diagnostic facilities, and universal health coverage for primary and specialists care. The diagnosis of IBD was made on the basis of endoscopic or radiologic evidence supported by mucosal biopsy or surgical pathology when possible. Over the 2-year period, the EC-IBD study found an incidence of 10.4 per 10^5 for UC and 5.6 per 10^5 for CD. The rates for UC in the northern centers were 40% higher than in the south (rate ratio [RR], 1.4; 95% CI, 1.2 to 1.5) and 80% higher for CD (RR, 1.8; 95% CI, 1.5 to 2.1). The increased incidence was not explained by differences in tobacco consumption or education level. Furthermore, there were no statistically significant differences in the presenting symptoms or severity of disease.

Although this study confirmed an increased occurrence of IBD in the north, the difference between northern and southern Europe is smaller than suggested by previous studies. While this may be secondary to the use of more stringent criteria for case ascertainment and the uniformity of data analysis, IBD may have an increased prevalence in southern Europe.

EASTERN EUROPE

Studies from eastern Europe have found an increasing incidence of both UC and CD. This region had been considered an area of low incidence and prevalence of IBD, although this viewpoint may reflect the paucity of studies and health care delivery issues. While not conventionally considered developing nations, these countries have undergone rapid political, social, and economic changes in recent decades, emerging closer to a western European lifestyle and health profile. A population-based epidemiologic survey from Hungary revealed an increasing incidence of UC from 1.7 per 10^5 (1977 to 1981) to 11.0 per 10^5 (1997 to 2001). During the same time period, the incidence of CD increased from 0.4 per 10^5 to 4.7 per 10^5.[41] A prospective population-based study of IBD in Zagreb, Croatia from 1980 to 1989 included inpatient and outpatient data as well as general practitioners' reports; all centers were contacted every 2 months. Over this time period, the investigators reported an unchanged incidence rate for UC of 1.5 per 10^5, and for CD the incidence rate was 0.7 per 10^5.[35,36]

Investigators in Croatia report much higher incidence and prevalence rates for both UC and CD. A retrospective study from 1995 to 2001 by Sincic et al, looking at the population in the Adriatic Sea coastal area, found an incidence rate of 3.88 per 10^5 for UC and 3.92 per 10^5 for CD.[42] These data, however, were based on the inpatient and outpatient records of a single hospital. A prospective follow-up of the same population in Croatia from 2000 to 2004 using the same methodology found even higher incidence rates for IBD, with 4.3 per 10^5 for UC and 7.0 per 10^5 for CD.[43] Reports from the Czech Republic also reveal a trend toward an increase in IBD. In 1967, Nedbal et al in a single hospital-based survey in Prague reported an incidence rate of 1.4 per 10^5 for UC.[44] A more recent prospective population-based survey by Bitter et al from 1975 to 1990 revealed a higher incidence rate of 3.1 per 10^5 for UC.[45]

Several reports, though with significant methodological limitations, have found a much lower burden of IBD in eastern Europe. A retrospective case series from a single hospital in Poland for the period between 1990 and 2003 estimated an incidence rate of 1.8 per 10^5 for UC and 0.1 per 10^5 for CD.[46] However, other centers in the same area also were treating patients with IBD, which clearly leads to underestimating the true incidence and prevalence of these diseases. In Romania, a nationwide epidemiologic survey of 18 secondary and tertiary centers between the period of June 2002 and June 2003 estimated the incidence of UC at 0.97 per 10^5 and 0.50 per 10^5 for CD.[47] However, this study appears to inappropriately extrapolate the region results as national data.

The increasing incidence of IBD in eastern Europe coincided with a change in the political environment and a trend toward a more Westernized way of living. Uncertain is whether this shift is evolving due to environmental exposures, making these populations more likely to develop IBD, or whether these increases reflect better diagnostic tools and increased physician awareness.

DEVELOPING NATIONS

Although the incidence and prevalence of IBD appears relatively low in developing nations when compared to North America and western Europe, recent trends reveal a dynamic epidemiology for IBD. Despite the paucity of epidemiologic data from many parts of the developing world, a number of studies in the past decade have reported an increasing incidence and prevalence of IBD in countries such as India, China, Japan, Argentina, and Puerto Rico (Table 2-3). Interpretation of these data remains challenging given the differences in study design, access to medical care, referral bias, experience at a particular center, and changing medical technologies among other factors.

ASIA

A review of CD in the Chinese population from Leong et al[48] reported an increased incidence from 0.3 per 10^5 in 1986 to 1989 to 1.0 per 10^5 in 1999 to 2001. Similarly, a retrospective study from Seoul, South Korea revealed a rise in incidence rates for UC from 0.2 per 10^5 in 1986 to 1988 to 1.23 per 10^5 in 1995 to 1997.[26] A nationwide survey in 1991 from Japan reported an incidence for UC of 1.95 per 10^5 and 0.51 per 10^5 for CD.[28]

Data from Singapore also suggested an increasing prevalence of these diseases. The overall prevalence of UC was 6 per 10^5 and 3.6 per 10^5 for CD. Ethnic groups demonstrated marked differences. The prevalence of UC was 4.8 per 10^5 for Malay, 6.2 per 10^5 for Chinese, and 16 per 10^5 for Indians. Similar variations were not seen for CD.

In the state of Punjab in northern India, a population-based, door-to-door survey for UC showed a prevalence of 42.8 per 10^5.[25] A follow-up study 1 year later found an incidence rate of 6.02 per 10^5. A random sample of 51,910 inhabitants was screened for symptoms suggestive of UC such as history of diarrhea with or without rectal bleeding or prolonged diarrhea (>4 weeks). A total of 147 suspected cases were identified and of these, 128 agreed to undergo further

Table 2-3

INCIDENCE RATES FOR ULCERATIVE COLITIS AND CROHN'S DISEASE FROM ASIA, MIDDLE EAST, AFRICA, AND LATIN AMERICA

Reference	Location	Case Ascertainment	Dates	Incidence of UC (per 10^5)	Incidence of CD (per 10^5)
Asia					
Sood et al[25]	Punjab, India	Survey	1999 to 2000	6.0	N/A
Yang et al[26]	Seoul, South Korea	Population	1986 to 1988 1995 to 1997	0.20 1.23	N/A
Morita et al[28]	Japan	Survey	1991	1.95	0.51
Middle East					
Odes et al[49]	Southern Israel	Population	1987 to 1992	N/A	4.2
Abdul-Baki et al[50]	Lebanon	HMO-cohort	2000 to 2004	4.1	1.4
Radhakrishnan et al[51]	Oman	Population	1987 to 1994	1.35	N/A
Al-Nakib et al[52]	Kuwait	Hospital	1977 to 1982	2.27	0.45
Africa					
Wright et al[24]	Cape Town, South Africa	Population: White Mixed race Black	1980 to 1984	 5.0 1.9 0.6	 2.6 1.8 0.3
Latin America					
Linares de la Cal et al[53]	Colon, Panama	Hospital	1987 to 1993	1.2	0
Appleyard et al[27]	Partido General de P, Argentina	Hospital	1987 to 1993	2.2	0.03
Edouard et al[54]	Puerto Rico	Population	1996 2000	1.96 3.32	0.49 1.96
	French West-Indies	Multicenter survey	1997 to 1999	2.44	1.94

investigation with video sigmoidoscopy and rectal biopsy. UC was confirmed in 15 cases (11.7% of the suspected cases). Repeat survey the following year identified an additional 3 cases for a crude incidence rate of 6.02 per 10^5.

MIDDLE EAST

The incidence of IBD appears low in the Middle East with the exception of Israel, though Arabs living in Israel are significantly less affected than Jews. A study by Fireman et al of CD in a Jewish population from central Israel from 1970 to 1980 revealed a prevalence of 7.08 per 10^5 in 1970 and 19.47 per 10^5 in 1980.[55] In 1970, the prevalence in immigrants from Europe and America was 13.27, while that of immigrants from Asia and Africa was 1.69.[55] Odes et al reviewed all the hospital and outpatient records for CD from 1968 to 1992 for a population in southern Israel.[49] The authors did not find a significant difference in the prevalence rates among Jews from different ethnic backgrounds. At the end of 1992, the prevalence rate of Asian/African-born Jews was 55.0 per 10^5 while European/American-born Jews had a prevalence of 58.7 per 10^5, suggesting that environmental influences superseded any potential greater genetic predisposition to balance out the initial differences in rates. The rate among Bedouin Arabs was only 8.2 per 10^5. Rising incidence rates have also been reported for UC in the Middle East. A study of the Jewish population of central Israel by Grossman et al found that the incidence rate rose from 2.67 per 10^5 in 1970 to 5.09 per 10^5 in 1979.[56] The age-adjusted prevalence in Israel-born Jews was 45.8, in Asian/African-born Jews 48.5, and in European/American-born Jews 52.7. By 1980, the differences among these groups had markedly diminished when compared to a previous study 10 years earlier. A 10-year follow-up community-based survey (1987 to 1997) of kibbutz residents in Israel reported an incidence of 5.04 per 10^5 for UC. The prevalence of UC increased from 121 per 10^5 to 167.2 per 10^5 from 1987 to 1999.[57]

Increasing numbers of case series have been reported from Arab countries, suggesting these diseases are no longer uncommon in these countries, but broader population-based studies are unavailable. A 6-year case series (1977 to 1982) from the Amiri Hospital in Kuwait, which serves 55% of the population of Kuwait, estimated an incidence rate of 2.27 per 10^5 for UC and 0.45 per 10^5 for CD.[52] In contrast, the incidence of UC in Turkey ranged only from 0.59 to 0.69 per 10^5 between 1998 and 2001.[58]

AFRICA

Data from the African continent are limited. However, a series of studies from Cape Town, South Africa showed an increasing burden of IBD in this population[24] similar to that seen in the rest of the world. From 1980 to 1984, a retrospective review of hospital records in addition to a survey of private practitioners in Cape Town was conducted to identify new cases of IBD. Whites were more commonly affected than Blacks. The incidence of CD for Whites increased from 1.1 per 10^5 in 1970 to 1974 to 2.6 per 10^5 in 1980 to 1984; for UC, the incidence rose from 2.7 per 10^5 to 5.0 per 10^5 in 1980 to 1984. For Blacks, there were no cases of CD or UC identified in 1970 to 1974. However, for the period from 1980 to 1984, there were 0.3 per 10^5 for CD and 0.6 per 10^5 for UC.[24]

CENTRAL AND SOUTH AMERICA, CARIBBEAN

The epidemiology of IBD in Central and South America has been minimally investigated. In 2004, Appleyard et al reported a significant increase in the incidence of IBD in the southwest part of Puerto Rico.[27] From 1996 to 2000, they used ICD codes in the medical records of private gastroenterologists to identify possible cases. Further evaluation of the medical records was used to confirm the diagnosis of UC, CD, or nonspecified IBD. The incidence of UC increased from 1.96 per 10^5 to 3.32 per 10^5 and for CD it increased from 0.49 per 105 to 1.96 per 10^5. The investigators noted that the majority of patients resided in one of the two main towns in the area.

In contrast, a 7-year study (1987 to 1993) looking at hospital-based registries in 2 communities from Panama and Argentina reported much lower incidence rates for IBD.[53] The incidence of UC was 1.2 per 10^5 in Panama and 2.2 per 10^5 in Argentina. In this particular study, there were no cases of CD identified in Panama and only one case was identified in Argentina. This type of study underestimates the actual incidence of disease because the majority of patients with UC or CD can be managed in an outpatient setting and would not be included in a hospital registry.

Possible Explanations for Changing Epidemiology

Investigations into factors explaining this apparent shift in epidemiology in IBD in the developing world have been few to date. The first studies have been descriptive to assess the magnitude of these changes. How this emerging trend can help reveal the forces that provoke IBD remains undetermined.[59] The changing patterns in the geographic distribution of IBD with increasing numbers of cases in parts of the world where these diseases used to be rare implies that environmental factors such as diet and urbanization themselves may play important roles in the development of these diseases. The importance of these influences is underscored by the fact that the genetic composition of the population has not changed significantly over the years.

Epidemiologic observations on the differences in incidence and prevalence of IBD among different populations, as well as familial aggregation, point to the existence of some predisposing genetic factors. Identical twin studies have shown a concordance rate of 50% to 60% for CD,[60,61] which is higher than that seen among first-degree relatives. At the same time, the absence of higher concordance rates points to the existence of other factors playing an important role in the development of the disease. While genetic predisposition appears central, particularly for CD, this likely shifting epidemiology of IBD in developing countries underscores the critical role of undetermined environmental factors.

Investigations done in the United Kingdom by Probert et al found that south Asian immigrants (mostly Indian) in Leicester had a greater risk of developing UC than the background English population (135 x 10^5 cases in south Asians versus 90.8 x 10^5 in the English).[62,63] An increased incidence of IBD in Asians, mostly Indians and Pakistanis, born in the United Kingdom was confirmed in a nationally representative birth cohort born in Britain in 1 week of 1970. By age 26, Asians were 6 times more likely to be diagnosed with IBD compared to the non-Asian population.[64] A further epidemiologic study in Leicester confirmed a higher risk of developing UC in the south Asian population.[65] Genetic factors associated with this possible increased risk have not yet been identified. Investigations of the *NOD2/CARD15*, a common mutation identified in Western populations, have essentially been absent in studies in CD patients from Korea,[66,67] China,[68,69] and Japan.[70] Furthermore, genetic factors do not explain the changing picture of IBD in these countries that is occurring in the same genetic background present before IBD emerged.

Some investigators have suggested that previous cases of CD may have been mistaken for intestinal tuberculosis (TB), which can mimic the clinical, histological, and immunologic features of CD. While reports from India[71] suggest distinguishing between CD and intestinal TB is not difficult in most cases, this still could be a confounding issue in understanding the shifting epidemiology of IBD. It is interesting to note that a recent paper from India[72] suggested that 50% of individuals with intestinal TB were positive for anti-*Saccharomyces cerevisiae* antibody, reducing the use of this potential diagnostic tool in the developing countries to identify cases of CD.

Few environmental risk factors for IBD have been explored in developing countries. However, multiple studies have described a strong association between cigarette smoking, appendectomy, and IBD in the west. Some studies in developing countries have confirmed a similar role for these environmental factors in developing countries. Smoking in the Western literature appears to have a protective effect against UC and is associated with fewer exacerbations of UC and decreased need for colectomy.[73-75] This finding has been validated by Jiang et al in a Chinese case-control study in which smoking was found to be protective for UC and smoking cessation was associated with an increased risk of UC.[76] Another Chinese study revealed that smoking did not influence the severity of UC and ex-smokers appeared at higher risk of developing CD, although current smokers did not.[48]

Several epidemiologic studies have noted that appendectomy might have a protective effect against developing UC. Studies from France and Australia revealed that patients who had appendectomy prior to the diagnosis of UC were less likely to require colectomy.[77,78] A study from Japan showed that UC patients with prior appendectomy presented with UC at an older age and had less recurring symptoms than those without appendectomy.[79] A study of patients from Iran suggests that appendectomy is a risk factor in CD but has a modest protective effect for development of UC.[80] In a study of a Chinese population, Jiang et al also found that appendectomy was associated with a low risk for UC.[76]

Other reasons for the increase in IBD in developing nations remain speculative and unstudied. Potential immunologic influences are postulated by the "hygiene hypothesis." The hygiene hypothesis proposes that zeal to assure a clean environment has led to a lack of exposure to certain infectious illnesses that influence the immune system critically. This lack of immune exposure has been proposed as central to the development of autoimmune diseases. The evidence that the hygiene hypothesis applies to the development of IBD is equivocal. A modification of the hygiene hypothesis suggests that elimination of helminths from the intestinal microbiome has been an essential permissive step in the development of IBD by removing a factor that regulates T-cell activity.[81,82] This hypothesis concerning IBD has not been detailed in the developing countries.

Diet, particularly a shift toward a Westernized diet, may be critical to the emergence of IBD in India. In studies in the United States and Europe, an increased intake of refined sugar has been consistently identified as significantly associated with CD although less consistently with UC.[83-86] A Japanese study similarly confirmed that an increase in refined sugar intake was a risk factor for CD.[87] Other dietary factors implicated, although not consistently, included ingestion of fast foods,[88] fats,[87,89] meat,[90] sulfur,[90] and alcohol, which was protective.[91] Some of these dietary changes may influence the immune response such as had been suggested in a shift in N-3/N-6 fatty acids ratios.[91] These have not been assessed in developing countries.

Epidemiological studies of Indian immigrants in Britain with IBD implicated several possible environmental exposures as contributors to their risk of IBD, with diet being the most likely suspect. A postal questionnaire suggested that a high intake of refined carbohydrates was found among Hindu patients with CD compared to ethnically matched patients with UC or healthy controls. Hindus with IBD were less likely to drink milk, use spices, or eat foods cooked with flour.[93] Reuse of cooking oil appeared as a risk as well.[94] Betel nut chewing, common in India, appeared protective against the development of UC among Indians in England.[95] The applicability of this data to an Indian population living in India is indirect and uncertain.

Broad changes in dietary habits have been striking during the expansion of industrialization in Western countries, and these changes may have important implications for the composition of gut microbiome. An appreciation of the enormity of the alterations in diet in the West in the past century may be obscured by the relative homogeneity of US society. A decrease in complex carbohydrate intake has occurred over the past century concomitantly with a sharp increase in refined sugar. A study of refined sugar intake in England found the per capita intake in 1815 to be 6.8 kg, increasing by 1970 to 55.5 kg. In the United States in 2000, the per capita intake in refined sugar was 69.1 kg.[96] These 2 factors, an increase in refined sugar and a decrease in complex carbohydrates, may account for much of the possible shift in gut flora over the past century. While these broad shifts have been suggested in the diet of the developing world, these factors have not been directly associated with development of IBD in these countries.

While the influence of diet on gut flora has been subject to limited study, the influence of complex carbohydrates as a food supplement has been extensively studied. Complex carbohydrates poorly digested in the small bowel, or probiotics, have been shown in numerous studies to have a profound effect on flora, increasing *Bifidobacterium* species in particular.[97] Indirect studies suggested that gut flora may have changed radically recently. Studies comparing gut flora from rural Africa (Nigeria), where IBD is rare, to an English population suggested that a preindustrial diet may influence a different intestinal flora. Only 16% of the adult Nigerian population was found to have *Bacteroides* in stool cultures compared to 100% in UK adults.[98] A similar pattern was seen with *Clostridia*. The capacity of a high refined sugar intake to influence gut flora has been demonstrated in rats, with an increase of *Bacteroides* with a high sucrose diet, and an increase in *Clostridia* in a high starch diet.[99] The immediate relevance of these alterations to IBD remains uncertain.

Other dietary or environmental factors may influence flora. *Bifidobacterium* compose the predominant species in breastfed infants, whereas *Bacteroides* was prevalent in bottle-fed infants.[100,101] More recent studies have suggested coliforms may be increased in breastfed infants while bottle-fed infants had similar amounts of *Bifidobacterium* with changes persisting over time.[102] Breastfeeding has been decreasing in the developing countries although a link to IBD in these countries has not been demonstrated.

Clinical Features and Treatment

Although there are marked differences in the prevalence of IBD between the West and the developing world, many clinical features are shared. A recent review of IBD in the Asian Pacific region by Ouyang et al suggests that age of onset is similar.[103] Smoking and previous appendectomy appear to have the same protective effect in UC as in the West. The distribution and extent of disease is also comparable, but with the exception of Northern Indians, disease severity is generally less. In contrast to European and North American reports where the distribution of IBD is roughly equal among men and women, reports from Japan, Singapore, and China suggest a slight male predominance of UC. A striking difference is the lack of association with mutations of the *NOD2/CARD15* gene in Asian patients with CD.[103] A recent study from India by Venkataraman et al found that the risk of developing colorectal cancer in Indian patients with UC is lower than that reported from the West.[104]

A study from Korea found that the rates of colectomy are much lower (2% after 1 year and 3.3% after 5 to 15 years) than in Western patients where rates range from 3% to 10% after 1 year and 8% to 34% after 10 years.[105] In contrast, a study from India showed that surgical intervention played a much larger role for UC patients than it did in the West. This was secondary to the severity of disease with which patients presented and the limited access to medical therapies to induce remission.[106]

The initial pharmacological approach to treating IBD in developing nations is similar to that of the West beginning with the use of sulfasalazine, 5-aminosalicylates, and steroids. However, the use of immune suppression and the availability of newer therapies such as the biologics may differ markedly among countries. Lastly, cultures with a rich heritage in traditional medicine, such as China, have almost 90% of people using traditional medicine combined with Western medicine.[103,107]

Summary

The incidence of IBD remains highest in North America and western Europe. However, epidemiological studies over the past 20 years have suggested an increasing burden of disease in the developing world. Environmental factors influencing the apparent emergence of IBD in these countries have not been established; however, likely culprits include changes in lifestyle with an increase in tobacco use and the adoption of a Westernized diet. Confounding factors for this suggested increase include an improving awareness and recognition of this diagnosis, improved diagnostic capacity, and changes in health care delivery.

Whether phenotypic differences exist between IBD in the developing world and Western countries has only begun to be examined. However, as some of the environmental and genetic factors may differ, it remains uncertain if the diseases may contrast in terms of disease presentation, fundamental disease behavior, and response to medications as well as risks. What appears likely is that countries in which IBD was considered rare until recently may overtake Western countries in incidence and prevalence of these diseases. In the decades ahead, China and India may be confronted with a larger IBD population than the United States and western Europe. This globalization of IBD does offer the possibility of identifying risk factors that may have been obscured by time or homogenization of society as has occurred in the West. However, the environmental, economic, and political differences present in developing countries present challenges in understanding and treating IBD in a different context and adapting our current knowledge, based largely on studies in the West, to the needs of patients in the developing world.

References

1. Pinchbeck BR, Kirdeikis J, Thomson AB. Inflammatory bowel disease in northern Alberta: an epidemiologic study. *J Clin Gastroenterol.* 1988;10(5):505-515.
2. Hiatt RA, Kaufman L. Epidemiology of inflammatory bowel disease in a defined northern California population. *West J Med.* 1988;149(5):541-546.
3. Stowe SP, Redmond SR, Stormont JM. An epidemiologic study of inflammatory bowel disease in Rochester, New York: hospital incidence. *Gastroenterology.* 1990;98(1):104-110.
4. Kurata JH, Kantor-Fish S, Frankl H, Godby P, Vadheim CM. Crohn's disease among ethnic groups in a large health maintenance organization. *Gastroenterology.* 1992;102(6):1940-1948.
5. Loftus EV Jr, Silverstein MD, Sandborn WJ, Tremaine WJ, Harmsen WS, Zinsmeister AR. Crohn's disease in Olmsted County, Minnesota, 1940-1993: incidence, prevalence, and survival. *Gastroenterology.* 1998;114(6):1161-1168.
6. Bernstein CN, Blanchard JF, Rawsthorne P, Wajda A. Epidemiology of Crohn's disease and ulcerative colitis in a central Canadian province: a population-based study. *Am J Epidemiol.* 1999;149(10):916-924.
7. Loftus EV Jr, Silverstein MD, Sandborn WJ, Tremaine WJ, Harmsen WS, Zinsmeister AR. Ulcerative colitis in Olmsted County, Minnesota, 1940-1993: incidence, prevalence, and survival. *Gut.* 2000;46(3):336-343.
8. Blanchard JF, Bernstein CN, Wajda A, Rawsthorne P. Small-area variations and sociodemographic correlates for the incidence of Crohn's disease and ulcerative colitis. *Am J Epidemiol.* 2001;154(4):328-335.
9. Loftus CG, Loftus EV Jr, Harmsen WS. Update on the incidence and prevalence of Crohn's disease and ulcerative colitis in Olmsted County, Minnesota, 1940-2000. *Inflamm Bowel Dis.* 2007;13(3):254-261.
10. Lapidus A, Bernell O, Hellers G, Persson PG, Löfberg R. Incidence of Crohn's disease in Stockholm County 1955-1989. *Gut.* 1997;41(4):480-486.
11. Shivananda S, Lennard-Jones J, Logan R. Incidence of inflammatory bowel disease across Europe: is there a difference between north and south? Results of the European Collaborative Study on Inflammatory Bowel Disease (EC-IBD). *Gut.* 1996;39(5):690-697.
12. Moum B, Vatn MH, Ekbom A. Incidence of ulcerative colitis and indeterminate colitis in four counties of southeastern Norway, 1990-1993: a prospective population-based study. The Inflammatory Bowel South-Eastern Norway (IBSEN) Study Group of Gastroenterologists. *Scand J Gastroenterol.* 1996;31(4):362-366.
13. Munkholm P, Langholz E, Nielsen OH, Kreiner S, Binder V. Incidence and prevalence of Crohn's disease in the county of Copenhagen, 1962-87: a sixfold increase in incidence. *Scand J Gastroenterol.* 1992;27(7):609-614.
14. Daiss W, Scheurlen M, Malchow H. Epidemiology of inflammatory bowel disease in the county of Tubingen (West Germany). *Scand J Gastroenterol Suppl.* 1989;170:39-43; discussion 50-55.
15. Roin F, Roin J. Inflammatory bowel disease of the Faroe Islands, 1981-1988: a prospective epidemiologic study: primary report. *Scand J Gastroenterol Suppl.* 1989;170:44-46; discussion 50-55.
16. Halme L, von Smitten K, Husa A. The incidence of Crohn's disease in the Helsinki metropolitan area during 1975-1985. *Ann Chir Gynaecol.* 1989;78(2):115-119.
17. Langholz E, Munkholm P, Nielsen OH, Kreiner S, Binder V. Incidence and prevalence of ulcerative colitis in Copenhagen county from 1962 to 1987. *Scand J Gastroenterol.* 1991;26(12):1247-1256.
18. Gower-Rousseau C, Salomez JL, Dupas JL, et al. Incidence of inflammatory bowel disease in northern France (1988-1990). *Gut.* 1994;35(10):1433-1438.
19. Stewénius J, Adnerhill I, Ekelund G, et al. Ulcerative colitis and indeterminate colitis in the city of Malmo, Sweden: a 25-year incidence study. *Scand J Gastroenterol.* 1995;30(1):38-43.

20. Moum B, Vatn MH, Ekbom A, et al. Incidence of Crohn's disease in four counties in southeastern Norway, 1990-93: a prospective population-based study. The Inflammatory Bowel South-Eastern Norway (IBSEN) Study Group of Gastroenterologists. *Scand J Gastroenterol.* 1996;31(4):355-361.

21. Russel MG, Dorant E, Volovics A, et al. High incidence of inflammatory bowel disease in The Netherlands: results of a prospective study. The South Limburg IBD Study Group. *Dis Colon Rectum.* 1998;41(1):33-40.

22. Björnsson S, Jóhannsson JH. Inflammatory bowel disease in Iceland, 1990-1994: a prospective, nationwide, epidemiological study. *Eur J Gastroenterol Hepatol.* 2000;12(1):31-38.

23. Björnsson S, Johannsson JH, Oddsson E. Inflammatory bowel disease in Iceland, 1980-89: a retrospective nationwide epidemiologic study. *Scand J Gastroenterol.* 1998;33(1):71-77.

24. Wright JP, Froggatt J, O'Keefe EA, et al. The epidemiology of inflammatory bowel disease in Cape Town 1980-1984. *S Afr Med J.* 1986;70(1):10-15.

25. Sood A, Midha V, Sood N, Bhatia AS, Avasthi G. Incidence and prevalence of ulcerative colitis in Punjab, North India. *Gut.* 2003;52(11):1587-1590.

26. Yang SK, Hong WS, Min YI, et al. Incidence and prevalence of ulcerative colitis in the Songpa-Kangdong District, Seoul, Korea, 1986-1997. *J Gastroenterol Hepatol.* 2000;15(9):1037-1042.

27. Appleyard CB, Hernández G, Rios-Bedoya CF. Basic epidemiology of inflammatory bowel disease in Puerto Rico. *Inflamm Bowel Dis.* 2004;10(2):106-111.

28. Morita N, Toki S, Hirohashi T, et al. Incidence and prevalence of inflammatory bowel disease in Japan: nationwide epidemiological survey during the year 1991. *J Gastroenterol.* 1995;30(Suppl 8):1-4.

29. Trallori G, Palli D, Saieva C, et al. A population-based study of inflammatory bowel disease in Florence over 15 years (1978-92). *Scand J Gastroenterol.* 1996;31(9):892-899.

30. Ladas SD, Mallas E, Giorgiotis K, et al. Incidence of ulcerative colitis in Central Greece: a prospective study. *World J Gastroenterol.* 2005;11(12):1785-1787.

31. Vind I, Riis L, Jess T, et al. Increasing incidences of inflammatory bowel disease and decreasing surgery rates in Copenhagen City and County, 2003-2005: a population-based study from the Danish Crohn colitis database. *Am J Gastroenterol.* 2006;101(6):1274-1282.

32. Ogunbi SO, Ransom JA, Sullivan K, Schoen BT, Gold BD. Inflammatory bowel disease in African-American children living in Georgia. *J Pediatr.* 1998;133(1):103-107.

33. Yapp TR, Stenson R, Thomas GA, Lawrie BW, Williams GT, Hawthorne AB. Crohn's disease incidence in Cardiff from 1930: an update for 1991-1995. *Eur J Gastroenterol Hepatol.* 2000;12(8):907-911.

34. Rubin GP, Hungin AP, Kelly PJ, Ling J. Inflammatory bowel disease: epidemiology and management in an English general practice population. *Aliment Pharmacol Ther.* 2000;14(12):1553-1559.

35. Vuceli B, Kora B, Senti M, et al. Epidemiology of Crohn's disease in Zagreb, Yugoslavia: a ten-year prospective study. *Int J Epidemiol.* 1991;20(1):216-220.

36. Vuceli B, Kora B, Senti M, et al. Ulcerative colitis in Zagreb, Yugoslavia: incidence and prevalence 1980-1989. *Int J Epidemiol.* 1991;20(4):1043-1047.

37. Manousos ON, Giannadaki E, Mouzas IA, et al. Ulcerative colitis is as common in Crete as in northern Europe: a 5-year prospective study. *Eur J Gastroenterol Hepatol.* 1996;8(9):893-898.

38. Manousos ON, Koutroubakis I, Potamianos S, et al. A prospective epidemiologic study of Crohn's disease in Heraklion, Crete: incidence over a 5-year period. *Scand J Gastroenterol.* 1996;31(6):599-603.

39. Maté-Jimenez J, Muñoz S, Vicent D, Pajares JM. Incidence and prevalence of ulcerative colitis and Crohn's disease in urban and rural areas of Spain from 1981 to 1988. *J Clin Gastroenterol.* 1994;18(1):27-31.

40. Tragnone A, Corrao G, Miglio F, Caprilli R, Lanfranchi GA. Incidence of inflammatory bowel disease in Italy: a nationwide population-based study. Gruppo Italiano per lo Studio del Colon e del Retto (GISC). *Int J Epidemiol.* 1996;25(5):1044-1052.

41. Lakatos L, Mester G, Erdélyi Z, et al. [Epidemiology of inflammatory bowel diseases in Veszprem county of Western Hungary between 1977 and 2001]. *Orv Hetil.* 2003;144(37):1819-1827.

42. Mijandrusic-Sincic B, Vucelic B, Stimac D, et al. The epidemiology of the inflammatory bowel diseases in Northern Costal County, Croatia. In: *Falk Symposium 140.* Berlin, Germany: Springer-Verlag; 2005:34-40.

43. Sinci BM, Vuceli B, Persi M, et al. Incidence of inflammatory bowel disease in Primorsko-goranska County, Croatia, 2000-2004: a prospective population-based study. *Scand J Gastroenterol.* 2006;41(4):437-444.

44. Nedbal J, Maratka Z. [Ulcerative colitis in Czechoslovakia]. *Vnitr Lek.* 1967;13(11):1054-1063.

45. Bitter J, Dyrhonova V, Komarkova O, et al. Nespecificke strevni sanety v Ceske republice. *Ceskoslovenska Gastroenterologia a Vyliva.* 1992;46:313-321.

46. Wiercinska-Drapalo A, Jaroszewicz J, Flisiak R, Prokopowicz D. Epidemiological characteristics of inflammatory bowel disease in North-Eastern Poland. *World J Gastroenterol.* 2005;11(17):2630-2633.

47. Gheorghe C, Pascu O, Gheorghe L, et al. Epidemiology of inflammatory bowel disease in adults who refer to gastroenterology care in Romania: a multicentre study. *Eur J Gastroenterol Hepatol.* 2004;16(11):1153-1159.

48. Leong RW, Lau JY, Sung JJ. The epidemiology and phenotype of Crohn's disease in the Chinese population. *Inflamm Bowel Dis.* 2004;10(5):646-651.

49. Odes HS, Locker C, Neumann L, et al. Epidemiology of Crohn's disease in southern Israel. *Am J Gastroenterol.* 1994;89(10):1859-1862.

50. Abdul-Baki H, ElHajj I, El-Zahabi LM, et al. Clinical epidemiology of inflammatory bowel disease in Lebanon. *Inflamm Bowel Dis.* 2007;13(4):475-480.

51. Radhakrishnan S, Zubaidi G, Daniel M, Sachdev GK, Mohan AN. Ulcerative colitis in Oman: a prospective study of the incidence and disease pattern from 1987 to 1994. *Digestion.* 1997;58(3):266-270.

52. Al-Nakib B, Radhakrishnan S, Jacob GS, Al-Liddawi H, Al-Ruwaih A. Inflammatory bowel disease in Kuwait. *Am J Gastroenterol.* 1984;79(3):191-194.

53. Linares de la Cal JA, Cantón C, Hermida C, Pérez-Miranda M, Maté-Jiménez J. Estimated incidence of inflammatory bowel disease in Argentina and Panama (1987-1993). *Rev Esp Enferm Dig.* 1999;91(4):277-286.

54. Edouard A, Paillaud M, Merle S, Orhan C, Chenayer-Panelatti Dagger M; COGEAG. Incidence of inflammatory bowel disease in the French West Indies (1997-1999). *Gastroenterol Clin Biol.* 2005;29(8-9):779-783.

55. Fireman Z, Grossman A, Lilos P, Eshchar Y, Theodor E, Gilat T. Epidemiology of Crohn's disease in the Jewish population of central Israel, 1970-1980. *Am J Gastroenterol.* 1989;84(3):255-258.

56. Grossman A, Fireman Z, Lilos P, Novis B, Rozen P, Gilat T. Epidemiology of ulcerative colitis in the Jewish population of central Israel 1970-1980. *Hepatogastroenterology.* 1989;36(4):193-197.

57. Niv Y, Abuksis G, Fraser GM. Epidemiology of ulcerative colitis in Israel: a survey of Israeli kibbutz settlements. *Am J Gastroenterol.* 2000;95(3):693-698.

58. Tezel A, Dökmeci G, Eskiocak M, Umit H, Soylu AR. Epidemiological features of ulcerative colitis in Trakya, Turkey. *J Int Med Res.* 2003;31(2):141-148.

59. Podolsky DK. Inflammatory bowel disease. *N Engl J Med.* 2002;347(6):417-429.

60. Orholm M, Binder V, Sørensen TI, Rasmussen LP, Kyvik KO. Concordance of inflammatory bowel disease among Danish twins: results of a nationwide study. *Scand J Gastroenterol.* 2000;35(10):1075-1081.

61. Halfvarson J, Bodin L, Tysk C, Lindberg E, Järnerot G. Inflammatory bowel disease in a Swedish twin cohort: a long-term follow-up of concordance and clinical characteristics. *Gastroenterology.* 2003;124(7):1767-1773.

62. Jayanthi V, Probert CS, Pinder D, Wicks AC, Mayberry JF. Epidemiology of Crohn's disease in Indian migrants and the indigenous population in Leicestershire. *Q J Med.* 1992;82(298):125-138.

63. Probert CS, Jayanthi V, Hughes AO, Thompson JR, Wicks AC, Mayberry JF. Prevalence and family risk of ulcerative colitis and Crohn's disease: an epidemiological study among Europeans and south Asians in Leicestershire. *Gut.* 1993;34(11):1547-1551.

64. Montgomery SM, Morris DL, Pounder RE, Wakefield AJ. Asian ethnic origin and the risk of inflammatory bowel disease. *Eur J Gastroenterol Hepatol.* 1999;11(5):543-546.

65. Carr I, Mayberry JF. The effects of migration on ulcerative colitis: a three-year prospective study among Europeans and first- and second-generation South Asians in Leicester (1991-1994). *Am J Gastroenterol.* 1999;94(10):2918-2922.

66. Lee GH, Kim CG, Kim JS, Jung HC, Song IS. [Frequency analysis of *NOD2* gene mutations in Korean patients with Crohn's disease]. *Korean J Gastroenterol.* 2005;45(3):162-168.

67 Croucher PJ, Mascheretti S, Hampe J, et al. Haplotype structure and association to Crohn's disease of *CARD15* mutations in two ethnically divergent populations. *Eur J Hum Genet.* 2003;11(1):6-16.

68. Guo QS, Xia B, Jiang Y, Qu Y, Li J. *NOD2* 3020insC frameshift mutation is not associated with inflammatory bowel disease in Chinese patients of Han nationality. *World J Gastroenterol.* 2004;10(7):1069-1071.

69. Leong RW, Armuzzi A, Ahmad T, et al. *NOD2/CARD15* gene polymorphisms and Crohn's disease in the Chinese population. *Aliment Pharmacol Ther.* 2003;17(12):1465-1470.

70. Inoue N, Tamura K, Kinouchi Y, et al. Lack of common *NOD2* variants in Japanese patients with Crohn's disease. *Gastroenterology.* 2002;123(1):86-91.

71. Amarapurkar DN, Patel ND, Rane PS. Diagnosis of Crohn's disease in India where tuberculosis is widely prevalent. *World J Gastroenterology.* 2008;14(5):741-746.

72. Ghoshal UC, Ghoshal U, Singh H, Tiwari S. Anti-*Saccharomyces cerevisiae* antibody is not useful to differentiate between Crohn's disease and intestinal tuberculosis in India. *J Postgrad Med.* 2007;53(3):166-170.

73. Calkins BM. A meta-analysis of the role of smoking in inflammatory bowel disease. *Dig Dis Sci.* 1989;34(12):1841-1854.

74. Boyko EJ, Perera DR, Koepsell TD, Keane EM, Inui TS. Effects of cigarette smoking on the clinical course of ulcerative colitis. *Scan J Gastroenterol.* 1998;23(9):1147-1152.

75. Boyko EJ, Koepsell TD, Perera DR, Inui TS. Risk of ulcerative colitis among former and current cigarette smokers. *N Engl J Med.* 1987;316(12):707-710.

76. Jiang L, Xia B, Li J, et al. Risk factors for ulcerative colitis in a Chinese population: an age-matched and sex-matched case-control study. *J Clin Gastroenterol.* 2007;41(3):280-284.

77. Radford-Smith GL, Edwards JE, Purdie DM, et al. Protective role of appendicectomy on onset and severity of ulcerative colitis and Crohn's disease. *Gut.* 2002;51(6):808-813.

78. Cosnes J, Carbonnel F, Beaugerie L, Blain A, Reijasse D, Gendre JP. Effects of appendicectomy on the course of ulcerative colitis. *Gut.* 2002;51(6):803-807.

79. Naganuma M, Iizuka B, Torii A, et al. Appendectomy protects against the development of ulcerative colitis and reduces its recurrence: results of a multicenter case-controlled study in Japan. *Am J Gastroenterol.* 2001;96(4):1123-1126.

80. Firouzi F, Bahari A, Aghazadeh R, Zali MR. Appendectomy, tonsillectomy, and risk of inflammatory bowel disease: a case control study in Iran. *Int J Colorectal Dis.* 2006;21(2):155-159.

81. Weinstock JV. Helminths and mucosal immune modulation. *Ann N Y Acad Sci.* 2006;1072:356-364.

82. Guarner F, Bourdet-Sicard R, Brandtzaeg P, et al. Mechanisms of disease: the hygiene hypothesis revisited. *Nat Clin Pract Gastroenterol Hepatol.* 2006;3(5):275-284.

83. Klein I, Reif S, Farbstein H, Halak A, Gilat T. Preillness non dietary factors and habits in inflammatory bowel disease. *Ital J Gastroenterol Hepatol.* 1998;30(3):247-251.

84. Riordan AM, Ruxton CH, Hunter JO. A review of associations between Crohn's disease and consumption of sugars. *Eur J Clin Nutr.* 1998;52(4):229-238.

85. Russel MG, Engels LG, Muris JW, et al. Modern life in the epidemiology of inflammatory bowel disease: a case-control study with special emphasis on nutritional factors. *Eur J Gastroenterol Hepatol.* 1998;10(3):243-249.

86. Tragnone A, Corrao G, Miglio F, Caprilli R, Lanfranchi GA. Dietary habits as risk factors for inflammatory bowel disease. *Eur J Gastroenterol Hepatol.* 1995;7(1):47-51.

87. Sakamoto N, Kono S, Wakai K, et al. Dietary risk factors for inflammatory bowel disease: a multicenter case-control study in Japan. *Inflamm Bowel Dis.* 2005;11(2):154-163.

88. Persson PG, Ahlbom A, Hellers G. Diet and inflammatory bowel disease: a case-control study. *Epidemiology.* 1992;3(1):47-52.

89. Geerling BJ, Dagnelie PC, Badart-Smook A, Russel MG, Stockbrügger RW, Brummer RJ. Diet as a risk factor for the development of ulcerative colitis. *Am J Gastroenterol.* 2000;95(4):1008-1013.

90. Jowett SL, Seal CJ, Pearce MS, et al. Influence of dietary factors on the clinical course of ulcerative colitis: a prospective cohort study. *Gut.* 2004;53(10):1479-1484.

91. Boyko EJ, Perera DR, Koepsell TD, Keane EM, Inui TS. Coffee and alcohol use and the risk of ulcerative colitis. *Am J Gastroenterol.* 1989;84(5):530-544.

92. Campos FG, Waitzberg DL, Habr-Gama A, et al. Impact of parenteral n-3 fatty acids on experimental acute colitis. *Br J Nutr.* 2002;87(Suppl 1):S83-S88.

93. Probert CS, Bhakta P, Bhamra B, Jayanthi V, Mayberry JF. Diet of South Asians with inflammatory bowel disease. *Arq Gastroenterol.* 1996;33(3):132-135.

94. Chuah SY, Jayanthi V, Lee CN, McDonald B, Probert CS, Mayberry JF. Dietary fats and inflammatory bowel disease in Asians. *Ital J Gastroenterol.* 1992;24(7):386-388.

95. Lee CN, Jayanthi V, McDonald B, Probert CS, Mayberry JF. Betel nut and smoking: are they both protective in ulcerative colitis? A pilot study. *Arq Gastroenterol.* 1996;33(1):3-5.

96. Cordain L, Eaton SB, Sebastian A, et al. Origins and evolution of the Western diet: health implications for the 21st century. *Am J Clin Nutr.* 2005;81(2):341-354.

97. Crociani F, Alessandrini A, Mucci MM, Biavati B. Degradation of complex carbohydrates by *Bifidobacterium spp. Int J Food Microbiol.* 1994;24(1-2):199-210.

98. Drasar BS, Montgomery F, Tomkins AM. Diet and faecal flora in three dietary groups in rural northern Nigeria. *J Hyg (Lond).* 1986;96(1):59-65.

99. Cresci A, Orpianesi C, Silvi S, Mastrandrea V, Dolara P. The effect of sucrose or starch-based diet on short-chain fatty acids and faecal microflora in rats. *J Appl Microbiol.* 1999;86(2):245-250.

100. Balmer SE, Wharton BA. Diet and faecal flora in the newborn: breast milk and infant formula. *Arch Dis Child.* 1989;64(12):1672-1677.

101. Harmsen HJ, Wildeboer-Veloo AC, Raangs GC, et al. Analysis of intestinal flora development in breast-fed and formula-fed infants by using molecular identification and detection methods. *J Pediatr Gastroenterol Nutr.* 2000;30(1):61-67.

102. Penders J, Vink C, Driessen C, London N, Thijs C, Stobberingh EE. Quantification of *Bifidobacterium spp., Escherichia coli* and *Clostridium difficile* in faecal samples of breast-fed and formula-fed infants by real-time PCR. *FEMS Microbiol Lett.* 2005;243(1):141-147.

103. Ouyang Q, Tandon R, Goh KL, Ooi CJ, Ogata H, Fiocchi C. The emergence of inflammatory bowel disease in the Asian Pacific region. *Curr Opin Gastroenterol.* 2005;21(4):408-413.

104. Venkataraman S, Mohan V, Ramakrishna BS, et al. Risk of colorectal cancer in ulcerative colitis in India. *J Gastroenterol Hepatol.* 2005;20(5):705-709.

105. Park SH, Kim YM, Yang SK, et al. Clinical features and natural history of ulcerative colitis in Korea. *Inflamm Bowel Dis.* 2007;13(3):278-283.

106. Duphare H, Misra SC, Patnaik PK, Mathur M, Tandon RK. Spectrum of ulcerative colitis in North India. *J Clin Gastroenterol.* 1994;18(1):23-26.

107. Jiang XL, Cui HF. An analysis of 10218 ulcerative colitis cases in China. *World J Gastroenterol.* 2002;8(1):158-161.

CHAPTER 3

IMMUNE DEVELOPMENT AND INFLAMMATORY BOWEL DISEASE

Lee A. Denson, MD

While the key structural components of the mucosal immune system are present at birth, they do not reach complete functional maturity until early adolescence. In contrast to the systemic immune system, the mucosal immune system in the gut must be able to mount vigorous responses to pathogens while maintaining tolerance to a tremendous variety of nonpathogenic antigens from diet and the commensal flora.

This is accomplished in part via compartmentalization of inductive and effector functions, and in part via a more "tolerogenic" skewing of cell populations, cell surface receptors, and local cytokine production. The inductive compartments are the organized lymphoid structures including Peyer's patches (PPs) in the small bowel and isolated lymphoid follicles (ILFs) in the small bowel and colon. The effector compartments include the T- and B-cell populations distributed throughout the lamina propria and in the intraepithelial location.

Individual variation in development of the mucosal immune system in the postnatal period is critically dependent upon environmental influences. The most important environmental influence is the mode of bacterial colonization, which may have a profound and lasting effect upon the functional properties of the mucosal immune system. During puberty, rapid changes in circulating growth factors and sex hormones also influence the function of the systemic and mucosal immune systems. These environmental influences may then combine with genetic susceptibility and discrete intrinsic stages in the development of the mucosal immune system to create windows of susceptibility for developing subtypes of Crohn's disease (CD) or ulcerative colitis (UC). This chapter will review development of the mucosal immune system in the context of the development of inflammatory bowel disease (IBD) in children and adolescents.

Scherl EJ, Dubinsky MC.
*The Changing World of Inflammatory Bowel Disease:
Impact of Generation, Gender, and Global Trends (pp 33-48)*
© 2009 SLACK Incorporated.

Clinical Subtypes of Inflammatory Bowel Disease Relative to Stages of Mucosal Immune Development

A recent report from 6 centers in North America has defined important clinical and demographic differences in pediatric IBD relative to adult-onset disease.[1] Of the 1370 children in the registry (54% male), the mean age of diagnosis was 10.3 ± 4.4 years. Fifteen percent of the patients presented before the age of 6, 48% between the ages of 6 to 12, and 37% at age 13 to 17. Twenty-nine percent had one or more family members with IBD. The highest frequency of affected first-degree family members (44%) was observed in the youngest children (age <3 years) with UC. This is in contrast to the relatively low concordance (10%) for UC in adult monozygotic twins and illustrates the importance of considering the effects of genetic variation upon the development of IBD during specific periods of immune development.

In contrast to adults, colonic involvement is predominant in children under the age of 8 with CD, while ileal involvement becomes more common later in life, reaching levels comparable to adulthood by adolescence. In the Heyman series, 63% of the children with IBD who were younger than 8 years old had isolated colonic disease, while only 35% of those age 8 and older had isolated colonic disease, when considering CD, UC, and indeterminate colitis (IC) combined.[1] The frequency of UC was comparable to the frequency of CD in children less than 6 years of age, with the frequency of CD exceeding UC in older children. Importantly, the majority of pediatric UC patients had pancolitis (>80%) compared with a minority of adult UC patients (25%).[2] Data from a European series show similar results, with the probability of ileal involvement at the age of 8 years being 0.19 (0.07 to 0.39), increasing to a maximum of 0.61 (0.54 to 0.68) at age 16.[3] The overall probability of ileal disease appeared to plateau at approximately 0.60 by age 12. A concurrent *CARD15* mutation at age 16 years in this study increased the probability of ileal involvement from 0.46 (0.34 to 0.58) to 0.75 (0.55 to 0.89) and reduced the age of ileal involvement by approximately 2 years. These clinical observations support the concept that susceptibility to the different subtypes of IBD in childhood and adolescence is influenced by factors unique to this period in life, of which a critical one is likely to be the stage of development of the mucosal immune system.

As shown in Figure 3-1, humoral mucosal immune responses are largely mature by age 5 to 6 years, while the full range of inductive and effector cellular mechanisms are not fully mature until age 10 to 12 years. Moreover, the overall Th1/Th2 skewing of the mucosal immune response varies over time, with Th2 responses more common at younger ages. If colonic IBD, Crohn's colitis, and UC are more dependent upon defects in epithelial function, Th2 responses, and activation of humoral immunity, while small bowel CD is more dependent upon activation of cellular immunity and Th1/Th17 responses, this may contribute to the different types of IBD observed at different ages. Pro- and anti-inflammatory effects of estrogen, progesterone, and androgens may further modify these responses during puberty, ultimately leading to the frequency and gender dependence of IBD subtypes observed in adulthood.

Development of the Mucosal Immune System

Most components of the mucosal immune system are functionally mature by 3 years of age. IBD remains uncommon in the first 3 years of life, although the frequency of younger cases is increasing. By comparison, food allergies that resolve with time are quite common during this period. This may be due in part to functional immaturity of the mucosal immune system during this period and in part to skewing toward a more tolerogenic and Th2 phenotype of responses. While the fundamental components of the mucosal immune system are present in the term neonate,

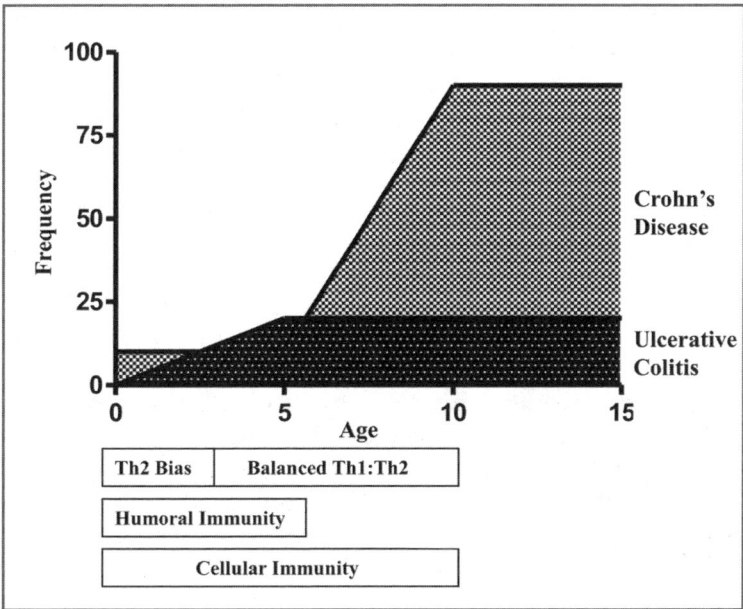

Figure 3-1. Maturation of mucosal immunity and development of IBD. The frequency of UC and CD as a function of age is shown, together with the time span over which the humoral and cellular components and Th1/Th2 skewing of the mucosal immune system become fully mature. Most components of the mucosal immune system mature over the first 3 years of life, under the influence of diet and bacterial colonization. During this period, the mucosal immune system exhibits a Th2 bias. Following this, a more balanced Th1/Th2 bias develops. The humoral immune system, including IgG- and IgA-producing lamina propria plasma cells, is fully mature by age 5. In comparison, specific inductive (eg, PPs) and effector (eg, oligoclonal T-cell receptor [TCR] repertoire) components of the cellular immune system are not fully mature until age 10 to 14 years.

substantial functional maturation influenced by the mode of feeding, circulating hormones, and the pattern of bacterial colonization occurs during the first year of life.[4] Aspects of this maturation specifically relevant to the pathogenesis of IBD will be reviewed in this section.

Epithelial Barrier Function

Alterations in epithelial barrier function are thought to contribute to increased susceptibility to IBD by increasing exposure of the mucosal immune system to antigens derived from the enteric flora. This increased antigen uptake could occur via the paracellular route because of alterations in the composition and function of the tight junction protein (TJP) complex or could occur via the transcellular route via endocytosis. In fact, both modes of excess antigen uptake have been demonstrated in the ileum in CD, and both have been shown to be secondary at least in part to local effects of tumor necrosis factor alpha (TNFα).[5]

In this regard, term infants exhibit a relative increase in epithelial permeability compared to adults.[4] While not well understood in humans, this may be due to incomplete development of TJP complexes and differences in mucus production, which in turn limit interaction between the enteric flora and the epithelium.[4] Under normal conditions, this increased permeability serves the function of exposing the mucosal adaptive immune system to the antigens associated with food and the enteric flora to which antigen-specific tolerance should ideally develop. However, this permeability is not associated with a high frequency of IBD in this age group, suggesting that either differences in the inductive or effector aspects of the immune response may be protective during this period or that proinflammatory mechanisms required for the development of IBD have not yet matured. Within several weeks of birth, intestinal permeability decreases in infants, in part under the influence of circulating glucocorticoids.[4]

Intestinal epithelial cells (IECs) are glycosylated. During infancy, most oligosaccharides attached to the epithelial surface contain terminal sialylation.[4] This changes to predominately terminal fucosylation and galactosylation with maturity; in rodents, this change occurs after weaning.[4] These changes in IEC glycosylation patterns may in turn affect bacterial colonization. For example, colonization with *Bacteroides thetaiotaomicron*, which exerts anti-inflammatory effects in the gut, is facilitated by fucosylation because it uses L-fucose as a nutrient source.[4] In this regard, several recent studies have identified differences in bacterial colonization of the gut in IBD patients.[6] Whether these differences are due in part to alterations in IEC glycosylation during infancy is not known.

In addition to the epithelial barrier provided by the tight junction complexes, a variety of secreted epithelial products limit access of the enteric flora to the mucosal immune system. These include mucins produced by epithelial goblet cells and defensins produced by epithelial Paneth cells. While production of mucins has been shown to be reduced in UC, and defensins in CD patients with *CARD15* single-nucleotide polymorphisms (SNP) carriage, whether developmental alterations in these in infancy or later in childhood contribute to the development of IBD is not known.[7-9]

Epithelial cells also actively participate in the inflammatory response in CD through the production of chemokines such as eotaxin, IL-8, and IP-10, which promote tissue recruitment of eosinophils, neutrophils, and effector T cells, respectively. The ability of IECs to produce nuclear factor kappa B (NFkB)-dependent chemokines including IL-8 in response to bacterial products such as flagellin is reduced as these mature postnatally; this has recently been attributed to increased levels of inhibitor kappa B.[10] IEC may also serve as antigen-presenting cells (APCs), leading to activation of CD8+ T cells.[7] Inappropriate upregulation of chemokine production and major histocompatibility complex class II expression on IEC in IBD may then promote T-cell recruitment and T-cell–dependent induction of IEC apoptosis, which further compromises barrier function.

Secretory IgA

The principal immune product that contributes to barrier function is secretory immunoglobulin A (sIgA) produced by plasma cells in the lamina propria. This prevents excessive antigen stimulation by binding bacterial antigens in the lumen of the gut and by actively mediating export of bound antigens from the lamina propria through IECs. The fetal lamina propria lacks sIgA-producing plasma cells. Following birth, antigenic stimulation from the enteric flora leads to a rapid increase in the numbers of lamina propria IgA and IgM plasma cells; by 6 months of age, the adult pattern of IgA predominance is seen.[4] The frequency of sIgA-producing plasma cells in the lamina propria is then fully mature by 3 years of age. By the age of 6, intestinal humoral immune responses would be expected to be comparable to that of adults.[11]

Phagocytic Cells

Macrophages, the principal phagocytic cells of the gut, are typically found in a subepithelial location and clustered in PPs.[4] Macrophages in the human intestine are normally relatively anergic in terms of activation of Toll-like receptor (TLR)-dependent inflammatory responses and proinflammatory cytokine production, while retaining active phagocytic function. This has been linked to transforming growth factor beta (TGFβ) production by neighboring stromal cells and absence of CD14 expression, which is required for lipopolysaccharide (LPS):TLR4 responses.[12] In CD, a paradoxical reduction in phagocytosis and other antimicrobial functions has been observed, combined with inappropriate TLR:NFkB activation and production of cytokines, including IL-12 and IL-23, which drive the expansion of Th1 and Th17 effector cells, respectively.[13] In this regard, mutations in *CARD15* in most studies have been shown to reduce inflammatory responses, including NFkB activation and chemokine and cytokine production, in response to the *CARD15* ligand muramyl dipeptide.[14]

Neutrophils are not observed in the intestine under basal conditions but are rapidly recruited with the onset of infection or injury. Antimicrobial functions of neutrophils, including migration, superoxide generation, and phagocytic function, are also paradoxically reduced in CD and in some patients with UC.[7,15] These reductions in phagocytic cell antimicrobial function may contribute to activation of cellular immunity in CD by reducing clearance of bacterial antigens from inductive sites in the small bowel and colon. It is not known whether differences in the development of intestinal macrophages or systemic neutrophils contribute to the ultimate development of CD, although current data suggest that this would be likely in patients with *CARD15* SNP carriage.

Dendritic Cell Maturation and the Development of Mucosal Tolerance

Dendritic cells (DCs) are the principal APCs in the intestine and play an active role in modulating the developing repertoire of mucosal activated/memory and regulatory T cells.[16] Under normal conditions, this leads to tolerance to dietary antigens and the enteric flora. Immature DCs take up and process antigens, both within the organized lymphoid follicles and throughout the epithelium. DC processes are in fact able to sample enteric antigens in the lumen without disrupting the epithelial TJP complexes. In infants, the predominant DC populations appear to be plasmacytoid DCs, which are much less potent in terms of stimulating a robust Th1 response to antigens, such as LPS stimulation of IL-12 production. The myeloid DCs that are present are also less effective in producing IL-12 and stimulating a Th1 response with interferon gamma (IFNγ) production than myeloid DCs from adults. These factors may combine to limit Th1 responses to the enteric flora in this age group. With increasing age, the myeloid DC becomes the predominant intestinal DC, which in turn is more likely to generate a Th1 response. As the mucosal T-cell response matures toward a more balanced Th1/Th2 profile in older children, this also may then contribute to the Th1 skewing observed in CD and the relative increase in the frequency of CD in children after age 8.[11]

The microenvironment within the neonatal intestine is well suited for the development of tolerance to a tremendous variety of dietary antigens and the enteric flora. The initial Th2 bias, with production of cytokines including IL-4 and IL-10 as well as TGFβ, promotes the expansion of regulatory T cells in an antigen-dependent manner, which can then suppress effector responses against gut flora and dietary antigens largely through local secretion of IL-10 and TGFβ.[17] This process is actively directed by immature DCs present in organized lymphoid tissues, including PPs and ILFs, which produce IL-10 but not IL-12 or IL-23. The net effect is the acquisition of tolerance driven by antigens present within the host flora.

Genetic effects upon DC function (eg, *CARD15* SNP carriage) or environmental factors such as breastfeeding that affect the composition of the flora may then have a lasting effect during this critical period for the acquisition of mucosal tolerance. Mutations in *CARD15* also would be expected to affect DC function and potentially the development of mucosal tolerance early in life.[18] An increased frequency of activated DCs expressing increased levels of TLR2 and TLR4 are observed in CD.[7] In CD and perhaps UC, tolerance to the enteric flora is lost; activated DC function then plays a critical role in generating proinflammatory populations of Th1, Th2, and/or Th17 cells reactive to bacterial products such as flagellin, which home to the gut and drive mucosal inflammation.

Development of the Gut Adaptive Immune System

The T-cell populations in the gut undergo significant changes following birth in response to the antigenic stimulation provided by diet and colonization with the enteric flora. Neonatal T cells overall are less responsive to stimulation. This may be due in part to a greater requirement for costimulatory signals, and in large part to the tolerogenic microenvironment of the infant's intestine provided by relatively high levels of IL-10 and TGFβ production.[4] In fact, regulatory T cells with functional ability to suppress effector T-cell expansion are already present in the periphery soon after birth.[19]

The majority of T cells in the human intestine express the αβ-TCR, while a smaller percentage of the intraepithelial lymphocytes express the γδ-TCR. Initially, T cells in the intestine of both the γδ and αβ-TCR lineages exhibit polyclonality. Beginning after birth, largely in response to antigenic stimulation by the enteric flora, the T-cell population undergoes expansion and restriction. By the age of 10 to 14 years, the intestinal αβ and γδ-TCR lineages are oligoclonal and resemble that of adults in their 60s.[20] Moreover, the mature TCR-δ repertoire is almost identical throughout the small intestine and colon and is unique in each individual.[20] While the function of these TCR-δ intraepithelial lymphocytes is not well defined, they may play a role in epithelial growth and function and antimicrobial defenses. Further restriction of the αβ-TCR repertoire consistent with clonal expansion in response to dominant enteric antigens has been identified by several groups in CD.[21] Whether the establishment of the mature repertoire for the αβ and γδ-TCR lineages in the intestine by age 10 to 14 years and the increased incidence of ileal CD at this age are related is not known. However, if these processes are related, it is likely that genetic variation combines with the effects of the mode of feeding, weaning, and bacterial colonization in the first year of life to play a significant part in the TCR repertoire that is ultimately observed at the onset of IBD.

Following antigen exposure in the inductive sites, memory/effector mucosal T cells then enter the circulation, with the vast majority homing back to the intestine. Instruction for this gut homing also is provided by intestinal DCs in the inductive sites. This process is regulated by a complex system of selectins, integrins, and chemokines.[22] Naïve lymphocytes that traffic to inductive sites in the PPs and ILFs are typically α4β7+/L-selectin+/CCR9+, while effector/memory cells that return to the intestinal lamina propria are typically α4β7+/L-selectin-/CCR9+. Upregulation of adhesion molecules and chemokines in IBD promotes increased intestinal recruitment of effector lymphocytes and neutrophils, and biologic agents targeting these pathways have entered clinical trials. However, whether age-dependent expression of specific selectins, integrins, or chemokines contributes to developmental susceptibility to IBD is not known. In general, the mechanisms for mucosal homing of T cells appear to be largely mature following the postnatal antigenic exposure from the enteric flora and diet that occurs over the first 2 to 3 years of life.

Bacterial Colonization and the Development of Mucosal Immunity

The principal components of the mucosal immune system initially develop within the sterile prenatal environment. The mode of feeding and bacterial colonization following birth play a critical role in the ensuing maturation of the mucosal immune system over the next 1 to 3 years. This section will review what is currently known regarding the effects of breastfeeding versus bottle or formula feeding upon colonization of the intestine in humans and the effect of bacterial colonization in turn upon development of the mucosal immune system.

Breastfeeding has been shown to have a profound influence upon bacterial colonization in infancy. Prebiotic oligosaccharides present in breast milk such as inulin-type fructans are fermented in the colon to produce short-chain fatty acids, which in turn promote colonization with bacteria, including lactobacilli and bifidobacteria.[23] By comparison, formula feeding leads to a relative reduction in these species and an increase in enterococci and enterobacteria. Both patient-based and animal studies have shown that bacterial species, including lactobacilli and bifidobacteria, may promote tolerogenic gut immune responses. For example, a recent animal study showed that PP lymphocytes produced significantly less IFNγ and TNFα after treatment with bifidobacteria.[23] Similar results have been shown when CD colon biopsies have been cocultured with lactobacilli species.[23] If bacterial colonization is stable over time, this may thereby influence the likelihood of developing IBD during critical windows of susceptibility.

Human milk contains several substances, including IgA and lactoferrin, that provide protection against enteric pathogens as the mucosal immune system matures over the first year of life. Human milk also contains growth factors, including epidermal growth factor, insulin-like growth factor 1, and TGFβ, that regulate enterocyte growth and maturation and so drive development of the epithelial barrier.[4] The TGFβ present in human milk may in addition exert immunomodulatory effects that promote tolerance to oral and enteric antigens.

Studies involving gnotobiotic mice have shown that bacterial colonization is essential for the development of a normal mucosal immune system. Colonization with the enteric flora has a net anti-inflammatory effect in the developing intestine.[4] In the absence of gut bacteria, both the inductive and effector compartments of the mucosal immune system are substantially underdeveloped. The PP are small and lack germinal centers, and the numbers of IgA plasma cells, CD4+ LP T cells, and CD8+ intraepithelial lymphocytes are greatly reduced.[24] The gut-associated lymphoid tissue of germ-free mice also resembles that of neonates in terms of exhibiting a Th2 bias.[25] Reconstitution with a relatively limited flora is sufficient to restore development of the mucosal immune system, including the development of the organized lymphoid tissues, the expansion of IgA plasma cells, and a shift toward a more balanced Th1/Th2 cytokine profile.

However, studies using germ-free mice have also shown that enteric flora are required for the development of experimental IBD and, by extension, human disease. Interestingly, the pattern of neonatal bacterial colonization has been shown to differ between normal and colitis-prone mice, suggesting that genetic variation in the host may influence early colonization, development of the mucosal immune system, and the later emergence of clinically apparent IBD.[26] Moreover, recent intriguing animal studies have shown that mono-association of genetically susceptible IL-10 deficient mice with different bacterial strains leads to disease in discrete segments of the small intestine or colon.[27]

A recent animal study also has demonstrated that a self-limited neonatal immune challenge may in fact increase the severity of colitis in adulthood.[28] In these experiments, neonatal or young adult rats were exposed to endotoxin and then challenged with trinitrobenzene sulfuric acid (a chemical agent that is well established as a trigger for acute colitis in rodents) later in adulthood. The severity of colitis induced by trinitrobenzene sulfuric acid was increased following LPS exposure in the neonatal but not young adult rats. This greater severity of colitis was associated with an increase in TNFα production but no differences in cortisol production. While the underlying mechanism was not identified, it was speculated that neonatal LPS challenge might lead to long-lasting differences in TLR4 expression and/or signaling, which might in turn affect the severity of colitis in response to a different environmental challenge in adulthood. Consistent with this, some studies have demonstrated an association between childhood bacterial infections and an earlier age of onset for both CD and UC.[29]

Alternately, several epidemiological studies have also suggested that the risk for CD is increased in children with higher socioeconomic status.[30] Specific factors associated with an increased risk for CD in this regard have included the presence of a hot water tap and a separate bathroom.[30] In this case, these environmental factors also are purported to affect early development of the mucosal immune system and susceptibility to CD later in life. Recently, Russell and colleagues found that the risk for CD associated with the *DLG5 R30Q* variant is highest in children with higher socioeconomic status.[30] This study provided for the first time a link between genetic and environmental variation relative to the risk of CD in children. Taken together, these patient-based and animal studies suggest that parameters that influence the composition of the enteric flora in humans—such as the mode of feeding during infancy, the use of antibiotics, the relative "cleanliness" of the environment, and the frequency of childhood infections—are likely to interact with genetic variation and have a profound influence upon the development of specific subtypes of IBD at older ages.

Genetic Polymorphisms Influencing Risk for Inflammatory Bowel Disease Subtypes

The genetic polymorphisms associated with increased susceptibility for IBD will be reviewed in another chapter and so will not be covered in detail here. This section will be limited to evidence of any specific effects of genetic polymorphisms upon early-onset disease or subtypes of disease observed with different frequencies in the pediatric age group. As a whole, loss of functional polymorphisms in genes involved in the innate response to the enteric flora, including *CARD15* and *ATG16L1*, have been associated with an increased risk for CD with small bowel involvement.[31,32] By comparison, a rare protective polymorphism in *IL-23R*, which would be predicted to influence primarily adaptive T-cell responses, has been associated with both CD and UC.[33] Patients with small bowel CD in turn exhibit increased serologic responses to the enteric flora and expansion of effector T cells directed against components of the flora such as flagellin. Taken together, these patient-based and animal studies suggest that the development of small bowel CD may require defects in innate immunity, which promotes induction of adaptive T cell responses to the enteric flora, mediated by interactions between APCs and naïve T cells in PPs, and subsequent recruitment of these activated/memory T cells to the ileal lamina propria. Interestingly, the inductive and effector components of mucosal immunity needed to mount this response are not fully developed until early adolescence when this form of CD reaches a frequency comparable to that observed in adulthood (see Figure 3-1).

Recent studies also have begun to explore the genetic basis for increased susceptibility to UC and Crohn's colitis. While not replicated to the same degree as the multiple studies examining *CARD15* and CD, studies in UC have identified susceptibility primarily due to genes involved in regulating colon epithelial cell function. These include *ABCB1*, an epithelial transport gene, and *MYO9B*, a component of the epithelial cytoskeleton.[34,35] Importantly, targeted deletion of *ABCB1/MDR1* in mouse models leads to spontaneous colitis resembling human UC.[36] These studies have suggested that alterations in the epithelial barrier or response to injury may be fundamental causes of UC, and so could conceivably play a role at the early age (3 to 8 years) when UC occurs at a comparable frequency to CD in children. However, an association between *CARD15* SNP carriage and disease in children less than age 6 with UC has been reported (27.6% in very early onset UC versus 7.8% in UC diagnosed after age 6 and 9.2% in controls).[37] This intriguing result awaits confirmation in additional cohorts. If confirmed, this would indicate a fundamental difference in the pathogenesis of UC in younger children.

Th1/Th2 Bias and Maturation of Mucosal Humoral Immunity Relative to the Development of Ulcerative Colitis and Colonic Crohn's Disease in Young Children

The infant normally exhibits a Th2 bias in the cytokine profile of potential effector cells in the gut, as well as a relatively high level of tolerogenic IL-10 and TGFβ production. This likely contributes to the much higher frequency of allergic gastrointestinal disease in this age group and the greatly reduced frequency of IBD. Preferential production of IL-4 and TGFβ during this period supports humoral IgG1 and IgE responses to exogenous antigens.[11] With a susceptible genetic background and environmental stimuli, this Th2 bias with IgE production will lead to the development of food allergies and atopic dermatitis in this age group.

With increasing age, infants and young children then normally evolve to a more balanced Th1/Th2 phenotype in the gut, which is felt to limit the development of allergic gastrointestinal disease. The important Th17 population has not yet been studied in this regard. While results have been mixed, most early studies in UC demonstrated a relative increase in the production of Th2 cytokines, including IL-5 and IL-13. In contrast, most studies in CD have demonstrated an increase in Th1 cytokines, including IL-12 and IFNγ. However, more recent studies have suggested a more mixed profile that may change over time, as well as what is likely a significant role for the recently characterized IL-23–dependent Th17 pathway. Nevertheless, a persistent skewing of the mucosal immune profile toward Th2 beyond age 3 to 5 years would be anticipated to promote the persistence of food allergy or development of UC, while a skewing toward a Th1/Th17 pathway would be expected to promote the development of CD. These intrinsic age-dependent differences in skewing of the Th1/Th2 pathways in the gut may therefore contribute to the increased frequency of UC in the youngest IBD patients and the consistent increase in the relative frequency of CD at ages older than 6 to 8 years.

In UC, an increase in IgG1-secreting B cells and increased IL-5 production by mucosal CD4+ T cells has been observed.[11] IgG1 coating of epithelial cells has in turn been shown to lead to complement activation, which likely contributes to epithelial injury.[38] While data have been mixed, a reasonable number of studies have demonstrated that the IgG-producing cells in UC may target true autoantigens. Tropomyosin isoform 5 has been identified as a putative UC autoantigen in this regard.[39] Importantly, research has suggested that autoantibodies against tropomyosin isoform 5 in UC mediate antibody and complement mediate lysis of colon epithelial cells.[40] Antineutrophil cytoplasmic antibodies (ANCA) have also been identified in the majority of UC patients and a substantial fraction of patients with Crohn's colitis. However, whether these antibodies exert a pathogenic effect is not known. A functional reduction in the production and secretion of IgA by tissue plasma cells and epithelial cells, which would be expected to promote increased exposure of the mucosal adaptive immune system to bacterial products, also may contribute to the chronic inflammatory response in UC. This type of mucosal humoral immune response would be expected to be fully matured by age 6, and so could account for the relative increased frequency of UC in younger children.

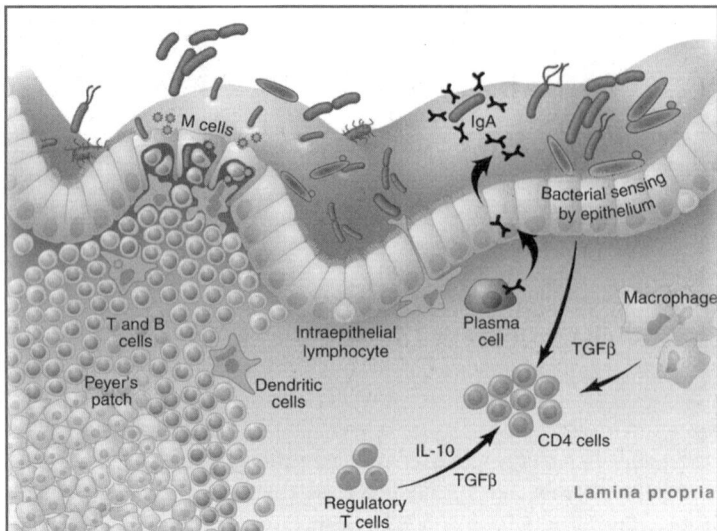

Figure 3-2. Organization of the gut-associated lymphoid tissue. The inductive sites (PP with overlying microfold [M] cells) are separated from the effector sites (lamina propria and intraepithelial T lymphocytes and plasma cells) in the mucosal immune system. Under normal conditions, the epithelial barrier, local regulatory T cells, and IgA-secreting plasma cells limit effector T-cell responses to the enteric flora. Dysregulation of these tolerogenic processes in CD is associated with activation of Th1/Th17 effector T-cell responses directed against enteric antigens. (From Macdonald TT, Monteleone G. Immunity, inflammation, and allergy in the gut. *Science.* 2005;307(5717):1920-1925. Reprinted with permission from AAAS.)

Organized Lymphoid Follicles and Induction of Th1/Th17 Adaptive Immune Responses Relative to the Development of Ileal Crohn's Disease in Older Children and Adolescents

In contrast to the systemic immune system, the inductive sites in the organized lymphoid tissue (PPs, ILFs) in the intestine are anatomically separated from the effector sites (LP, epithelium) (Figure 3-2).[24] PP contain B-cell lymphoid follicles and interfollicular populations of CD4 and CD8 T cells. Following activation by mucosal DCs, these T cells can then recirculate to the intestinal lamina propria, where they may mediate both antigen-specific protective responses against pathogens, and in the case of CD, inappropriate responses directed against the enteric flora. In this regard, mucosal DCs provide instruction to naïve PP T cells for both antigen specificity of responses and subsequent homing to the intestinal lamina propria. Both an intact thymus and bacterial colonization are required for complete development of the PPs.[4] Microfold cells, or M cells, are specialized epithelial cells that overly the organized lymphoid follicles in the gut and mediate antigen uptake to these tissues. These cells differentiate in parallel with the development of the underlying PPs and ILFs due to the combined effects of the enteric flora and the germinal center B cells.[4]

Current data suggest that the organized lymphoid follicles in the gut represent critical sites for activation of adaptive immune responses to the enteric flora in CD. As recently summarized by Meinzer et al, these data include 1) the most frequent sites of involvement for CD are in the segments (ileum, PPs and colon, ILFs) where the lymphoid follicles are most frequent; 2) CD lesions are discontinuous, as is the distribution of the lymphoid follicles; and 3) detailed morphological analyses have localized early CD lesions to areas where lymphoid follicles are most abundant.[3,26] Of course, the ileum and colon also contain the highest concentrations of enteric flora, and therefore potential antigenic load, in the body. Importantly, a recent animal study has demonstrated increased numbers of M cells, specialized epithelial cells overlying follicle-associated epithelium (FAE) and designed for antigen uptake, combined with increased CD4+ T cells, in PPs of *CARD15*-deficient mice.[41] These data have for the first time provided a reasonable mechanistic basis for increased antigen uptake and T-cell activation in patients with CD and *CARD15* SNP carriage.

While the principal inductive sites for antigen processing in the small bowel, the PPs, are present in infants, these do not reach adult levels of frequency and size until adolescence.[3] Van Kruiningen et al compared the frequency of PP and the incidence of CD and found these to be quite similar, with the peak in PP formation preceding the peak in CD incidence by 5 to 10 years.[42] Term infants have approximately 80 to 120 PPs. This increases to a maximum of 250 in midadolescence and then progressively decreases to 100 by age 90.[43] In comparison, the frequency of ILFs in the colon is relatively constant with age.[3] Isolation of T cells from human PPs has demonstrated a Th1 bias dominated by IFNγ production, with relatively little IL-4, IL-5, or TGFβ production. This appears to be secondary to increased PP expression of IL-12p40, which drives Th1 responses.[44] It has been speculated that this overall difference in the abundance of inductive sites may contribute to the higher frequency of colonic CD in younger children and the increasing frequency of ileal involvement after age 8 to 10.

Support for this concept has been shown in a mouse model of multiple sclerosis. In this Th17-dependent autoimmune disease model, experimental autoimmune encephalomyelitis, increased expression of the self-antigen, in this case myelin basic protein during puberty, led to a window of increased susceptibility for disease.[45] It will be important in the future to define the relative IL-23/Th17 versus IL-12/Th1 bias in PPs from individuals with CD and healthy controls and to determine whether data support increased antigen exposure and T-cell activation during the age range when PP reach a maximal size. This will have implications for future strategies to restore mucosal tolerance and potentially prevent disease in genetically susceptible individuals.

Thymic Expansion and Involution

With the exception of a small population of intraepithelial lymphocytes, intestinal T lymphocytes originate in the thymus. Within the thymus, the CD4+ and CD8+ T lymphocytes are selected through a carefully regulated process that ordinarily protects against the development of autoreactive clones. The thymus is well developed at birth and continues to increase in size until around age 10. Interestingly, this parallels the increase in size of the ileal PPs and the increasing frequency of ileal involvement with CD (see Figure 3-1). However, in contrast to the PPs, the thymus then begins to involute around the time of puberty, perhaps in response to the effect of growth factors and/or sex steroids.[46] Despite this relative reduction in size, the thymus is still able to increase T lymphocyte production in adulthood in response to severe lymphopenia, such as that observed with cytoablative chemotherapy. The contribution of age-dependent variation in thymic T lymphocyte clonal selection or production to susceptibility for different subtypes of IBD is not known.

Gender Differences, Puberty, and the Mucosal Immune System

CD, but not UC, is more common in males than females prior to puberty. Population-based studies have demonstrated a 2:1 male-to-female ratio in pediatric-onset cases. After puberty, the gender frequency approaches that observed in adulthood. Overall, data have suggested a somewhat more severe course for females with CD, with higher rates of surgery.[47] This has suggested that circulating levels of growth factors and sex hormones that change around the time of puberty might influence mucosal immunity and susceptibility to CD. Both patient-based and animal studies have demonstrated that estrogen exerts a proinflammatory effect in this regard, while androgens, including testosterone, may exert an anti-inflammatory effect. Moreover, in some autoimmune diseases such as systemic lupus erythematosus, both male and female patients have increased levels of biologically potent estrogen and lower levels of androgens.[48] Whether this is also the case with IBD during puberty is not known.

Nonpregnant women tend to exhibit more pronounced Th1 responses to infection and other stimuli compared to men or pregnant women.[49] Prior to puberty, young females actually have low levels of estrogen compared to males, while after puberty, this is reversed.[50] Greater post-pubertal Th1 responses in females in part may involve effects of estrogen upon TLR4 activation of NFkB and production of proinflammatory cytokines, including IL-12. The effects of estrogen are antagonized by androgens. Moreover, estrogen in other settings has been shown to promote expansion of autoreactive CD4+ effector cells and the production of IgG class autoantibodies. A recent animal study demonstrated that postpubertal female mice exhibit an increased expression of genes regulating adaptive immunity, while male mice showed increased expression of genes involved in innate responses. In this study, estrogen was shown to promote CD8+ T cell-derived B cell help and increased immunoglobulin production in postpubertal females.[51] In comparison, androgens have been shown to promote IL-2 production by Th1 cells, which reduces Th2 activity and drives expansion of CD8+ suppressor T cells with a generalized anti-inflammatory effect.[48] In this regard, it is intriguing to note that estrogen increases the expression of Bcl-2; this antiapoptotic gene has now been implicated in the resistance of mucosal effector T cells to apoptosis in CD.[48,52]

Demonstration of direct effects of pubertal hormones upon the mucosal immune system have largely been limited to animal studies. The severity of colitis due to trinitrobenzene sulfuric acid in rats has been shown to vary during the menstrual cycle, with more severe disease when progesterone levels are highest. This has been linked to increased expression of macrophage migration inhibitory factor in the colon and increased proinflammatory cytokine levels.[53] Susceptibility to trinitrobenzene sulfuric acid colitis in female mice has been linked to TLR4 signaling genetically while this has not been the case for male mice.[54] Whether alterations in estrogen or progesterone production around the time of puberty directly regulate proinflammatory TLR4 or macrophage migration inhibitory factor-dependent pathways in the gut in humans is not known.

Genetic variance in *DLG5*, an epithelial scaffolding protein, has recently been linked to gender differences in CD susceptibility.[2] The *DLG5 R30Q* variant has been shown to confer risk for CD in adult males, while this has not been the case for adult females. In comparison, Biank et al found that the *DLG5 R30Q* variant appeared to exert a protective effect in North American female children.[55] Consistent with this, a study in a cohort of Scottish children also showed association with the *DLG5 R30Q* variant and male gender in CD.[30] This study extended prior studies regarding gender by finding that *DLG5* SNP carriage was also associated with higher socioeconomic status. It is intriguing to note that *DLG5* has been shown to be regulated by progesterone in breast cancer cells.[56] Further genetic and functional studies will be required to define exactly how *DLG5* may influence mucosal immunity and risk for CD in an age-, gender-, and potentially socioeconomic status-dependent fashion.

Effectiveness and Potential Adverse Effects of Inflammatory Bowel Disease Therapy Relative to Stages of Mucosal Immune Development

The stage of development of the mucosal immune system might in theory influence the effectiveness of specific therapies, although to date this has not been evident. However, as younger children are diagnosed and treated at earlier stages of the disease, this may become more apparent. In general, it would be expected that therapies that target the epithelial barrier or the mucosal humoral immune response might be fully effective in younger children age 5 to 6 years and above, as these aspects of the mucosal immune system are fully mature at this stage. By comparison, therapies specifically targeting the inductive and effector aspects of cellular immunity might not fully match the maturational stage of the mucosal immune system until age 10. Likewise, therapies targeting modulation of mucosal inflammation by growth factors, sex steroids, or immune pathways regulated by sex steroids might be most applicable in postpubertal patients. However, current therapies used to induce or maintain remission, including corticosteroids, enteral nutrition, immunomodulators, and/or anticytokine monoclonal antibodies, do not act in a manner that can be anticipated to have an age-dependent window of maximal efficacy. This will become more of an issue as strategies to induce mucosal tolerance enter clinical trials, in which specific aspects of mucosal immunity may be required to observe a maximal effect.

Of more immediate concern is the potential for these agents to interact during critical windows of mucosal immune development to incur long-term adverse events, including malignancies. It would appear the incidence of lymphoma in conjunction with the use of the immunomodulator 6-mercaptopurine (6-MP) in children with IBD is likely comparable to that observed in adults. In comparison, the increasing reports of hepatosplenic T-cell lymphoma primarily in adolescent and young adult males with CD treated with both 6-MP and the monoclonal anti-TNFα antibody infliximab may represent the emergence of a rare malignancy during a vulnerable period of immune development.[57] Further study and increased vigilance will be required to determine whether this is in fact the case.

References

1. Heyman MB, Kirschner BS, Gold BD, et al. Children with early-onset inflammatory bowel disease (IBD): analysis of a pediatric IBD consortium registry. *J Pediatr.* 2005;146(1):35-40.
2. Biank V, Broeckel U, Kugathasan S. Pediatric inflammatory bowel disease: clinical and molecular genetics. *Inflamm Bowel Dis.* 2007;13(11):1430-1438.
3. Meinzer U, Idestrom M, Alberti C, et al. Ileal involvement is age dependent in pediatric Crohn's disease. *Inflamm Bowel Dis.* 2005;11(7):639-644.
4. Teitelbaum JE, Allan Walker W. The development of mucosal immunity. *Eur J Gastroenterol Hepatol.* 2005;17(12):1273-1278.
5. Soderholm JD, Streutker C, Yang PC, et al. Increased epithelial uptake of protein antigens in the ileum of Crohn's disease mediated by tumour necrosis factor alpha. *Gut.* 2004;53(12):1817-1824.
6. Bibiloni R, Mangold M, Madsen KL, Fedorak RN, Tannock GW. The bacteriology of biopsies differs between newly diagnosed, untreated, Crohn's disease and ulcerative colitis patients. *J Med Microbiol.* 2006;55(Pt 8):1141-1149.
7. Latinne D, Fiasse R. New insights into the cellular immunology of the intestine in relation to the pathophysiology of inflammatory bowel diseases. *Acta Gastroenterol Belg.* 2006;69(4):393-405.
8. Moehle C, Ackermann N, Langmann T, et al. Aberrant intestinal expression and allelic variants of mucin genes associated with inflammatory bowel disease. *J Mol Med.* 2006;84(12):1055-1066.
9. Wehkamp J, Wang G, Kubler I, et al. The Paneth cell {alpha}-defensin deficiency of ileal Crohn's disease is linked to Wnt/Tcf-4. *J Immunol.* 2007;179(5):3109-3118.

10. Claud EC, Lu L, Anton PM, Savidge T, Walker WA, Cherayil BJ. Developmentally regulated IkappaB expression in intestinal epithelium and susceptibility to flagellin-induced inflammation. *Proc Natl Acad Sci U S A.* 2004;101(19):7404-7408.
11. Winter HS, Russell GJ. Development immunology and inflammatory bowel disease. *Inflamm Bowel Dis.* 1998;4(2):107-108.
12. Smythies LE, Sellers M, Clements RH, et al. Human intestinal macrophages display profound inflammatory anergy despite avid phagocytic and bacteriocidal activity. *J Clin Invest.* 2005;115(1):66-75.
13. Caradonna L, Amati L, Lella P, Jirillo E, Caccavo D. Phagocytosis, killing, lymphocyte-mediated antibacterial activity, serum autoantibodies, and plasma endotoxins in inflammatory bowel disease. *Am J Gastroenterol.* 2000;95(6):1495-1502.
14. van Heel DA, Hunt KA, King K, et al. Detection of muramyl dipeptide-sensing pathway defects in patients with Crohn's disease. *Inflamm Bowel Dis.* 2006;12(7):598-605.
15. Marks DJ, Harbord MW, MacAllister R, et al. Defective acute inflammation in Crohn's disease: a clinical investigation. *Lancet.* 2006;367(9511):668-678.
16. Niess JH, Reinecker HC. Dendritic cells: the commanders-in-chief of mucosal immune defenses. *Curr Opin Gastroenterol.* 2006;22(4):354-360.
17. Iweala OI, Nagler CR. Immune privilege in the gut: the establishment and maintenance of non-responsiveness to dietary antigens and commensal flora. *Immunol Rev.* 2006;213:82-100.
18. Kramer M, Netea MG, de Jong DJ, Kullberg BJ, Adema GJ. Impaired dendritic cell function in Crohn's disease patients with NOD2 3020insC mutation. *J Leukoc Biol.* 2006;79(4):860-866.
19. Dujardin HC, Burlen-Defranoux O, Boucontet L, Vieira P, Cumano A, Bandeira A. Regulatory potential and control of Foxp3 expression in newborn CD4+ T cells. *Proc Natl Acad Sci U S A.* 2004;101(40):14473-14478.
20. Holtmeier W, Witthoft T, Hennemann A, Winter HS, Kagnoff MF. The TCR-delta repertoire in human intestine undergoes characteristic changes during fetal to adult development. *J Immunol.* 1997;158(12):5632-5641.
21. Probert CS, Saubermann LJ, Balk S, Blumberg RS. Repertoire of the alpha beta T-cell receptor in the intestine. *Immunol Rev.* 2007;215:215-225.
22. Salmi M, Jalkanen S. Lymphocyte homing to the gut: attraction, adhesion, and commitment. *Immunol Rev.* 2005;206:100-113.
23. Forchielli ML, Walker WA. The role of gut-associated lymphoid tissues and mucosal defence. *Br J Nutr.* 2005;93(Suppl 1):S41-S48.
24. Macdonald TT, Monteleone G. Immunity, inflammation, and allergy in the gut. *Science.* 2005;307(5717):1920-1925.
25. Nagler-Anderson C. Tolerance and immunity in the intestinal immune system. *Crit Rev Immunol.* 2000;20(2):103-120.
26. Kucharzik T, Maaser C, Lugering A, et al. Recent understanding of IBD pathogenesis: implications for future therapies. *Inflamm Bowel Dis.* 2006;12(11):1068-1083.
27. Kim SC, Tonkonogy SL, Albright CA, et al. Variable phenotypes of enterocolitis in interleukin 10-deficient mice monoassociated with two different commensal bacteria. *Gastroenterology.* 2005;128(4):891-906.
28. Spencer SJ, Hyland NP, Sharkey KA, Pittman QJ. Neonatal immune challenge exacerbates experimental colitis in adult rats: potential role for TNF-alpha. *Am J Physiol Regul Integr Comp Physiol.* 2007;292(1):R308-R315.
29. Wurzelmann JI, Lyles CM, Sandler RS. Childhood infections and the risk of inflammatory bowel disease. *Dig Dis Sci.* 1994;39(3):555-560.
30. Russell RK, Drummond HE, Nimmo ER, et al. The contribution of the DLG5 113A variant in early-onset inflammatory bowel disease. *J Pediatr.* 2007;150(3):268-273.
31. Russell RK, Drummond HE, Nimmo EE, et al. Genotype-phenotype analysis in childhood-onset Crohn's disease: NOD2/CARD15 variants consistently predict phenotypic characteristics of severe disease. *Inflamm Bowel Dis.* 2005;11(11):955-964.
32. Rioux JD, Xavier RJ, Taylor KD, et al. Genome-wide association study identifies new susceptibility loci for Crohn disease and implicates autophagy in disease pathogenesis. *Nat Genet.* 2007;39(5):596-604.
33. Dubinsky MC, Wang D, Picornell Y, et al. IL-23 receptor (IL-23R) gene protects against pediatric Crohn's disease. *Inflamm Bowel Dis.* 2007;13(5):511-515.
34. Ho GT, Soranzo N, Nimmo ER, Tenesa A, Goldstein DB, Satsangi J. ABCB1/MDR1 gene determines susceptibility and phenotype in ulcerative colitis: discrimination of critical variants using a gene-wide haplotype tagging approach. *Hum Mol Genet.* 2006;15(5):797-805.
35. van Bodegraven AA, Curley CR, Hunt KA, et al. Genetic variation in myosin IXB is associated with ulcerative colitis. *Gastroenterology.* 2006;131(6):1768-1774.
36. Resta-Lenert S, Smitham J, Barrett KE. Epithelial dysfunction associated with the development of colitis in conventionally housed mdr1a-/- mice. *Am J Physiol Gastrointest Liver Physiol.* 2005;289(1):G153-G162.
37. Ferraris A, Torres B, Knafelz D, et al. Relationship between CARD15, SLC22A4/5, and DLG5 polymorphisms and early-onset inflammatory bowel diseases: an Italian multicentric study. *Inflamm Bowel Dis.* 2006;12(5):355-361.

38. Brandtzaeg P, Carlsen HS, Halstensen TS. The B-cell system in inflammatory bowel disease. *Adv Exp Med Biol.* 2006;579:149-167.

39. Onuma EK, Amenta PS, Ramaswamy K, Lin JJ, Das KM. Autoimmunity in ulcerative colitis (UC): a predominant colonic mucosal B cell response against human tropomyosin isoform 5. *Clin Exp Immunol.* 2000;121(3):466-471.

40. Ebert EC, Geng X, Lin J, Das KM. Autoantibodies against human tropomyosin isoform 5 in ulcerative colitis destroys colonic epithelial cells through antibody and complement-mediated lysis. *Cell Immunol.* 2006;244(1):43-49.

41. Barreau F, Meinzer U, Chareyre F, et al. *CARD15*/NOD2 is required for Peyer's patches homeostasis in mice. *PLoS ONE.* 2007;2:e523.

42. Van Kruiningen HJ, Ganley LM, Freda BJ. The role of Peyer's patches in the age-related incidence of Crohn's disease. *J Clin Gastroenterol.* 1997;25(2):470-475.

43. Cornes JS. Peyer's patches in the human gut. *Proc R Soc Med.* 1965;58(9):716.

44. Newberry RD, Lorenz RG. Organizing a mucosal defense. *Immunol Rev.* 2005;206:6-21.

45. Huseby ES, Sather B, Huseby PG, Goverman J. Age-dependent T cell tolerance and autoimmunity to myelin basic protein. *Immunity.* 2001;14(4):471-481.

46. Min H, Montecino-Rodriguez E, Dorshkind K. Reassessing the role of growth hormone and sex steroids in thymic involution. *Clin Immunol.* 2006;118(1):117-123.

47. Gupta N, Cohen SA, Bostrom AG, et al. Risk factors for initial surgery in pediatric patients with Crohn's disease. *Gastroenterology.* 2006;130(4):1069-1077.

48. Ackerman LS. Sex hormones and the genesis of autoimmunity. *Arch Dermatol.* 2006;142(3):371-376.

49. Whitacre CC, Reingold SC, O'Looney PA. A gender gap in autoimmunity. *Science.* 1999;283(5406):1277-1278.

50. Sandborg C. Expression of autoimmunity in the transition from childhood to adulthood: role of cytokines and gender. *J Adolesc Health.* 2002;30(4 Suppl):76-80.

51. Lamason R, Zhao P, Rawat R, et al. Sexual dimorphism in immune response genes as a function of puberty. *BMC Immunol.* 2006;7:2.

52. Ina K, Itoh J, Fukushima K, et al. Resistance of Crohn's disease T cells to multiple apoptotic signals is associated with a Bcl-2/Bax mucosal imbalance. *J Immunol.* 1999;163(2):1081-1090.

53. Houdeau E, Moriez R, Leveque M, et al. Sex steroid regulation of macrophage migration inhibitory factor in normal and inflamed colon in the female rat. *Gastroenterology.* 2007;132(3):982-993.

54. Bouma G, Kaushiva A, Strober W. Experimental murine colitis is regulated by two genetic loci, including one on chromosome 11 that regulates IL-12 responses. *Gastroenterology.* 2002;123(2):554-565.

55 Biank V, Friedrichs F, Babusukumar U, et al. DLG5 R30Q variant is a female-specific protective factor in pediatric onset Crohn's disease. *Am J Gastroenterol.* 2007;102(2):391-398.

56. Purmonen S, Ahola TM, Pennanen P, et al. HDLG5/KIAA0583, encoding a MAGUK-family protein, is a primary progesterone target gene in breast cancer cells. *Int J Cancer.* 2002;102(1):1-6.

57. Rosh JR, Gross T, Mamula P, Griffiths A, Hyams J. Hepatosplenic T-cell lymphoma in adolescents and young adults with Crohn's disease: a cautionary tale? *Inflamm Bowel Dis.* 2007;13(8):1024-1030.

Financial disclosure: This work was supported in part by NIH grants DK068164 and DK078683.

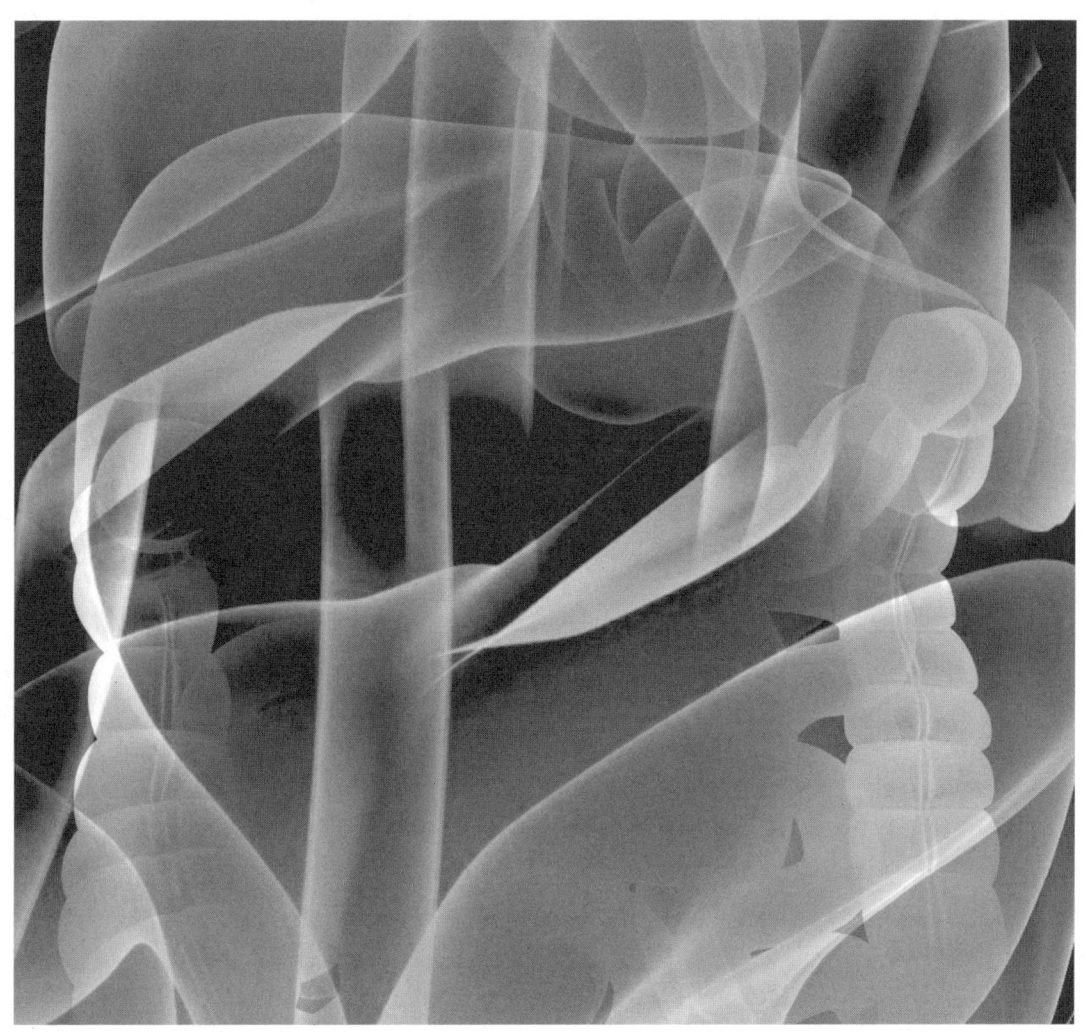

SECTION II

INFLAMMATORY BOWEL DISEASE AND THE PEDIATRIC PATIENT

WHY CHILDREN GET INFLAMMATORY BOWEL DISEASE

Ernest G. Seidman, MD and Devendra K. Amre, MD

A simplistic, yet not inaccurate answer to the question as to why so many children get inflammatory bowel disease (IBD) is that it "runs in the family." One might then ask whether such a statement entails genetic or environmental risk factors or both. It is well accepted that IBD represents a multi-factorial disease with contributions both from the environment as well as genes (Figure 4-1). Epidemiological, clinical, and animal studies have provided valuable clues to the etiology and management of these highly perplexing diseases. However, despite the many inroads, the etiology and pathogenesis of IBD remain enigmas. It is not clear which environmental or genetic factors cause these chronic inflammatory disorders.[1] Linkage and association studies have implicated several potential genes in multiple chromosomal regions in diverse populations. Similarly, the risks from dietary, infectious, and other environmental factors have been inconsistent across studies. In the absence of definitive information on specific causative agents, it has been difficult to recommend or apply any preventive or curative measures that could lessen the considerable public health burden of IBD.

It is generally estimated that IBD manifests during childhood or adolescence in about 25% of cases.[2] Population-based studies have revealed that the incidence and prevalence of IBD in Canada is the highest yet reported in the world.[3] The incidence of Crohn's disease (CD) reported in that study was particularly high during the second decade of life. Not all adults with IBD have necessarily had long-standing disease, and not all pediatric patients have very recent onset disease. Nevertheless, the investigation of pediatric-onset IBD is of particular interest in terms of elucidating the complex etiology and pathogenesis of these disorders. Children and adolescents with IBD are habitually closer to disease initiation and thus to the causal factors in the processes underlying the chronic intestinal inflammation. Young patients have fewer comorbid conditions and confounding factors such as smoking and medication use. Moreover, first-degree relatives of pediatric probands are more often accessible for genetic studies. In this chapter, we review the data concerning genetic variants and environmental risk factors reported to confer susceptibility to IBD that relate to pediatric onset.

Scherl EJ, Dubinsky MC.
The Changing World of Inflammatory Bowel Disease:
Impact of Generation, Gender, and Global Trends (pp 51-66)
© 2009 SLACK Incorporated.

Figure 4-1. Although the pathogenesis of IBD is incompletely understood, the consensus of opinions center on aberrant immune responses to microbial factors in genetically predisposed individuals. Among persons with susceptibility genes, yet unidentified environmental factors are thought to initiate onset of disease and to contribute to disease exacerbations.

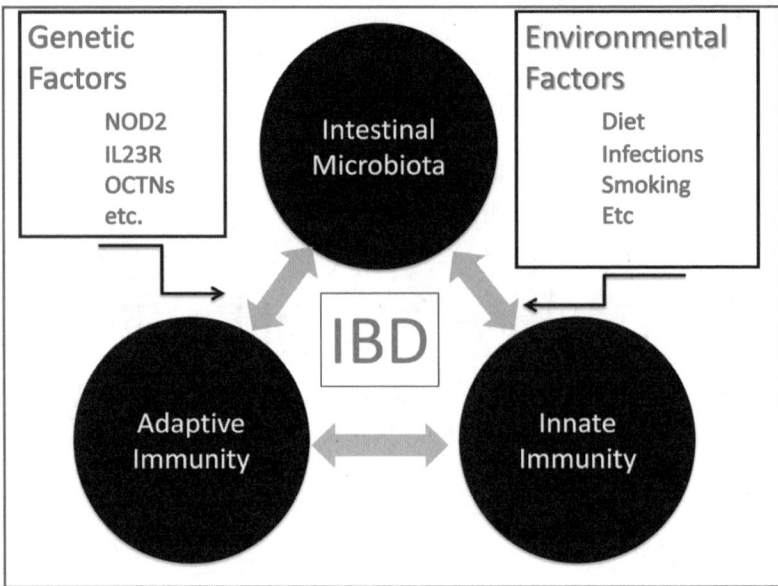

Genetic Contributions to Pediatric Inflammatory Bowel Disease

A significant role for genetic factors in IBD was established from epidemiologic studies and, more recently, the identification of well-established disease associations, notably that of *NOD2* (*CARD15*) polymorphisms with CD.[4] In contrast to the environmental risk factors discussed next, the identification of which is much more challenging and for which evidence for risk is less apparent, it is increasingly clear that genetic factors contribute to the development of IBD in children as in adults. In general, genetic factors play a larger role in the pathogenesis of complex disorders with onset early compared to later in life. It is thus of interest to discern whether IBD with onset early in life differs from that diagnosed during adulthood and whether these differences are related to divergent genetic risks.

It is now evident that individuals diagnosed with IBD in the pediatric age group may represent a distinct subset of susceptible individuals. Pediatric patients differ in clinical presentation, disease location, behavior, and—to a certain extent—in the clinical course of disease.[2,5] Given these distinguishing attributes in disease characteristics, one may speculate that genetic factors contributing to susceptibility may vary according to the patient's period of life at diagnosis. Details on the genetic epidemiology of pediatric IBD have been provided in an accompanying chapter (see Chapter 5). In this section, we summarize and highlight differences between pediatric- and adult-onset disease vis-à-vis genetic contributions to disease pathogenesis.

FAMILY HISTORY OF INFLAMMATORY BOWEL DISEASE

The degree of contribution of genetic factors to the etiology of any disease can be assessed by examining its prevalence among the proband's family members. In the context of pediatric IBD, studies suggest that up to 30% of affected children have a first-degree relative affected with IBD.[6-9] These rates of familial occurrence are higher than those observed for adult-onset IBD, reported to range from 5% to 15%.[8,9] Ethnicity would appear to play a role as demonstrated by the observation that a positive family history of IBD in any relative(s) was reported by 45.6% of Jewish probands with pediatric-onset IBD compared to 26.7% of non-Jewish probands.[2]

In the same report, 30.7% of the Jewish children had one or more first-degree relative(s) with IBD compared with 12.8% of non-Jewish probands. It is not known whether this reflects a distinct pattern of genetic susceptibility or simply an increased frequency of IBD-associated alleles in Jewish populations.

Clear interpretation of these findings is hampered by the fact that the definition of family history (first versus second degree) varies between studies. Moreover, although a family history of IBD may implicate sharing of common genetic risk factors, it certainly could also reflect shared environmental influences. Additionally, these differences are confounded by the unequal "disease-free intervals" between childhood- and adult-onset IBD. Given that first-degree relatives of individuals who acquire adult-onset IBD have a longer disease-free interval, their chances of acquiring IBD are comparatively higher vis-à-vis the relatives of individuals who acquire IBD at an earlier age. In addition, these differences in rates could reflect the influence of selection factors that apply differently between pediatric-onset and adult-onset disease. Families of children with a known family history of disease are likely to seek medical advice if they suspect that the child has symptoms suggestive of IBD. On the other hand, adults with or without a family history of IBD may equally seek medical attention. Thus, although findings of potential differences in the rates of disease in the family are of interest, they are limited in their ability to provide insights or biological clues for genetically mediated disease mechanisms.

GENES/GENETIC REGIONS ASSOCIATED WITH BOTH PEDIATRIC AND ADULT ONSETS OF INFLAMMATORY BOWEL DISEASE

IBD is polygenic with modest contributions from multiple genes required to increase susceptibility. As observed from most investigations for complex diseases, the literature on genetic susceptibility for IBD has yielded some inconsistent findings with lack of replication for some associations. Over the past decade, considerable research efforts have been and continue to be carried out in order to identify potential genes that increase susceptibility for IBD. The recent emphasis on large-scale investigations in well-defined homogeneous cohorts has seen an explosion in the detection of associations with greater validity.[4,10] Earlier linkage analysis methods paved the way for candidate gene association studies. With advances in technology and development of high-throughput genotyping platforms, genome-wide association studies have now become feasible. Much emphasis has been placed on delineating genetic risk factors for adult-onset IBD given the higher incidence. Increasing awareness of IBD in children is expected to lead to increased research focused on this population. In the sections that follow, we outline the major genes for which associations have been extensively validated for IBD affecting children and that might be involved in the etiopathogenesis of early-onset IBD.

NOD2/CARD15-IBD1

The mapping to CD of *NOD2* variants that alter protein function represents one of the earliest and best-established associations in complex genetic disorders. Since the initial discovery, genotype-phenotype correlations, definition of *NOD2* expression and signaling pathways, association studies in other related disorders, and features of *NOD2* deficiency in murine models have been reported.[4,10] Three common variants in the gene (*R702W*, *G908R*, and *L1007fs*) each independently confer risk for CD. The risk among individuals who possess at least one of these variants is high. Although the majority of the studies do not suggest associations with ulcerative colitis (UC), a few studies do indicate that common variants in the gene may be associated with UC, albeit the strength of the associations is lower.[11-13] Of particular interest are observations that the frequency of the 3 variants varies among populations that have a similar incidence of IBD.[14] We have recently observed that in the ethnically heterogeneous population in the north of India, the 3 common *NOD2* variants are either absent or rare.[15] Yet, the incidence of UC in this population is comparable to that reported among White populations.[16] In order to further explore these findings, we resequenced the exons of the gene to identify other potentially susceptibility variants. We found that *SNP5*, another common variant (12%), was significantly associated with UC among north Indians.[15] *SNP5*, also common in Whites, is associated with CD as well, but only in the presence of SNP *L1007fs*. These findings point to allelic heterogeneity among associations between *NOD2* and IBD.

Increased linkages of early-onset CD to the *NOD2* gene are also well-established.[17-19] The magnitude of the associations is generally similar for pediatric and adult CD.[20] However, the association between *NOD2* and CD was found to be even stronger among Jewish children[21] compared to Jewish adults, suggesting that age of onset is associated with carriage of *NOD2* risk alleles in this population. These findings could also be a consequence of the lower contribution of confounding or interacting factors, in particular those related to the environment. Other possibilities to consider in interpreting these observations are discussed next.

Another interesting aspect regarding the contribution of *NOD2* to susceptibility for pediatric-onset CD is the strength of the associations with each of the 3 common single nucleotide polymorphisms (SNPs). We observed that although *SNP8* and *SNP13* are strongly associated with CD in children,[22,23] associations with *SNP12* are less obvious. These findings may be related to the lower frequency of *SNP12* and requirement for larger sample sizes to detect association. On the other hand, it is possible that the contribution of *SNP12* may take longer to impact on disease pathogenesis and hence associations may not be observed as frequently in children as in adults. Alternatively, it can be postulated that the effects of *SNP12* may require different contributions from environmental exposures to influence susceptibility. At present, there is no evidence that *NOD2* variants are associated with pediatric-onset UC.

5q31 Locus-IBD5

The IBD5 locus spans an 18 cM region of chromosome 5q31. Linkages with IBD were first reported in 2000 in a sample of Canadian sibling-affected pairs using microsatellite markers.[24] In extensive follow-up studies using haplotype-tagging SNPs, the risk-conferring variants were defined within a 250-kb region. However, multiple haplotype-tagging SNPs appeared to be equally conferring risk for CD, and identifying the causal variant has proven to be challenging.[25] The IBD5 region contains many putative genes that may well be implicated in the pathogenesis of IBD. The 2 most commonly studied are the genes for the organic cation transporters OCTN1 and OCTN2.[26] Proof as to whether these genes are the ones conferring risk remains imprecise. Much of the difficulty in replicating findings across seemingly homogeneous populations is the extensive linkage disequilibrium between markers with the IBD5 risk region. It is increasingly accepted that associations between the OCTN genes are not present in the absence of a 5-marker risk haplotype, indicating that other genes within the region may be implicated.[27] It is also possible that interactions between markers may be necessary to confer significant disease risk. Investigation of larger groups would be required to delineate these effects with certainty. In studies that have focused on pediatric patients,[28-31] the evidence for associations is by and large similar to that observed among adults, with risk generally present only among individuals harboring the IBD5-risk haplotype.

IL-23 Receptor

The IL-23R gene is located on chromosome 1p31. Its ligand IL-23 is a key element in the regulation of host immune response pathways. It is intricately linked to the development of the subset of Th17 cells implicated in mechanisms underlying gut-related inflammation.[32] This gene was the first to be identified as associated with IBD using the genome-wide association strategy. At least 10 SNPs in the gene were significantly associated with CD in the North American population.[33] Associations were also evident with UC. These findings have been subsequently replicated in other adult White populations.[34,35]

We[23] and others[36,37] have replicated associations between the IL-23R gene and pediatric-onset CD. Using both the case-control and case-parent designs, we investigated associations between 10 SNPs in the gene in a cohort of Canadian children. We observed significant associations between at least 4 SNPs in the gene. The findings were consistent between the case-parent and case-control designs, thus confirming that the IL-23R gene is also associated with pediatric-onset CD. Of relevance were findings that the IL-23R variants were associated with CD in the absence of the 3 common *NOD2* susceptibility variants, highlighting that IL-23R independently confers risk for CD.

There is limited information on whether IL-23R variants are also associated with UC in children. A study in a US cohort[36] based on a small sample showed marginally nonsignificant (p = 0.06) association with IL-23R risk-conferring variant (R381Q). In a Scottish cohort, however, an association with the gene and UC was not observed.[37]

OTHER GENES POTENTIALLY ASSOCIATED WITH PEDIATRIC-ONSET INFLAMMATORY BOWEL DISEASE

Paraoxonase

Considerable evidence suggests that an increase in oxidative stress is involved in the pathogenesis of IBD.[38] It has been postulated that cellular detoxification systems in IBD may be unable to adequately control the amplified generation of reactive oxygen species, put a stop to free-radical injury, and repair damaged cellular elements. Such a deficiency in defenses against free-radical injury may be due to environmental (dietary) and/or genetic factors. Human paraoxonase family members (PON1, PON2, and PON3) possess important antioxidant and anti-inflammatory properties. We recently carried out an investigation on the 8 common variants in PON1, PON2, and PON3 by genotyping, using polymerase chain reaction allele-specific oligonucleotide hybridization assays in 192 incident cases of childhood IBD.[39] We found evidence supporting a potential role for genetic variants in PON2 contributing to the risk of developing childhood IBD. Additional studies are needed to ascertain the potential role of PON2 polymorphisms in childhood IBD in view of their potential effect on the expression of PON2 activity as an antioxidant.

Chemokine CXCL9

CXCL9 belongs to the CXC group of chemokines mainly expressed on the surface of epithelial, endothelial, and hematopoietic cells that participate in immune and inflammatory responses via chemoattraction and activation of polymorphonuclear neutrophils, T cells, and B cells.[40-42] CXCL9 interacts with the receptor CXCR3, which also binds 2 other structurally related ligands: IFN-gamma-inducible protein (IP-10/CXCL10) and IFN-inducible T-cell alpha chemoattractant (I-TAC/CXCL11).[42] A recent study revealed an association of a CXCL9 polymorphism with pediatric-onset CD.[43] CXCL9 was overexpressed in colonic tissue of both CD and UC patients compared to healthy controls. SNP genotyping for the 77147452GfiA polymorphism of the CXCL9 gene in a cohort of pediatric IBD patients and ethnically matched unaffected adults detected a minor allele frequency of 20.3% in CD patients compared to 31.3% controls (p = 0.016). Interestingly, children with homozygosity for the wild-type allele had a significant earlier onset of CD than heterozygous individuals. This report is the first noting an inverse association of the CXCL9 77147452GfiA polymorphism with pediatric CD.

Pregnane-X Receptor (NR1I2) Gene

Another potential candidate gene for CD is the *NR1I2* gene (3q12-3q13.3) that codes for the pregnane-X receptor (PXR). PXR is a nuclear receptor that has a broad range of substrate specificity that includes endogenous and exogenous compounds.[44] Expressed in the small intestine, it is a key regulator of the xenobiotic metabolizing enzyme CYP3A4.[45] The latter is responsible for the regulation and metabolism of >60% of pharmaceutical substrates encountered in the intestine. Recent studies have shown that DNA variants in the *NR1I2* gene influence the expression of the CYP3A4 enzyme[46,47] and that PXR influences xenobiotic metabolic processes by regulating the expression of the multi-drug resistance 1 gene (MDR1) that is involved in cellular transport of substrates. The latter is particularly relevant to CD as a strong correlation between the expression of MDR1 and PXR has been observed in the intestine.[48] The *NR1I2* gene encoding PXR may thus confer susceptibility for CD, but evidence for associations is conflicting. We recently carried out a case-control and family-based (case-parent) study at 3 pediatric IBD clinics across Canada.[49] For determination of gene associations, parents of the cases and unrelated controls were evaluated. Eight tag-SNPs across the gene were genotyped for allelic or genotypic associations. For 7, single SNP analysis using case-control or case-parent data did not reveal associations with development of CD and none of the SNPs were significantly associated with disease location or disease behavior at diagnosis. One SNP rs2461823 (p = 0.05) was nominally associated with CD. No overall haplotype association (omnibus p-value = 0.61) or association with individual haplotypes was evident. Overall, our gene-wide analysis in a pediatric cohort using both the case-control and case-parent designs did not suggest that the NR1I2 gene is associated with CD in Canadian children.[49]

OTHER DIFFERENCES IN GENES ASSOCIATED WITH ADULT-ONSET COMPARED TO PEDIATRIC-ONSET INFLAMMATORY BOWEL DISEASE

The clinical phenotypes of pediatric-onset IBD are reported to be different from that of adult-onset IBD. Children with CD have more frequent ileocolonic disease and those with UC more extensive disease (pancolitis).[5] In contrast, adults more frequently have ileal CD and left-sided UC. Similarly, there are gender-based differences in the incidence of IBD. In adults, the incidence is higher in females whereas in children a higher incidence in males has been reported. These findings suggest that the genetic mechanisms underlying pediatric-onset IBD may differ from that in adult IBD. In general, genetic influences are considered to be more likely an important risk factor in pediatric-onset IBD. Although genes associated with adult-onset IBD also seem to be associated with pediatric-onset IBD, recent studies suggest the potential for age-dependent genetic heterogeneity. de Ridder et al[50] investigated whether genes such as NOD2, TLR4, OCTN1/OCTN2, and DLG5 were differentially associated with pediatric-onset IBD. A cohort of 103 pediatric-onset IBD (mean age 12.0 years) and 612 adult-onset (mean age 35.3 years) IBD patients from Amsterdam was studied. There were 72 pediatric-onset CD and 368 adult-onset CD patients. For the NOD2 gene, they observed that the frequency of the G908R mutant allele did not differ between the CD cases (both pediatric and adult onset) from that among controls, suggesting lack of association between this variant and CD. The 3020insC variant was more common among the pediatric-onset CD patients compared to both the adult-onset CD patients and the controls, implying a stronger association between this variant and CD in children. For the TLR4 gene, no associations with 2 variants (Asp299Gly and Thr399Ile) were observed with pediatric-onset IBD, but associations were significant among the adult patients. For the OCTN1/2 gene variants, the authors reported that the frequency of variant rs3792876 was higher among the pediatric-onset CD patients (12.1%) compared to that in adult-onset CD patients (8.3%) and controls (6.8%).[50] Five other variants in the gene were associated with neither pediatric-onset IBD nor with adult-onset IBD. For the DLG5 gene, variant rs2165047 was associated with adult-onset but not with pediatric-onset IBD, whereas 3 other variants in the gene were associated with neither pediatric-onset nor adult-onset IBD.

In addition to the above-mentioned genes, there were suggestions that other genetic associations may differ between pediatric- and adult-onset IBD. An important example is the ATG16L1 gene. Associations between this gene and CD have been recently confirmed in multiple adult cohorts.[51] However, in a comprehensive investigation on both pediatric and adult cohorts, Van Limbergen et al[52] did not observe associations between the risk variant (rs2241880A/G) and pediatric-onset CD, both in a case-control as well as a case-parent analysis. However, associations between the variant and adult-onset CD were evident.

WHY DO THE SAME GENETIC FACTORS DIFFERENTIALLY AFFECT PEDIATRIC- AND ADULT-ONSET INFLAMMATORY BOWEL DISEASE?

The above findings raise many intriguing questions. Why would the same susceptibility genes have different magnitudes of association for pediatric- versus adult-onset IBD? Why, for certain susceptibility genes, should risks be observed for either pediatric- or adult-onset IBD? Currently, answers to these questions are not easily forthcoming. Many of the observed differences in genetic associations between adult and pediatric IBD could be related to the allelic and/or genetic heterogeneity and the influence of potential epigenetic or nongenetic factors involved in the pathogenesis of IBD. These differences might underlie the observed differences in clinical phenotypes, disease localization, severity, and course between pediatric- and adult-onset IBD. It has to be appreciated, however, that investigation of these differences may be limited using case-control methodologies. In order to understand the genetic mechanisms (if any) that underlie age-of-onset effects, a birth cohort design would be ideal.[53-55] This design includes the follow-up over time of a group of individuals born during the same calendar time period. A variant of the prospective cohort design, individuals could be stratified according to whether they possess variants of the genes of interest, and their risks for acquiring IBD either in childhood or adulthood could be measured and compared. This design would overcome many of the limitations of the current methods used to ascertain genetic contributions to age-of-onset effects, in particular age-period effects and generation effects. Relevant exposures of interest could be measured at different times of follow-up as the cohort ages. This approach would enable the understanding of why certain individuals are more susceptible to acquire IBD in childhood.[56] It would assist in understanding why certain individuals who have the same risk-conferring mutations escape acquiring IBD in childhood but acquire it in adulthood. Finally, it would also help discern which environmental factors influence the development of IBD in childhood and adulthood and whether they differ.

Although an ideal design to explore genetic contributions to age-of-onset effects given the relative low incidence of IBD, very large birth cohorts would need to be established and followed over a long period of time. Such birth cohorts have been established to assess contributions of genetic and environmental factors and are currently being followed up for more than 50 years.[55] These cohorts have provided valuable information on the pathogenesis of many chronic diseases. Given the high morbidity related to IBD and its increasing incidence and prevalence in certain geographic regions, implementing such a birth cohort would be worthwhile.

Environmental Risk Factors and Pediatric Inflammatory Bowel Disease

The incidence of CD is high in Western countries[57] and is emerging in other developing regions of the world.[58] Not long ago, CD was thought to be relatively rare among children and adolescents. Recent estimates from a population-based study in several Canadian provinces indicate that the incidence of CD among children between 9 and 20 years of age now approaches that seen in adults.[3] The current paradigm suggests that CD is a disease of complex etiopathogenesis, wherein genetic, environmental, and immunological factors interact in unknown ways to induce intestinal inflammation (see Figure 4-1). As reviewed previously, considerable progress has recently been made in determining the genetic basis for susceptibility to IBD. At the same time, understanding the contribution of potential environmental risk factors has proven to be challenging.[55] Research efforts of several teams, including ours, have focused on potential gene-environment interactions as causal pathways leading to IBD in the pediatric age group.[1,22] In this section, we critically review some insights into the plausible environmental factors that could be implicated in these processes (Table 4-1). We will discuss the contribution of hygiene, specific dietary factors, smoking and other environmental "insults," and vaccines and infections most commonly implicated in IBD.

THE HYGIENE HYPOTHESIS

Exposure to infections as risk factors has been the focus of interest of many studies. Akin to other autoimmune diseases, some epidemiological studies have suggested a role for the "hygiene

Table 4-1

ENVIRONMENTAL FACTORS POTENTIALLY IMPLICATED IN PEDIATRIC-ONSET INFLAMMATORY BOWEL DISEASE

- "Hygiene" hypothesis
- Diet, breastfeeding
- Smoking
- Medications
  * Oral contraceptives
  * Non-steroidal anti-inflammatory drugs
- Microbes and vaccines
- Appendectomy
- Geography and social status
- Stress

hypothesis," whereby exposure to infections in childhood confers protection against disease.[59] On the other hand, several studies have suggested that infections early in life could increase risk for disease.[60-65] Thus, the exact role of infections in the etiology of CD remains unclear. We recently reported[66] our findings on the relationship between various infection-related exposures and their role in the etiology of pediatric CD. A hospital-based case-control study was carried out in newly-diagnosed cases of pediatric CD (n = 194) in Montreal, Canada. Orthopedic patients without gastrointestinal symptoms and pair matched (n = 194) for timing of diagnosis and area of residence were recruited as controls. Information on infection-related exposures between birth and disease diagnosis was ascertained using a structured questionnaire to the mother and the index subject. The relationship between the frequency and timing of infection-related exposures with CD was studied. In multivariate conditional logistic regression, family history of IBD (odds ratio [OR], 4.6; 95% confidence interval [CI], 1.6 to 13.3], age (OR, 1.2; 95% CI, 1.1 to 1.3), and owning a pet (OR, 2.0; 95% CI, 0.9 to 4.5) were associated with risk for CD, whereas regular use of a personal towel (OR, 0.5; 95% CI, 0.2 to 0.9) and lesser crowding in homes (OR, 0.3; 95% CI, 0.1 to 0.8) were found to be protective. Day-care attendance during the first 6 months of life and physician-diagnosed infections between the ages of 5 to 10 were associated with increased risks for CD. In conclusion, findings from our study suggested that hygiene-related characteristics that are markers of exposure to infections could be associated with increased risk for CD in children.[66] There were suggestions that the timing of infection during childhood may be relevant to the etiology of pediatric-onset CD. We did not find any support for the hygiene hypothesis. Nonetheless, the relationship between infection exposures and CD is likely to be more complex and the pattern, type, and frequency at different time periods in childhood may be important. Future studies using prospectively collected primary or secondary data, such as information on infection exposures acquired from relevant provincial or national databases, are needed to further clarify the role of infections in the pathogenesis of pediatric IBD.

DIETARY FACTORS

The role of dietary factors in the etiology of IBD is inconsistent largely due to difficulties in acquiring valid information on consumption habits. We recently reported[67] the results of our study on the impact of diet on new-onset CD in children using a validated food-frequency questionnaire (FFQ). A case-control study was carried out in newly diagnosed patients with CD recruited from

3 Canadian pediatric IBD centers. Population or hospital controls were selected matched to cases for time of diagnosis (6 months) and area of residence. Overall, 130 CD patients and 202 controls were included for study. Dietary consumption 1 year prior to disease diagnosis was evaluated using a validated FFQ, administered within 1 month of diagnosis. Conditional logistic regression analysis was carried out, adjusting for potential confounding variables (energy intake, age, gender, body mass index). Comparing the highest to the lowest levels of consumption, higher amounts of vegetables (OR, 0.69; 95% CI, 0.33 to 1.44; p = 0.03), fruits (OR, 0.49; 95% CI, 0.25 to 0.96; p = 0.02), fish (OR, 0.46; 95% CI, 0.20 to 1.06; p = 0.02), and dietary fiber (OR, 0.12; 95% CI, 0.04 to 0.37; p<0.001) protected from pediatric-onset CD. Consumption of long-chain omega-3 fatty acids (LCN-ω-3) was negatively associated with CD (OR, 0.44; 95% CI, 0.19 to 1.00; p<0.001). A higher ratio of LCN-ω-3/ω-6 fatty acids was significantly associated with lower risks for CD (OR, 0.32; 95% CI, 0.14 to 0.71; p = 0.02). In conclusion, we observed that imbalances in dietary consumption of fatty acids, vegetables, and fruits could predispose children to CD.[67] From the public health perspective, dietary patterns are likely to be more amenable to intervention. Therefore, further studies on larger incident cohorts that assess associations between specific dietary patterns and CD would be important. The ratio of LCN-ω-3 fatty acids to ω-6 fatty acids (arachidonic acid) may be particularly relevant to the etiology of CD, especially in view of our recent studies on polymorphisms of genes involved in antioxidant metabolism we recently described for paraoxonase.[39] It would thus be of considerable potential interest to now expand upon these studies using the gene-environmental interaction concept[1] by examining which susceptibility genes impact on these dietary risks.

We recently reported the results of a more extensive case-control study on dietary patterns and risk for CD in Canadian children.[68] Factor analyses and unconditional logistic regression (adjusted) were used to determine gender-specific dietary patterns and assess associated risks for CD (n = 149 CD cases and 251 controls). Specific dietary patterns each were observed among both boys and girls. Pattern 1 in girls, characterized by meats, fatty foods, and desserts, was positively associated with CD (OR, 4.7; 95% CI, 1.6 to 14.2). Pattern 2, common to both boys and girls, was characterized by vegetables, fruits, olive oil, fish, grains, and nuts and was inversely associated with CD among both genders (girls: OR, 0.3; 95% CI, 0.1 to 0.9; boys: OR, 0.2; 95% CI, 0.1 to 0.5).

A number of studies have previously examined the role of diet in the etiology of CD (reviewed in reference 67). Barring one study by Gilat et al,[69] which mainly included young adults, most studies were restricted to adult populations. Evidence across these studies has been inconsistent, likely due to methodological limitations inherent on relying on retrospective assessment of diet. Moreover, most of the data were based on patients with long-standing disease, making differentiation between preillness and postillness diet difficult. Moreover, most studies were hospital based and used other diseased patients as controls.

Although the exact constituents in vegetables or fruits that confer protection are not known, we speculated that the ability of vegetables and fruits to modify xenobiotic metabolizing enzymes—in particular enzymes involved in the clearance of reactive oxygen species—may be relevant.[1] Previous in vivo and in vitro studies have suggested an important protective role for ω-3 fatty acids against inflammation.[38] Although some clinical trials have shown that diets richer in ω-3 fatty acids could reduce CD-related inflammation,[70] a large recent trial did not confirm clinical benefits of supplementation.[71]

Although previous studies have reported positive associations with consumption of refined sugars and CD risk, these findings were likely due to changes in diet of the CD patients postillness.[72] We observed that carbohydrate consumption was somewhat lower among CD patients.[67] However, this tendency for protection was entirely due to a lower consumption of dietary fiber by these patients. The negative associations between carbohydrates and CD risk disappeared when fiber consumption was included in the regression analysis. With regards to vitamins and minerals, positive associations with overall intake of retinol, vitamin D, and niacin were noted.[67] These associations were no longer evident when restricted to consumption from foods only. Similarly, no association between overall consumption of vitamin E and CD was observed. However, when supplements were excluded, significant negative association was evident. The same pattern was observed for consumption of minerals. These patterns suggested that consumption of supplemental vitamins or minerals was higher among cases. This may reflect that children predisposed to CD may manifest nutritional deficiencies early on, prompting parents or physicians to administer supplements.

SMOKING AND OTHER ENVIRONMENTAL "INSULTS"

Smoking has been repeatedly shown to have positive associations with adult-onset CD and to be protective for UC.[73] Never smoking and formerly smoking increase the risk of UC, whereas smoking exacerbates the course of CD. A recent study[74] observed that ex-smokers make up an increasing percentage of older patients diagnosed with UC, accounting for more than 35% of the attributable risk of late-onset (>45 years) UC. Current smokers accounted for a large percentage of patients diagnosed at a younger adult age with familial CD but not with sporadic CD. The authors suggested that families with IBD should be counseled that early tobacco use significantly increases the risk of developing CD or, if an ex-smoker, UC at a young age.[74] However, smoking is uncommon in children less than 15 years of age, an age at which new-onset pediatric CD is relatively common.[3] Hence, smoking may not be as important an influence on risk for CD in pediatrics. However, acquiring information on smoking from young children is generally unreliable. Theoretically, maternal smoking or even second-hand smoke may also be important. We[66] and others[75] have reported that maternal smoking is not associated with CD in children.

In addition to smoking, other environmental risk factors that could be important in pediatrics are a history of breastfeeding and the use of oral contraceptive medications (in female adolescents). A case control study of adult IBD patients in Italy[76] again showed that being a former smoker was the factor with the highest attributable risk of UC both in males and females. Smoking was the factor with the highest attributable risk for CD in males. Lack of breastfeeding accounted for the highest proportion of CD in females (attributed risk 11%). Despite this observation, breastfeeding in the more recent "Generation X"-ers was far more frequent than for the post-World War II "baby boomers," yet the incidence of CD is higher among the former group. Our study did not find any effect of breastfeeding on risk for pediatric IBD.[66] In the Italian study, oral contraceptive use accounted for 7% of attributed risk for UC and for 11% of CD.[76]

A small pediatric study in New York reported that breastfeeding was negatively associated with CD ($p = 0.04$) and UC ($p = 0.07$), with relative risk point estimates around 0.5 and with evidence of duration-dependent trends in both instances.[77] There was no evidence of association of either disease with maternal age at birth, birth order, maternal smoking, or season of birth. On the other hand, another small pediatric matched case-control study[78] found that passive smoking exposure at birth was significantly associated with the development of IBD (OR, 3.02; 95% CI, 1.28 to 7.06). The effect was greater for CD (OR, 5.32) than UC (OR, 2.19). Maternal smoking at birth was also significantly associated with the development of IBD (OR, 2.09; 95% CI, 1.02 to 4.29), an effect that also was greater in CD than in UC. There was a dose-response relationship between packs smoked per day and IBD and packs smoked at home per day and IBD.[78]

VACCINES AND INFECTIONS

Measles virus infection or vaccination has been proposed as a potential environmental factor increasing the risk of pediatric IBD. Wakefield et al[79] proposed that CD results from a chronic infection of intestinal submucosal endothelium with measles virus. The authors suggested that this infection generated a granulomatous reaction and intestinal microinfarctions,[80] leading to the inflammation characteristic of CD. This theory was buttressed with a number of pathologic and epidemiologic investigations, including elevated titers to measles in some studies of CD and presumed paramyxovirus identified in granulomas from CD tissue.[81-83] Epidemiologic studies suggested that perinatal exposure to measles virus increased the risk of the development of CD.[84,85] Wakefield's group contended that exposure to the attenuated measles vaccine was associated with an increased risk of the development of CD.[84,86] This led to considerable media hype and substantial public concern over use of live measles vaccine, as well as other vaccines. Indeed, herd immunity was unfortunately compromised in several countries, resulting in an increased number of deaths from wild measles virus infections. Other studies countered these claims, finding that titers to measles were not increased in CD, granulomas were not found in the intestinal endothelium, measles virus particles were not observed in intestinal granulomas, and the measles vaccine was not associated with an increased risk of CD.[87-93] Our recent study was perhaps the final nail in the coffin for the measles virus story as a cause of IBD.[94] We developed a highly specific real-time assay targeting the fusion gene using novel primers and an internal fluorescent probe. All positive reactions were then rigorously evaluated and the amplicons were sequenced. None of the IBD or control intestinal samples yielded positive results using the probe-based, fusion gene assay. The study showed that there is no evidence of measles virus persistence in intestinal biopsy specimens of patients with IBD.[94]

Future Directions

It is apparent that pediatric-onset IBD constitutes a distinct phenotype with differences from adult-onset disease. However, it remains unclear as to whether these disparities are related to genetic and/or environmental factors. There is some evidence that genetic factors contribute to age-of-onset effects, whereby the same genetic markers are more strongly associated with pediatric-onset IBD compared to adult-onset IBD. However, most of the studies investigating age-of-onset effects are based on cross-sectional samples of pediatric and adult IBD cases. These studies are not ideal for investigating age-of-onset effects, as findings could be confounded by cohort effects, population substructure, or gene-environmental interactions. Currently, most association studies, including genome-wide association analyses, are predominantly based on adult IBD cohorts. In order to delineate the genetic and environmental factors unique to pediatric-onset IBD, efforts need to be made to implement studies specifically focused on these populations. Similarly, much emphasis has been placed on identifying genetic associations with CD based on the putative larger contribution of genetics factors to its pathogenesis. However, recent studies[56] have shown that—in particular for pediatric-onset UC and specifically for very early-onset disease (<5 years of age)—genetic contributions, as assessed by history of IBD in first-degree relatives, may be greater than that for CD. Thus, continued efforts to identify potential genetic contributions to pediatric-onset UC are also needed. The Crohn's and Colitis Foundation of Canada has recently embarked upon a large prospective "GEM" study in first-degree relatives of CD probands in an effort to prospectively identify the genetic, environmental, and microbial factors related to early-onset CD (see Figure 4-1).

References

1. Amre D, Seidman E. Etiopathogenesis of pediatric Crohn's disease: biologic pathways based on interactions between genetic and environmental factors. *Med Hypotheses.* 2003;60:344-350.
2. Griffiths AM. Specificities of inflammatory bowel disease in childhood. *Best Pract Res Clin Gastroenterol.* 2004;18:509-523.
3. Bernstein CN, Wajda A, Svenson LW, et al. The epidemiology of inflammatory bowel disease in Canada: a population-based study. *Am J Gastroenterol.* 2006;101(7):1559-1568.
4. Cho JH, Abraham C. Inflammatory bowel disease genetics: NOD2. *Ann Rev Med.* 2007;58:401-416.
5. Nieuwenhuis EES, Escher JC. Early onset IBD: what's the difference? *Dig Liver Dis.* 2008;40:12-15.

6. Weinstein TA, Levine M, Petteti MJ, et al. Age and family history at presentation of pediatric inflammatory bowel disease. *J Pediatr Gastroenterol Nutr.* 2003;37:609-613.

7. Heyman MB, Kirschner BS, Gold BD, et al. Children with early-onset inflammatory bowel disease (IBD): analysis of a pediatric IBD consortium. *J Pediatr.* 2005;146:35-40.

8. Polito II JM, Childs B, Mellits ED, et al. Crohn's disease: influence of age at diagnosis on site and clinical type of disease. *Gastroenterology.* 1996;111:580-586.

9. Halme L, Paavola-Sakki P, Turunen U, et al. Family and twin studies in inflammatory bowel disease. *World J Gastroenterol.* 2006;12:3668-3672.

10. Van Limbergen J, Russell RK, Nimmo ER, Satsangi J. The genetics of inflammatory bowel disease. *Am J Gastroenterol.* 2007;102(12):2820-2831.

11. McGovern DP, van Heel DA, Negoro K, et al. Further evidence of IBD5/CARD15 (NOD2) epistasis in the susceptibility to ulcerative colitis. *Am J Hum Genet.* 2003;73:1465-1466.

12. Andriulli A, Annese V, Latiano A, et al. The frame-shift mutation of the NOD2/CARD15 gene is significantly increased in ulcerative colitis: an *IG-IBD study. *Gastroenterology.* 2004;126:625-627.

13. Brant SR, Wang M-H, Rawsthorne RN, et al. A population-based case-control study of CARD15 and other risk factors in Crohn's disease and ulcerative colitis. *Am J Gastroenterol.* 2007;102:313-323.

14. Cavanaugh J. NOD2: ethnic and geographic differences. *World J Gastroenterol.* 2006;12:3673-3677.

15. Juyal G, Amre D, Midha V, et al. Evidence of allelic heterogeneity for associations between the NOD2 gene and ulcerative colitis among North Indians. *Aliment Pharm Ther.* 2007;26:1325-1332.

16. Sood A, Midha V, Sood N, Bhatia AS, Avasthi G. Incidence and prevalence of ulcerative colitis in Punjab, North India. *Gut.* 2003;52:1587-1590.

17. Brant SR, Panhuysen CI,, Bailey-Wilson JE, et al. Linkage heterogeneity for the IBD1 locus in Crohn's disease pedigrees by disease onset and severity. *Gastroenterology.* 2000;119:1483-1490.

18. Akolkar PN, Gulwani-Akolkar B, Lin XY, et al. The IBD1 locus for susceptibility to Crohn's disease has a greater impact in Ashkenazi Jews with early onset disease. *Am J Gastroenterol.* 2001;96:1127-1132.

19. De Mesquita MB, Civitelli F, Levine A. Epidemiology, genes and inflammatory bowel diseases in childhood. *Digest Liver Dis.* 2008;40:3-11.

20. Vermeire S, Wild G, Kocher K, et al. CARD15 genetic variation in a Quebec population: prevalence, genotype-phenotype relationship, and haplotype structure. *Am J Hum Genet.* 2002;1(1):74-83.

21. Weiss B, Shamir R, Bujanover Y, et al. NOD2/CARD15 mutation analysis and genotype-phenotype correlation in Jewish pediatric patients compared with adults with Crohn's disease. *J Pediatr.* 2004;45:208-212.

22. Amre DK, Seidman EG. DNA variants in cytokine and NOD2 genes, exposures to infections and risk for Crohn's disease in children. *Paediatr Perinat Epidem.* 2003;17:302-312.

23. Amre DK, Mack DM, Morgan K, et al. Association between genetic variants in the IL-23R gene and early-onset Crohn's disease: results from a case-control and family-based study among Canadian children. *Am J Gastroenterol.* 2008;103:615-620.

24. Rioux JD, Silverberg MS, Daly MJ et al. Genomewide search in Canadian families with inflammatory bowel disease reveals two novel susceptibility loci. *Am J Hum Genet.* 2000;66:1863-1870.

25. Reinhard C, Rioux J. Role of the IBD5 susceptibility locus in inflammatory bowel diseases. *Inflamm Bowel Dis.* 2006;12:227-238.

26. Qureshi I, Elimrani I, Seidman E, Mitchell G. Organic cation/carnitine transporters (OCTNs). In: You G, Morris ME, eds. *Drug Transporters: Molecular Characterization and Role in Drug Disposition.* New York, NY: John Wiley & Son, Inc; 2007:35-50.

27. Silverberg M. OCTNs: will the real gene stand out? *World J Gastroenterol.* 2006;12:3678-3681.

28. Babusukumar U, Wang T, McGuire E, et al. Contribution of OCTN variants within the IBD5 locus to pediatric onset Crohn's disease. *Am J Gastroenterol.* 2006;101:1354-1361.

29. Ferraris A, Torres B, Knafelz D, et al. Relationship between CARD15, SLC22A4/5, and DLG5 polymorphisms and early-onset inflammatory bowel diseases: an Italian multicentric study. *Inflamm Bowel Dis.* 2006;12:355-361.

30. Russell RK, Drummond HE, Nimmo ER, et al. Analysis of the influence of OCTN1/2 variants within the IBD5 locus on disease susceptibility and growth indices in early-onset inflammatory bowel disease. *Gut.* 2006;55:1114-1123.

31. Cucchiara S, Latiano A, Palmieri O, et al. Role of CARD15, DLG5 and OCTN genes polymorphisms in children with inflammatory bowel diseases. *World J Gastroenterol.* 2007;13(8):1221-1229.

32. Neurath MF. IL-23: a master regulator in Crohn's disease. *Nature Med.* 2007;13:26-28.

33. Duerr RH, Taylor KD, Brant SR, et al. A genome-wide association study identifies IL-23R as an inflammatory bowel disease gene. *Science.* 2006;314:1461-1463.

34. Tremelling M, Cummings SA, Fisher J, et al. IL-23R variation determines susceptibility but not disease phenotype in inflammatory bowel disease. *Gastroenterology.* 2007;132(5):1657-1664.

35. Roberts RL, Gearry RB, Hollis-Moffatt JE, et al. IL-23R R381Q and ATG16L1 T300A are strongly associated with Crohn's disease in a study of New Zealand Caucasians with inflammatory bowel disease. *Am J Gastroenterol.* 2007;102:2754-2761.

36. Dubinsky MC, Wang D, Picornell Y, et al. IL-23 receptor (IL-23) gene protects against pediatric Crohn's disease. *Inflamm Bowel Dis.* 2007;13(5):511-515.

37. Van Limbergen JE, Russell RK, Nimmo ER, et al. IL-23R Arg381Gln is associated with childhood onset inflammatory bowel disease in Scotland. *Gut.* 2007;56:1173-1174.

38. Seidman EG, Bernotti S, Levy E. Nutritional modulation of gut inflammation. In: Labadarios D, Pichard C, eds. *Clinical Nutrition: Early Intervention.* Nestlé Nutrition Workshop Series, Clinical & Performance Programme, Volume 7. Basel, Switzerland: 2002; 41-61.

39. Sanchez R, Levy E, Seidman E, Amre D, Costea F, Sinnett D. Paraoxonase 1, 2 and 3 DNA variants and susceptibility to childhood inflammatory bowel disease. *Gut.* 2006;55;1820-1821.

40. Baggiolini M, Dewald B, Moser B. Interleukin-8 and related chemotactic cytokines—CXC and CC chemokines. *Adv Immunol.* 1994;55:97-179.

41. Baggiolini M. Chemokines and leukocyte traffic. *Nature.* 1998;392:565-568.

42. Luster AD. Chemokines-chemotactic cytokines that mediate inflammation. *N Engl J Med.* 1998;338:436-445.

43. Lacher M, Kappler R, Berkholz F, Baurecht H, von Schwienitz D, Koletzko S. Association of a CXCL9 polymorphism with pediatric Crohn's disease. *Biochem Biophy Res Commun.* 2007;363:701-707.

44. Urquhart BL, Tirona RG, Kim RB. Nuclear receptors and the regulation of drug metabolizing enzymes and drug transporters: implications for interindividual variability in response to drugs. *J Clin Pharmacol.* 2007;47:566-578.

45. Cheng X, Klaassen CD. Regulation of mRNA expression of xenobiotic transporters by the pregnane x receptor in mouse liver, kidney, and intestine. *Drug Metab Dispos.* 2006;34:1863-1867.

46. Lamba J, Lamba V, Strom S, et al. Novel single nucleotide polymorphisms in the promoter and intron 1 of human pregnane X receptor/ NR1I2 and their association with CYP3A4 expression. *Drug Metab Dispos.* 2008;36:169-181.

47. Zhang J, Kuehl P, Green ED, et al. The human pregnane X receptor: genomic structure and identification and functional characterization of natural allelic variants. *Pharmacogenetics.* 2001;11:555-572.

48. Albermann N, Schmitz-Winnenthal FH, Z'graggen K, et al. Expression of the drug transporters MDR1/ABCB1, MRP1/ABCC1, MRP2/ABCC2, BCRP/ABCG2, and PXR in peripheral blood mononuclear cells and their relationship with the expression in intestine and liver. *Biochem Pharmacol.* 2005;70:949-958.

49. Amre DK, Mack DR, Israel D, et al. Investigation of associations between the pregnane-X receptor gene (NR1I2) and Crohn's disease in Canadian children using a gene-wide haplotype-based approach. *Inflamm Bowel Dis.* 2008;14(9):1214-1218.

50. de Ridder L, Weersma RK, Dijkstra G, et al. Genetic susceptibility has a more important role in pediatric-onset Crohn's disease than in adult-onset Crohn's disease. *Inflamm Bowel Dis.* 2007;13:1083-1092.

51. Achkar JP. IL-23R and ATG16L1 SNPs in IBD: alphabet soup or something more? *Am J Gastroenterol.* 2008;103:628-630.

52. Van Limbergen J, Russell RK, Nimmo ER, et al. Autophagy gene ATG16L1 influences susceptibility and disease location but not childhood-onset in Crohn's disease in Northern Europe. *Inflamm Bowel Dis.* 2008;14:338-346.

53 Lewis SJ, Brunner EJ. Methodological problems in genetic association studies of longevity—the apoprotein E gene as an example. *Int J Epidemiol.* 2004;33:962-970.

54. Lasky-Su J, Lyon HN, Emilsson V, et al. On the replication of genetic associations: timing can be everything. *Am J Human Genet.* 2008;82:849-858.

55. Frank J, Di Ruggiero E, McInnes RR, et al. Large life-course cohorts for characterizing genetic and environmental contributions: the need for more thoughtful designs. *Epidemiology.* 2006;17:595-598.

56. Thankam P, Birnbaum A, Pal DK, et al. Distinct phenotype of early childhood inflammatory bowel disease. *J Clin Gastroenterol.* 2006;40:583-586.

57. Loftus EV Jr. Clinical epidemiology of inflammatory bowel disease: incidence, prevalence, and environmental influences. *Gastroenterology.* 2004;126:1504-1517.

58. Ouyang Q, Tandon R, Goh KL, et al. The emergence of inflammatory bowel disease in the Asian Pacific region. *Curr Opin Gastroenterol.* 2005;21:408-418.

59. Rook GA. The hygiene hypothesis and the increasing prevalence of chronic inflammatory disorders. *Trans R Soc Trop Med Hyg.* 2007;101:1072-1074.

60. Gilat T, Hacohen D, Lilos P, et al. Childhood factors in ulcerative colitis and Crohn's disease: an international collaborative study. *Scand J Gastroenterol.* 1987;22:1009-1024.

61. Ekbom A, Adami HO, Helmick CG, et al. Perinatal risk factors for inflammatory bowel disease: a case-control study. *AJE.* 1990;132:1111-1119.

62. Baron S, Turck D, Leplat C, et al. Environmental risk factors in pediatric inflammatory bowel diseases: a population based case-control study. *Gut.* 2005;54:357-363.

63. Feeney MA, Murphy M, Clegg A, et al. A case-control study of childhood environmental risk factors for the development of inflammatory bowel disease. *Eur J Gastroenterol Hepatol.* 2002;14(5):529-534.

64. Van Kruiningen HJ, Joossens M, Vermiere S, et al. Environmental factors in familial Crohn's disease in Belgium. *Inflamm Bowel Dis.* 2005;11(4):360-365.

65. Thompson NP, Pounder RE, Wakefield AJ. Perinatal and childhood risk factors for inflammatory bowel disease: a case-control study. *Eur J Gastroenterol Hepatol.* 1995;7:385-390.

66. Amre DK, Lambrette P, Law L, et al. Investigating the hygiene hypothesis as a risk factor in pediatric onset Crohn's disease: a case-control study. *Am J Gastroenterol.* 2006;101:1005-1011.

67. Amre DK, D'Souza S, Morgan K, et al. Imbalances in dietary consumption of fatty acids, vegetables and fruits are associated with risk for Crohn's disease in children. *Am J Gastroenterol.* 2007;102(9):2016-2025.

68. D'Souza S, Levy E, Mack D, et al. Dietary patterns and risk for Crohn's disease in children. *Inflamm Bowel Dis.* 2008;14:367-373.

69. Gilat T, Hacohen D, Lilos P, et al. Childhood factors in ulcerative colitis and Crohn's disease: an international co-operative study. *Scand J Gastroenterol.* 1987;22:1009-1024.

70. Belluzi A. N-3 fatty acids for the treatment of inflammatory bowel diseases. *Proc Nutr Soc.* 2002;61:391-395.

71. Feagan BG, Sandborn WJ, Mittmann U, et al. Omega-3 free fatty acids for the maintenance of remission in Crohn disease: the EPIC Randomized Controlled Trials. *JAMA.* 2008;299(14):1690-1697.

72. Riordan AM, Ruxton CHS, Hunter JO. A review of associations between Crohn's disease and consumption of sugars. *Eur J Clin Nutr.* 1998;52:229-238.

73. Birrenbach T, Böcker U. Inflammatory bowel disease and smoking: a review of epidemiology, pathophysiology, and therapeutic implications. *Inflamm Bowel Dis.* 2004;10:848-859.

74. Tuvlin JA, Raza SS, Bracamonte S, et al. Smoking and inflammatory bowel disease: trends in familial and sporadic cohorts. *Inflamm Bowel Dis.* 2007;13(5):573-579.

75. Baron S, Turck D, Leplat C, et al. Environmental risk factors in pediatric inflammatory bowel diseases: a population based case-control study. *Gut.* 2005;54:357-363.

76. Corrao G, Tragnone A, Caprilli R, et al. Risk of inflammatory bowel disease attributable to smoking, oral contraception and breastfeeding in Italy: a nationwide case-control study. *Int J Epidemiol.* 1998;27(3):397-404.

77. Rigas A, Rigas B, Glassman M, et al. Breast-feeding and maternal smoking in the etiology of Crohn's disease and ulcerative colitis in childhood. *Ann Epidemiol.* 1993;3(4):387-392.

78. Lashner BA, Shaheen NJ, Hanauer SB, Kirschner BS. Passive smoking is associated with an increased risk of developing inflammatory bowel disease in children. *Am J Gastroenterol.* 1993;88(3):356-359.

79. Wakefield AJ, Ekbom A, Dhillon AP, et al. Crohn's disease: pathogenesis and persistent measles virus infection. *Gastroenterology.* 1995;108:911-916.

80. Wakefield AJ, Sawyerr AM, Dhillon AP, et al. Pathogenesis of Crohn's disease: multifocal gastrointestinal infarction. *Lancet.* 1989;2:1057-1062.

81. Wakefield AJ, Sim R, Akbar AN, et al. In situ immune responses in Crohn's disease: a comparison with acute and persistent measles virus infection. *J Med Virol.* 1997;51:90-100.

82. Wakefield AJ, Montgomery SM. Immunohistochemical analysis of measles related antigen in IBD. *Gut.* 2001;48:136-137.

83. Lewin J, Dhillon AP, Sim R, et al. Persistent measles virus infection of the intestine: confirmation by immunogold electron microscopy. *Gut.* 1995;36:564-569.

84. Ekbom A, Wakefield AJ, Zack M, et al. Perinatal measles infection and subsequent Crohn's disease. *Lancet.* 1994;344:508-510.

85. Ekbom A, Daszak P, Kraaz W, et al. Crohn's disease after in-utero measles virus exposure. *Lancet.* 1996;348:515-517.

86. Thompson NP, Montgomery SM, Pounder RE, et al. Is measles vaccination a risk factor for inflammatory bowel disease? *Lancet.* 1995;345:1071-1074.

87. Matson AP, Van Kruiningen HJ, West AB, et al. The relationship of granulomas to blood vessels in intestinal Crohn's disease. *Mod Pathol.* 1995;8:680-685.

88. Afzal MA, Armitage E, Ghosh S, et al. Further evidence of the absence of measles virus genome sequence in full thickness intestinal specimens from patients with Crohn's disease. *J Med Virol.* 2000;62:377-382.

89. Feeney M, Ciegg A, Winwood P, et al. A case-control study of measles vaccination and inflammatory bowel disease: the East Dorset Gastroenterology Group. *Lancet.* 1997;350:764-766.

90. Seagroatt V, Goldacre MJ. Crohn's disease, ulcerative colitis, and measles vaccine in an English population, 1979-1998. *J Epidemiol Community Health.* 2003;57:883-887.

91. Ghosh S, Armitage E, Wilson D, et al. Detection of persistent measles virus infection in Crohn's disease: current status of experimental work. *Gut.* 2001;48:748-752.

92. Davis RL, Kramarz P, Bohlke K, et al. Measles-mumps-rubella and other measles-containing vaccines do not increase the risk for inflammatory bowel disease: a case-control study from the Vaccine Safety Datalink project. *Arch Pediatr Adolesc Med.* 2001;155:354-359.

93. Robertson DJ, Sandler RS. Measles virus and Crohn's disease: a critical appraisal of the current literature. *Inflamm Bowel Dis.* 2001;7:51-57.

94. D'Souza Y, Dionne S, Seidman E, Bitton A, Ward BJ. No evidence of persisting measles virus in tissue from children with inflammatory bowel disease. *Gut.* 2007;56:886-888.

CHAPTER 5

GENETIC INFLUENCES OF EARLY-ONSET INFLAMMATORY BOWEL DISEASE

Robert James Pattison and Subra Kugathasan, MD

The occurrence of Crohn's disease (CD) and ulcerative colitis (UC), known in a broad sense as inflammatory bowel disease (IBD), is increasingly prevalent in children. Pathogenesis of IBD, as currently understood, is a complex interaction between environmental factors and promoting or modifying genetic determinants, resulting in the clinical expression of the disease in the gastrointestinal (GI) tract of genetically prone individuals.[1] The specific mutations occurring in disease-promoting genes influence the development of specific clinical phenotypes, while mutations in modifying genes influence the intricate parts of disease phenotype such as disease severity, progression, or response to treatment. IBD is therefore a complex disease involving multiple genetic and environmental risk factors that interact and evolve together into a clinical phenotype (Figure 5-1).[2] When examining the nature of pediatric- and adult-onset IBD, multiple phenotypic differences are observed, raising questions regarding the pathogenesis and significance of age of onset in the phenotypic progression of the disease. Using tools such as whole genome association (WGA) studies, researchers have attempted to identify susceptibility loci that influence the onset and prevalence of CD. The genes interleukin-23 receptor (*IL-23R*)[3] and autophagy-related 16-like 1 (*ATG16L1*)[4] discovered by WGA in adults have recently been confirmed in pediatric-onset CD.[5] These genes join the already confirmed IBD susceptibility genes, *NOD2/CARD15*, *IBD5*, and *DLG5*. More recent WGA scans have revealed many more single nucleotide polymorphisms (SNPs) from several different chromosomes found to be associated with IBD.[3,4]

In the complex model of genetic and environmental interactions, it is hypothesized that early-onset IBD development is rooted more strongly in genetic interactions due to the relatively small amount of time for additive environmental factors to have a strong effect. While the novel susceptibility genes identified to date have been discovered using mainly adult cohorts, it is valid to postulate that these as well as many more susceptibility genes will be shared in the early-onset IBD cohorts. While this theory has yet to be supported by studies, it is evident that in the search for genetic susceptibility loci the genetic make-up of pediatric patients is likely to cast the greatest light on disease pathogenesis since children are affected less by environment or modifying determinants compared with adults. The identification of more susceptibility genes and environmental

Scherl EJ, Dubinsky MC.
*The Changing World of Inflammatory Bowel Disease:
Impact of Generation, Gender, and Global Trends (pp 67-78)*
© 2009 SLACK Incorporated.

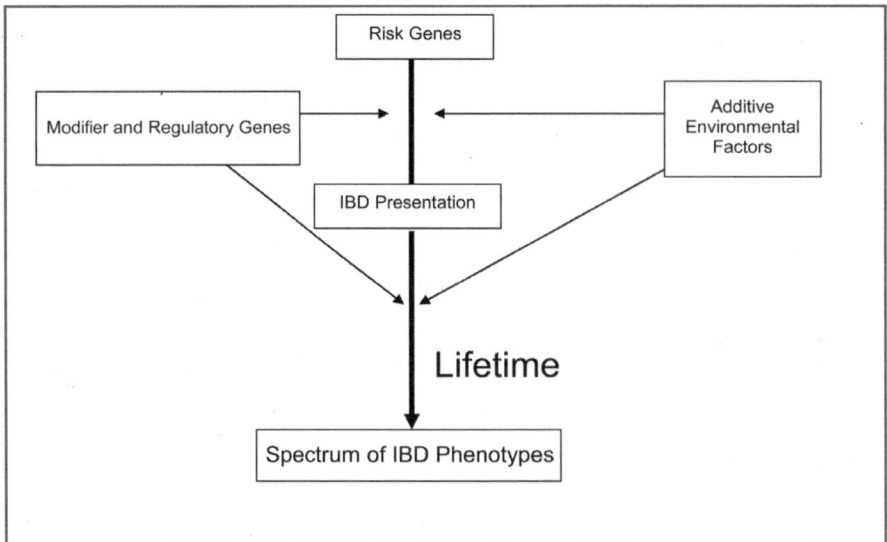

Figure 5-1. A combination of a predisposed genetic make-up (novel susceptibility loci associated with IBD) and the additive genetic modification of the environment throughout time can culminate into a spectrum of biological phenotypes in IBD.

stimuli will require specific clinical studies in specific phenotype population-based cohorts to identify the lifetime gene-gene and gene-environment interactions that determine the susceptibility and eventual outcome of IBD. Studies such as the International HapMap Consortium[5] and WGA scans to localize the risk genes followed by functional studies will likely lead to major advances over the next decade. Optimistic in the growing success of such studies, genetic research is searching for answers to the many open-ended questions in IBD.

Genetic Overview

Within the nucleus of a human cell, deoxyribonucleic acid (DNA) serves as a biological road map for all actions. Organized into 46 human chromosomes, the sets of chromosomes within a cell comprise the genome. Chromosomes are composed of genes. A gene is a set of segments of nucleic acids that code a functional ribonucleic acid (RNA) product when transcribed. The DNA sequences that code for genes are called alleles and occupy a given locus (position) on a specific chromosome. The central dogma of genetics follows directional steps of protein construction with DNA transcribed into RNA, which is then translated into specific proteins. The inherited variation of genetic material through the mechanisms of meiosis is the most fundamental aspect of medical genetics. Mutations are changes in the base pair sequence of DNA, potentially leading to a diseased phenotype. One specific type of mutation, an SNP, is a variation in a single nucleotide within a gene. This is commonly studied in the search for the genetic influence of disease pathogenesis. Due to the principles of meiosis, everyone has 2 copies of a gene, inheriting one from each parent. As a result, a mutated allele on a gene may or may not be expressed in an individual's phenotype. Some diseases such as IBD are influenced by polygenic inheritance, meaning a combined effect of multiple different genes that together form a specific phenotype. Modifying and regulatory genes can have an effect on how other genes function. Modifying genes change how a separate gene is expressed in a phenotype. Regulatory genes mediate gene translation by initiating blockage of gene expression. While these routes explain the inheritable characteristics of genes, they do not provide any information as to what genes may be causing disease onset.

From the 30,000 genes in the human genome, medical researchers attempt to locate specific genes and SNPs causing susceptibility to disease. This process becomes even more daunting with the coinciding levels of gene expression and controls mediating chromosome replication, gene structure, transcription, and translation. Technology plays a key role in this process. With the completion of the Human Genome project[6] in 2003 and the International HapMap Consortium in 2005,[5] researchers have been given the tools to "compare and contrast" the genotype of diseased individuals to "controls." The Human Genome project defined the complete DNA sequence of a set of human chromosomes of which only 1.5% is coded into genes. Although the remaining DNA is noncoding, it is important in the regulation of gene expression. Subsequently, the International HapMap Consortium has recently developed a map of the human genome-describing patterns of genetic variation. Together, these tools have set the path for genome-wide association (GWA) scans or, in other words, scanning of the entire genome of both diseased and control populations and comparing and contrasting variations and similarities. Shared associations and patterns are looked for within the genetic variations (SNPs) of the diseased individuals, which are then compared with that of the controls. When a genetic variant is significantly more recurrent in diseased individuals, the location of this variant on the genome is highlighted and marked as possibly containing a regulatory sequence or novel susceptibility gene predisposing the patient to the disease. Although the human genome's genetic make-up only differs by 0.1%, this small bit of variation can dictate an individual's susceptibility to disease. Computerized databases containing the reference human genome sequence, a map of human genetic variation, and a set of new chip technologies can precisely analyze whole genome samples for genetic variations involved in the onset of a disease by examining the entire genome. As a result, new advanced genotyping technologies such as the Illumina (Illumina, Inc, Santa Clara, CA) or Affymetrix (Affymetrix, Inc, San Diego, CA) are designing chips with up to 500,000 SNPs for fast comparison and will, therefore, facilitate the discovery of new pediatric-onset IBD genes. An understanding of the genetic determinants to IBD could mean the ability to treat more patients effectively and possibly even cure the disease.

Base Genetic Evidence for Inflammatory Bowel Disease

FAMILY CONCORDANCE

When determining the prevalence of genetic components to the susceptibility of a disease, concordance rates among direct family members are the strongest and most basic evidence. Familial aggregation studies have documented this, with statistics pointing to a significantly greater risk of first-degree family of affected individuals developing IBD versus the general population. This evidence was first recognized by Kirsner and Spencer[7] who summarized the familial aggregation for IBD in 1963. From this time, research findings have continually shown a significant link in IBD development and family history of the disease. Looking at the relative risk of IBD for offspring of 2 affected parents, rates of over 30% have been demonstrated.[8] This evidence points to family history as the strongest single risk factor for the development of IBD. When studying the sibling risk ratio (the rate of a sibling of an affected individual contracting IBD to that of the general population), the ratio ranges from 30% to 40% for CD and 10% to 20% for UC.[9] Additional evidence suggests that early-onset disease corresponds to a more distinct, more aggressive phenotype than a similar disease in patients older than 20 years.[10] When compared to older age groups, early onset was associated with a greater family history of disease, a greater need for surgery, and a greater occurrence of small bowel disease.[11] In addition, it has been recognized that these familial cases of CD occur with greater severity and with earlier onset.[12] Furthermore, concordance rates have been observed within disease location and behavior among affected relations with CD.[13] Familial aggregation studies have therefore demonstrated that genetic influences play a substantial role in the development of IBD because there is an increased risk of disease for a related individual as a result of his or her genetic similarity. However, the vast majority of cited studies were performed in the adult cohorts rather than pediatrics; this has resulted in the need for similar comprehensive studies to be conducted in pediatric cohorts.

TWIN INVESTIGATIONS

The most prominent evidence to suggest that the pathogenesis of IBD is genetic is the disease rate among twins. Monozygotic twins are formed when one egg is fertilized and the resulting zygote divides into 2 independent embryos that have the same DNA make-up but with different phenotypes due to environmental stimuli. Dizygotic twins result when 2 separate eggs are fertilized by separate sperm, forming twins that are genetically and phenotypically different. Predicting the rates of disease in monozygotic and dizygotic twins, a significantly higher rate of IBD in monozygotic twins would be expected because they contain the same DNA. In one of the largest twin studies by Orholm et al, disease concordance was 58% for monozygotic CD twins and 18% for monozygotic UC twins compared to dizygotic twins among whom the concordance rate for CD and UC was 0% and 4.5%, respectively.[14] Other reviews have replicated these findings, documenting concordance for CD ranging from 20% to 50% for monozygotic twins and 0% to 10% among dizygotic twins.[8,13,15,16] Lower rates were found with UC, ranging from 15% to 20% in monozygotic twins and 0% to 7% in dizygotic twins. In addition, monozygotic twins commonly have similar forms of IBD, suggesting that specific genotypes point to specific phenotypic expressions of CD and UC regarding onset, anatomical location, and severity.[14,16-18] Higher concordance rates among individuals with the identical genetic make-up is indisputable evidence for the genetic significance in the pathogenesis of IBD and specifically CD. Having verified a link between genotype and susceptibility of IBD, the next task is finding trends in specific genes and alleles in affected individuals and controls.

Gene-Specific Strategies Finding Prevalent Genes and Single Nucleotide Polymorphisms

PEDIATRIC COHORTS ARE CRITICAL TO INFLAMMATORY BOWEL DISEASE GENETIC INVESTIGATIONS

The rise in incidence of pediatric IBD over the last several decades is well recognized. This dramatic increase in disease incidence is unlikely to be explained by genetic susceptibility alone since the human genetic pool is unlikely to have drastically changed in such a short period of time. Therefore, it is hypothesized that the likely cause for this increase in pediatric incidence is environmental interactions in genetically susceptible individuals. In other words, pre-existing genetic risks are influenced by the effects of a rapidly changing environment. We must look at both genetic and environmental factors in an attempt to find a specific source of the disease pathogenesis.

Compared to adult-onset IBD, pediatric-onset IBD is presumed to be influenced greater by genetics as there is less time for the environment to have influenced disease in pediatric patients. Adult-onset IBD has a greater likelihood of being confounded by numerous environmental exposures when compared with pediatric-onset IBD, simply in the fact that adults have had more time to experience the additive environmental factors. For example, smoking has been investigated as a factor contributing to the adult onset of IBD yet has been ignored in pediatrics due to limited pediatric exposure. Such would be the case with many other environmental factors, ranging from various antigens and bacteria to different types of food, with the constant principle that as age increases so does the accumulation of additive triggers and a higher likelihood of coming into contact with specific environmental triggers of IBD.

Conveniently, patients with early-onset IBD are logistically easier to follow in genetic-based studies of IBD pathogenesis and behavior. As the parents frequently are present at the time of diagnosis and during subsequent clinic visits, it is relatively easy to collect parental DNA. Parental DNA is significantly important in family-based association studies, which are more advantageous than case-control studies as they bypass the potential problems of population stratification and reduce the risk of population heterogeneity when comparing various study populations.[19] These family-based studies take advantage of transmission disequilibrium testing, a powerful test for significant genetic associations that can be performed easily with DNA from family trios and siblings, giving results that are not influenced by population stratification. Additionally, even environmental exposure in children can be measured as many parents keep a diligent record of events such as infections, immunizations, other intercurrent illnesses, and even travel. Children are therefore the ideal genetic cohorts for genetic investigation.

IDENTIFICATION OF INFLAMMATORY BOWEL DISEASE GENES; FROM LINKAGE TO WHOLE GENOME ASSOCIATION

Until 2006, the search for IBD genes was primarily based on linkage mapping without taking advantage of linkage disequilibrium (LD) mapping on a genome-wide scale. LD describes different situations in which some combinations of alleles or genetic markers occur more or less frequently in a population than expected from the random construction of haplotypes from allelic frequencies. When loci are identified by linkage mapping studies, they span larger chromosomal segments and contain a larger number of candidate genes. Consequently, there is a need to develop further mapping strategies to overcome these limitations. On the other hand, LD mapping is not guaranteed to identify susceptibility variants if multiple rare susceptibility alleles exist within a given disease locus or if there is extensive LD around the disease locus. This has been the case for the *IBD5* locus in CD, where it is difficult, if not impossible, to distinguish one SNP as the etiological variant over others in strong LD with it. Using a high-density set of markers, a GWA study is likely to have greater power to localize genes with small-to-moderate effects. It is indeed evident that the vast precisions of GWA analyses are likely to be a powerful approach for disease mapping.[20]

The Genetic Determinants Behind Inflammatory Bowel Disease

GENETIC DISCOVERIES AND THEIR CLINICAL SIGNIFICANCE IN INFLAMMATORY BOWEL DISEASE

To review, complex diseases such as IBD are controlled by multiple risk factors that include a combination of genetic predispositions and additive environmental stimuli. Hypothesizing that specific genes and mutations are the pathogenesis of IBD, researchers have set out to find these genetic triggers in the genomes of IBD patients. Specific mutations occurring in disease-promoting genes influence the development of distinct clinical phenotypes whereas mutations in the modifying and regulatory genes influence specific features of the disease phenotype such as disease behavior or response to treatment. Mutations in the genes *NOD2/CARD15* have been studied extensively in genotype-phenotype of IBD patients in correlation studies. Patients with *NOD2/CARD15* variants were associated with a younger age at onset, the presence of ileal involvement, and a tendency to develop strictures or fistulas.[21,22] For instance, at least 95% of the patients homozygous for $NOD_2/CARD_{15}$ mutations present with ileal lesions.[23] Existing data are inconclusive as to whether $NOD_2/CARD_{15}$ carriage is associated with a more severe disease course, suggesting that this feature depends on modifying genes and environmental risk factors. Looking at specific mutations and SNPs within these genes, researchers have shown that stricturing complications leading to early surgery were found more frequently in patients with the 1007fs mutation within the $CARD_{15}$ gene compared with those children without mutations.[24] Children with this mutation had an almost 7-fold increased risk for developing a stricturing phenotype requiring surgery.[24] A stricturing phenotype results in abnormal narrowing of the digestive tract due to scarring and inflammation, necessitating surgery. Knowing the genetic make-up of the patients at presentation of disease may identify patients at risk for more rapid development of complications, and hence allow the selection of patients who would benefit from the early use of more aggressive therapies. With this genetic knowledge, the physician could select a medication based on the genetic make-up of the patient and the corresponding specific phenotypic presentation of disease. The results from genotype-phenotype analysis using other IBD susceptibility genes are ongoing. In a study by Newman and colleagues, the $SLC_{22}A_4$-TC diplotype did not influence the age of disease diagnosis.[25] Given the epistatic effect (ie, the interaction of 2 or more genes controlling the expression of a phenotype) between $NOD_2/CARD_{15}$ and $SLC_{22}A_4$-TC with ileal involvement in CD, genetic effects of this $SLC_{22}A_4$-A_5 and $NOD_2/CARD_{15}$ mutation may result from a common mechanism in the ileum. The presence of the $SLC_{22}A$-TC diplotype was not associated with UC in the presence or absence of $NOD_2/CARD_{15}$ risk alleles. Newman and colleagues[25] showed that the $SLC_{22}A$-TC diplotype constitutes a CD-specific variation that acts together with $CARD_{15}/NOD_2$ risk alleles to induce a predisposition to CD and ileal involvement among patients who have CD.

A correlation between the genes $NOD_2/CARD_{15}$ and the onset of CD understood, animal studies were used for more specific results. In mice lacking $NOD_2/CARD_{15}$, a defect in defense against a common bacterium (*Listeria monocytogenes*) was paralleled by a decreased expression of a specific Paneth cell.[26] Paneth cells contribute to the GI barrier of the GI tract by providing defense against microbes in the small intestine. Interestingly, CD patients homozygous for the $NOD_2/CARD_{15}$ mutations show a similar decreased expression of Paneth cells.[234] These results have opened the door to a better understanding of disease pathogenesis in suggesting that the immune system has a role in preventing inflammation from common bacteria and pathogens passing through the GI tract. Given the nature of this CD susceptibility gene, it seems reasonable to postulate that impaired bacterial sensing is a major event leading to local inflammation or hyper-responsiveness of the natural immune system or abnormal activation of the immune responsive T and B cells.

IBD5, DLG5, AND TLR

In addition to the $NOD_2/CARD_{15}$ gene, an additional gene of interest is the IBD_5 gene located on chromosome 5. The locus was identified in a genome-wide linkage scan, and the association of the IBD_5-risk haplotype with CD was subsequently confirmed by 3 other independent groups.[27-29] Looking at 2 novel polymorphisms in the solute carrier family, 22A4/22A5 ($SLC_{22}A_4$-A_5) genes within this region were identified in a Canadian population. These 2 CD-associated alleles carried by the same haplotype, $SLC_{22}A$-TC, $SLC_{22}A_4$, and $SLC_{22}A_5$, encode the organic cation transporters 1 and 2, respectively. Rioux et al[30] found that the IBD_5 locus was associated most strongly with the early onset of CD (maximum logarithm {base 10} of odds [LOD]) score of 3.9 in CD children under 16 years at disease onset), with a lesser effect when adult-onset CD was included (maximum LOD score 2.4).[30] It can be hypothesized from these results that IBD_5 may represent an early-onset CD susceptibility gene.[30] However, subsequent studies of pediatric-onset CD cohorts have shown that the effect of IBD_5 risk is only modest and lower compared with adult-onset CD. The inconsistent correlation between pediatric and adult cohorts highlights an important difference in the disease determinants based on age of onset.

Another gene of interest is discs large homologue 5 (DLG_5) genes located on chromosome 10. Using a positional cloning approach, Stoll and colleagues[31] identified disease-associated variants responsible for the linkage of CD with chromosome 10q23. A total of 3 IBD-associated genetic variations in the *DLG5* gene were found. This gene encodes for a scaffolding protein involved in maintaining normal epithelial death or growth. The authors also studied the gene-to-gene interaction between *DLG5* and *CARD15*, showing an association between the 113A variant and the presence of *CARD15* variants. Findings by Daly and colleagues[32] support the conclusion that *DLG5* relates to IBD susceptibility. Friedrichs and colleagues[33] published a report using multivariate logistic regression analysis to examine several large IBD cohorts from Germany, Italy, and Quebec, finding that the *DLG5* variant is a modest susceptibility risk factor for CD (odds ratio [OR], 1.5). However, they found that a dramatic increase in risk was seen for men (OR, 2.49) but not for women (OR, 1.0) with the gene.

Toll-like receptors (TLRs) are single membrane-spanning, noncatalytic receptors. They are crucial parts in the body's normal immune response to microbes in the GI tract that have breached the physical barriers of the intestinal tract mucosa, stimulating a cellular response. Located on the surface of monocytes, macrophages, and dendritic and epithelial cells, they serve as a type of pattern recognition receptor. Recognizing pathogenic micro-organisms, they are also essential in the identification of commensal microflora and maintenance of homeostasis within the GI tract. Despite the critical protective role of certain TLRs at the intestinal mucosal boundary, there have only been minor genetic variations affecting the TLR-signaling pathway identified in IBD.[34] It has been observed that *TLR4* is overexpressed in CD epithelial cells and *TLR3* is down regulated, while *TLR2* and *TLR5* remain unchanged.[35] Polymorphisms have been described in IBD in regard to the *TLR4* and *TLR9* genes; however, it is not know whether this correlates to any functional significance.[36,37] Due to TLRs' significance in the recognition and response to the various types of bacteria, it has been hypothesized that they may play a key function in a biological inter-relationship that could be dysfunctional in IBD. Despite the critical protective role of certain TLRs at the intestinal mucosal interface, only minor genetic variations affecting the TLR-signaling pathway have been identified in IBD.[35,38] In addition, a complex intronic polymorphism of the *CARD4/NOD1* gene recently was linked to CD development.[39] The *CARD4/NOD1* gene confers cellular responsiveness to the unique peptidoglycan (PGN) motif, suggesting a more general involvement of bacterial component sensing in this inflammatory disease rather than the specific TLR response.

The Recently Discovered Genes

IL-23R

The advancement in genome analysis studies has come with the greater understanding and documentation of the human genome. We have identified the human genome's 3 billion[5] base-pair DNA sequence and most of the 30,000 human genes via the International Human Genome Sequencing Consortium, and 4 million common human SNPs have been catalogued through the use of the International HapMap Consortium with correlations between linked SNPs. This is combined with the selection of nonredundant tag SNPs for genetic association studies.[5] The development of technologies for rapid and cost-effective genome-wide analysis of genetic differences between people with illness and controls has facilitated the potential for rapid progress in identifying the genetic factors underlying common inheritable diseases. Some of the first studies to take advantage of this knowledge and technology were the GWA studies in CD cohorts.[3,40-42]

In one of the first studies of this advanced technology, Duerr et al[40] found a highly significant variation in the gene encoding the *IL-23R* among CD patients using the WGA approach. These results were successfully replicated by numerous independent investigators, further advancing the results of Duerr et al.[40] *IL-23* is a heterodimeric cytokine composed of 2 different subunits, one called p40 (which is shared with the cytokine *IL-12*) and another called p19 (the *IL-23* alpha subunit). *IL-23* is an important part of early inflammatory response against bacteria, but more specifically in regard to natural immunity and the primal compilation of adaptive immune response mechanisms. This specific gene is correlated with inflammatory cytokines related to the *IL-12*, which is the fuel behind many pathologic inflammatory reactions. When this study was first commenced, the cohort was limited to adults with ileal CD in adults; however, these findings have been replicated in pediatric patients with CD.[40] *IL-23* activity is classically presented in the terminal ileum and its expression is increased in CD patients.[44] Mouse models have been used to define the role of *IL-23* as an activator of both the innate immune response and effector T cells, also orchestrating organ-specific inflammatory responses.[44,45] These findings are particularly prevalent due to its association with the innate inflammatory response in IBD.

Based on the functional nature of both the *IL-12* and *IL-23* pathways, it is feasible to assume that variations might negatively affect the immune response to microbial agents during childhood. *IL-12* transforms CD4+ T cells into a *Th1* phenotype and in the company of the *IL-23* sum into a TH17 phenotype.[46,47] This TH17 phenotype is characterized by the production of other inflammatory agents such as *IL-17, TNF,* and *IL-6*.[13,48] The immune role associated with TH17 has been shown to target many specific autoimmune inflammatory responses in various types of animals. In mouse models without the *IL-23* gene, there was no development of diverse autoimmune disease such as arthritis or chronic intestinal inflammation correlating to the absence of the *IL-17* to the absence of the TH17 in specific organs.[15,48,49] Various bacteria-specific components such as PGN were found to exercise a regulatory effect on the antigen-presenting cells, increasing the *IL-23* expression without affecting the *IL-12*.[50] This further illustrates how crucial even the smallest variation in *IL-12*– and *IL-23*–dependent inflammatory mechanisms may be on the impact of a specific phenotype.

Autophagy in the Pathogenesis of Crohn's Disease

Branching from the recent genetic strategies used in the exploration of IBD pathogenesis is the identification of the role of autophagy in the susceptibility of CD. A highly significant association with CD in 2 separate autophagy genes, *ATG16L1* and *IRGM*, was identified and replicated, confirming the suspected link. Autophagy is a recycling behavior of the cells in which they recycle surplus organelles. This process is thought to play a significant role in the normal defense against micro-organisms within the cytoplasm of the cells. Therefore, autophagy serves as the mechanism to engulf and eliminate any harmful bacteria within the cell membrane. After the antigen has been engulfed, various inflammatory responses involving lysosomes are used to destroy the invader.[52] In some specific cases, autophagy also has been prevalent in the connection of an antigen into a major histocompatibility complex (MHC)-binding groove presented on the cell surface.[53] Due to their tremendous inflammatory role in the recognition and destruction of an antigen, it is reasonable to speculate their role in the IBD inflammatory pathway.

ATG16L1

One loci identified in a GWA connecting CD with autophagy interactions has been the *ATG16L1* gene on chromosome 2q37. The signal of this gene is identified as coding for a nonsynonymous single nucleotide polymorphism (nsSNP) changing the amino-acid sequence coding for a threonine to alanine substitution, subsequently changing the production of the protein. This strong association has been confirmed by other independent studies from western Europe and North America.[3,41] While it is not known what this actually means in terms of protein function, it is understood that the *ATG16L1* protein is a key component in autophagy, the specific T300A substitution occurs in an evolutionarily conserved domain,[41] and it is expressed in the GI track but particularly strongly in CD4+ T lymphocytes. It is also understood that the gene diminishes the autophagy related to the intracellular pathogen *Salmonella typhimurium*.[3]

IRGM

The *IRGM* gene is another key contributor in autophagy. Using the Wellcome Trust Case Control Consortium (WTCCC) GWA scan, a highly significant association was found between variation in the *IRGM* gene and susceptibility to CD. This was originally found in the WTCCC scan and then replicated strongly in an independent CD panel.[4] When using animal testing to fortify these findings, it was found that mice without the homologue for this gene had an impaired ability to destroy the pathogens *Toxoplasma gondii* and *Listeria monocytogenes* within the cell 25. In human macrophages with a knockdown of the *IRGM* gene, there was significantly prolonged survival of the *Mycobacteria tuberculosis* in recent studies.[53] This study not only provided indisputable evidence of the *IL-23R* pathway in the pathogenesis of CD but also revealed the power of a GWA scan to produce reproducible data.

The genetic data for *ATG16L1* and *IRGM* clearly implicate defects in the mechanisms of autophagy with a predisposition to CD. Showing lengthened survival times of intracellular micro-organisms within macrophages altered has a clear reverberation with the hypothesis of *Mycobacterium avium subsp. paratuberculosis* (MAP) in the pathogenesis of CD.[54] These findings also may explain the presence of subpathogenic organisms such as adherent invasive *Escherichia coli* within intestinal epithelial cells and macrophages from individuals with CD. It has long been hypothesized that commensal intestinal bacteria play a role in the predisposition to CD; however, there is not an understanding of how they might do this. Therefore, an understanding of the defects in autophagy might provide this mechanism and be a key part of the pathogenic pathway. The question as to whether chronic intestinal inflammation is a consequence of impaired viability of epithelial cells, from the inappropriate activation of adaptive immune pathways causing "collateral damage," or to another mechanism altogether, will be answered in further specific studies.

Summary

The complex model of IBD is controlled by promoting/modifying genetic determinants and environmental risk factors that progress and interact into a specific IBD phenotype. It is postulated that specific mutations occurring in disease-promoting genes influence the development of the distinct clinical phenotypes while the mutations in the modifying genes influence specific features of the disease phenotype such as disease location, progression, severity, and response to treatment. Due to the unique characteristics of pediatric-onset IBD, children make an ideal subject of study in the analysis of the genetic components behind this complex disease. Therefore, while the genetic studies to this point have made great strides in the understanding of the genetic pathways to susceptibility in the predominately adult cohorts, the most promising information about genetic susceptibility is on the horizon using pediatric cohorts.

The successes to date in the search for susceptibility loci in adults have been the product of a GWA approach identifying strong evidence for novel susceptibility loci. While success to this point is promising, it is likely that very few of the genetic risk factors identified to date will remain significant among the hundreds of thousands of SNPs studies in GWA studies. It is likely that many of the true associations among the thousands of SNP loci will provide only weak evidence for association in individual GWA studies. Therefore, the genetic advances made in the past few years have marked the beginning of a new age in the understanding of the genetics of IBD in children. As the pediatric population is characterized with unique phenotypes, it is suggested that their genes may uniquely or more effectively play a role in risk. Despite the various phenotypic differences, the existence of an early-onset susceptibility gene remains a hypothesis. The identification of early-onset susceptibility genes will be facilitated with the rapid growth of technology in the use of GWA studies using phenotypically classified, exclusively early-onset cohorts.

Structural and functional studies of the candidate genes also will play a part in the understanding of susceptibility. Evaluating genes that are coexpressed under conditions as well as carrying out additional expression studies of the candidate genes in healthy tissues and diseased tissues will give an understanding of the genes that may alter which proteins are expressed when and what their function will be. As a result, animal models will play a key role in assessing the function and role of these newly discovered genes.

References

1. Strober W, Fuss I, Mannon P. The fundamental basis of inflammatory bowel disease. *J Clin Invest.* 2007;117:514-521.
2. Kugathasan S, Amre D. Inflammatory bowel disease: environmental modification and genetic determinants. *Pediatr Clin North Am.* 2006;53:727-749.
3. Rioux JD, Xavier RJ, Taylor KD, et al. Genome-wide association study identifies new susceptibility loci for Crohn's disease and implicates autophagy in disease pathogenesis. *Nat Genet.* 2007;39:596-604.
4. Parkes M, Barrett JC, Prescott NJ, et al. Sequence variants in the autophagy gene IRGM and multiple other replicating loci contribute to Crohn's disease susceptibility. *Nat Genet.* 2007;39:830-832.
5. The International HapMap Consortium. A haplotype map of the human genome. *Nature.* 2005;437:1299-1320.
6. International Human Genome Sequencing Consortium. Finishing the euchromatic sequence of the human genome. *Nature.* 2004;431:931-945.
7. Kirsner JB, Spencer JA. Family occurrences of ulcerative colitis, regional enteritis, and ileocolitis. *Ann Intern Med.* 1963;59:133-144.
8. Halme L, Paavola-Sakki P, Turunen U, Lappalainen M, Farkkila M, Kontula K. Family and twin studies in inflammatory bowel disease. *World J Gastroenterol.* 2006;12:3668-3672.
9. Satsangi J. Genetics of inflammatory bowel disease: from bench to bedside? *Acta Odontol Scand.* 2001;59:187-192.
10. Polito JM 2nd, Childs B, Mellits ED, Tokayer AZ, Harris ML, Bayless TM. Crohn's disease: influence of age at diagnosis on site and clinical type of disease. *Gastroenterology.* 1996;111:580-586.
11. Annese V, Andreoli A, Andriulli A, et al. Familial expression of anti-*Saccharomyces cerevisiae* Mannan antibodies in Crohn's disease and ulcerative colitis: a GISC study. *Am J Gastroenterol.* 2001;96:2407-2412.
12. Colombel JF, Grandbastien B, Gower-Rousseau C, et al. Clinical characteristics of Crohn's disease in 72 families. *Gastroenterology.* 1996;111:604-607.
13. Duerr RH. Update on the genetics of inflammatory bowel disease. *J Clin Gastroenterol.* 2003;37:358-367.
14. Orholm M, Binder V, Sorensen TI, Rasmussen LP, Kyvik KO. Concordance of inflammatory bowel disease among Danish twins: results of a nationwide study. *Scand J Gastroenterol.* 2000;35:1075-1081.
15. Bonen DK, Ogura Y, Nicolae DL, et al. Crohn's disease-associated NOD2 variants share a signaling defect in response to lipopolysaccharide and peptidoglycan. *Gastroenterology.* 2003;124:140-146.
16. Thompson NP, Driscoll R, Pounder RE, Wakefield AJ. Genetics versus environment in inflammatory bowel disease: results of a British twin study. *BMJ.* 1996;312:95-96.
17. Tysk C, Lindberg E, Jarnerot G, Floderus-Myrhed B. Ulcerative colitis and Crohn's disease in an unselected population of monozygotic and dizygotic twins: a study of heritability and the influence of smoking. *Gut.* 1988;29:990-996.
18. Halfvarson J, Bodin L, Tysk C, Lindberg E, Jarnerot G. Inflammatory bowel disease in a Swedish twin cohort: a long-term follow-up of concordance and clinical characteristics. *Gastroenterology.* 2003;124:1767-1773.
19. Halme L, Turunen U, Helio T, et al. Familial and sporadic inflammatory bowel disease: comparison of clinical features and serological markers in a genetically homogeneous population. *Scand J Gastroenterol.* 2002;37:692-698.
20. Risch N, Merikangas K. The future of genetic studies of complex human diseases. *Science.* 1996;273:1516-1517.
21. Ahmad T, Armuzzi A, Bunce M, et al. The molecular classification of the clinical manifestations of Crohn's disease. *Gastroenterology.* 2002;122:854-866.
22. Abreu MT, Taylor KD, Lin YC, et al. Mutations in NOD2 are associated with fibrostenosing disease in patients with Crohn's disease. *Gastroenterology.* 2002;123:679-688.
23. Chamaillard M, Iacob R, Desreumaux P, Colombel JF. Advances and perspectives in the genetics of inflammatory bowel diseases. *Clin Gastroenterol Hepatol.* 2006;4:143-151.
24. Kugathasan S, Collins N, Maresso K, et al. CARD15 gene mutations and risk for early surgery in pediatric-onset Crohn's disease. *Clin Gastroenterol Hepatol.* 2004;2:1003-1009.
25. Newman B, Gu X, Wintle R, et al. A risk haplotype in the Solute Carrier Family 22A4/22A5 gene cluster influences phenotypic expression of Crohn's disease. *Gastroenterology.* 2005;128:260-269.
26. Kobayashi KS, Chamaillard M, Ogura Y, et al. NOD2-dependent regulation of innate and adaptive immunity in the intestinal tract. *Science.* 2005;307:731-734.

27. Giallourakis C, Stoll M, Miller K, et al. IBD5 is a general risk factor for inflammatory bowel disease: replication of association with Crohn's disease and identification of a novel association with ulcerative colitis. *Am J Hum Genet.* 2003;73:205-211.

28. Negoro K, McGovern DP, Kinouchi Y, et al. Analysis of the IBD5 locus and potential gene-gene interactions in Crohn's disease. *Gut.* 2003;52:541-546.

29. Mirza MM, Fisher SA, King K, et al. Genetic evidence for interaction of the 5q31 cytokine locus and the CARD15 gene in Crohn's disease. *Am J Hum Genet.* 2003;72:1018-1022.

30. Rioux JD, Silverberg MS, Daly MJ, et al. Genomewide search in Canadian families with inflammatory bowel disease reveals two novel susceptibility loci. *Am J Hum Genet.* 2000;66:1863-1870.

31. Stoll M, Corneliussen B, Costello CM, et al. Genetic variation in DLG5 is associated with inflammatory bowel disease. *Nat Genet.* 2004;36:476-480.

32. Daly MJ, Pearce AV, Farwell L, et al. Association of DLG5 R30Q variant with inflammatory bowel disease. *Eur J Hum Genet.* 2005;13:835-839.

33. Friedrichs F, Brescianini S, Annese V, et al. Evidence of transmission ratio distortion of DLG5 R30Q variant in general and implication of an association with Crohn disease in men. *Hum Genet.* 2006;119:305-311.

34. Torok HP, Glas J, Tonenchi L, Mussack T, Folwaczny C. Polymorphisms of the lipopolysaccharide-signaling complex in inflammatory bowel disease: association of a mutation in the Toll-like receptor 4 gene with ulcerative colitis. *Clin Immunol.* 2004;112:85-91.

35. Cario E, Podolsky DK. Differential alteration in intestinal epithelial cell expression of toll-like receptor 3 (TLR3) and TLR4 in inflammatory bowel disease. *Infect Immun.* 2000;68:7010-7017.

36. Franchimont D, Vermeire S, El Housni H, et al. Deficient host-bacteria interactions in inflammatory bowel disease? The toll-like receptor (TLR)-4 Asp299gly polymorphism is associated with Crohn's disease and ulcerative colitis. *Gut.* 2004;53:987-992.

37. Torok HP, Glas J, Tonenchi L, Bruennler G, Folwaczny M, Folwaczny C. Crohn's disease is associated with a toll-like receptor-9 polymorphism. *Gastroenterology.* 2004;127:365-366.

38. Cario E. Bacterial interactions with cells of the intestinal mucosa: toll-like receptors and NOD2. *Gut.* 2005;54:1182-1193.

39. McGovern DP, Hysi P, Ahmad T, et al. Association between a complex insertion/deletion polymorphism in NOD1 (CARD4) and susceptibility to inflammatory bowel disease. *Hum Mol Genet.* 2005;14:1245-1250.

40. Duerr RH, Taylor KD, Brant SR, et al. A genome-wide association study identifies IL-23R as an inflammatory bowel disease gene. *Science.* 2006;314:1461-1463.

41. Hampe J, Franke A, Rosenstiel P, et al. A genome-wide association scan of nonsynonymous SNPs identifies a susceptibility variant for Crohn disease in ATG16L1. *Nat Genet.* 2007;39:207-211.

42. Libioulle C, Louis E, Hansoul S, et al. Novel crohn disease locus identified by genome-wide association maps to a gene desert on 5p13.1 and modulates expression of PTGER4. *PLoS Genet.* 2007;3:e58.

43. Achkar JP, Dassopoulos T, Silverberg MS, et al. Phenotype-stratified genetic linkage study demonstrates that IBD2 is an extensive ulcerative colitis locus. *Am J Gastroenterol.* 2006;101:572-580.

44. Fujino S, Andoh A, Bamba S, et al. Increased expression of interleukin 17 in inflammatory bowel disease. *Gut.* 2003;52:65-70.

45. Maul J, Loddenkemper C, Mundt P, et al. Peripheral and intestinal regulatory CD4+ CD25(high) T cells in inflammatory bowel disease. *Gastroenterology.* 2005;128:1868-1878.

46. Hue S, Ahern P, Buonocore S, et al. Interleukin-23 drives innate and T cell-mediated intestinal inflammation. *J Exp Med.* 2006;203:2473-2483.

47. Murphy CA, Langrish CL, Chen Y, et al. Divergent pro- and antiinflammatory roles for IL-23 and IL-12 in joint autoimmune inflammation. *J Exp Med.* 2003;198:1951-1957.

48. Bonen DK, Cho JH. The genetics of inflammatory bowel disease. *Gastroenterology.* 2003;124:521-536.

49. Lazaridis KN, Petersen GM. Genomics, genetic epidemiology, and genomic medicine. *Clin Gastroenterol Hepatol.* 2005;3:320-328.

50. Begum NA, Ishii K, Kurita-Taniguchi M, et al. Mycobacterium bovis BCG cell wall-specific differentially expressed genes identified by differential display and cDNA subtraction in human macrophages. *Infect Immun.* 2004;72:937-948.

51. Radtke AL, O'Riordan MX. Intracellular innate resistance to bacterial pathogens. *Cell Microbiol.* 2006;8:1720-1729.

52. Munz C. Autophagy and antigen presentation. *Cell Microbiol.* 2006;8:891-898.

53. Collazo CM, Yap GS, Sempowski GD, et al. Inactivation of LRG-47 and IRG-47 reveals a family of interferon gamma-inducible genes with essential, pathogen-specific roles in resistance to infection. *J Exp Med.* 2001;194:181-188.

54. Shanahan F, O'Mahony J. The mycobacteria story in Crohn's disease. *Am J Gastroenterol.* 2005;100:1537-1538.

NATURAL HISTORY AND PROGNOSIS OF PEDIATRIC-ONSET INFLAMMATORY BOWEL DISEASE

William Faubion, MD

Understanding the natural history of inflammatory bowel disease (IBD) is important to the clinician for 2 reasons: 1) to feel confident discussing future expectations with a newly diagnosed patient and family and 2) to consider early effective intervention in those patients predicted to be at highest risk of a complicated disease course. Quality natural history data exist for both Crohn's disease (CD) and ulcerative colitis (UC) describing the frequency of firm endpoints such as surgery, hospitalization, neoplasia, and death. The data of highest quality are derived from population-based analyses of predominantly adult patients. The term *population based* means that the population under study is drawn from a representative sample of patients with a centralized medical resource (thus avoiding referral bias). This chapter will explore the public health burden of IBD, the available natural history data focusing where available on data unique to the pediatric population, and finally the potential to alter this natural history with effective medical therapy. The goal of the chapter is to answer the following 5 questions:

1. How common is pediatric IBD?
2. How does pediatric IBD typically present?
3. What is the prognosis specifically relating to surgery, neoplasia, and mortality?
4. Is it possible to predict which patients will experience aggressive disease leading to complications?
5. Can early, effective therapy alter an anticipated poor prognosis?

How Common Is Pediatric Inflammatory Bowel Disease?

Investigators from the Medical College of Wisconsin performed a statewide study over 2 years of incident cases of pediatric IBD. Despite a lack of centralized medical resources, this study

Scherl EJ, Dubinsky MC.
*The Changing World of Inflammatory Bowel Disease:
Impact of Generation, Gender, and Global Trends (pp 79-90)*
© 2009 SLACK Incorporated.

approximates the recent true incidence of pediatric IBD from a large, predominately White North American population. In 2003, the incidence of pediatric CD and UC in Wisconsin was estimated to be 4.56 and 2.14 per 100,000.[1] Northern European population-based incidence rates are similar but notably demonstrate a sharp increase in the incidence of CD over the past decade. Incidence rates for CD described to be approximately 1 to 2 per 100,000 in Sweden, Finland, Norway, and France prior to 1990 have roughly doubled within the last decade.[2-5] Pediatric IBD cases generally represent 5% to 10% of the overall IBD population.[2,6] Thus, extrapolating from a recent estimate of the number of people in the United States with IBD (1.1 million),[7] there are approximately 50,000 to 100,000 pediatric patients with IBD in the United States.

Within this pediatric population, the majority of incident cases occur between the ages of 11 and 17, with 20% of patients being less than 6 and only 5% less than 3.[3,8,9] Incident cases of familial IBD tend to be younger at diagnosis than either parents or grandparents were at the time of their diagnosis, yet differentiating true genetic anticipation from bias such as length of follow-up or recent temporal changes in the risk of IBD has proven difficult.[10] One notable observation is the high frequency of a positive family history in those very young patients (less than 3) diagnosed with UC (44%).[8]

How Does Pediatric Inflammatory Bowel Disease Typically Present?

While not extensively studied, it would appear that pediatric UC tends to present with more extensive colonic disease in children than adults.[11,12] As demonstrated in a prospectively acquired population from northern France, CD presents in a similar fashion in children as in adults with the majority of incident cases being ileocecal with roughly 10% presenting as pure Crohn's colitis and 20% small bowel only.[2] A retrospective analysis from a US tertiary care center suggested that young-onset (<5 years old) CD frequently presents as colitis with significant perianal features,[13] and this observation may explain the high frequency of an initial diagnosis of indeterminate colitis established in both referral center[14] and population-based studies.[3] The majority of these indeterminate cases presenting with linear growth failure ultimately declare themselves as having CD.[13] Growth failure continues to be a major problem in pediatric IBD, affecting adult height in approximately one-third of pediatric-onset patients with CD and one-tenth pediatric-onset patients with UC.[15] The severity of gastrointestinal symptoms is the major factor influencing linear growth,[16] underscoring the importance of understanding the natural history of disease behavior in pediatric-onset IBD.

Over the lifetime of a patient with IBD, the majority of the time is spent in remission; however, long-term remission is very uncommon (<10%), with the majority of patients oscillating between multiple disease activity states (active disease, medically induced remission, or surgically induced remission).[11,17-19] IBD is also an expensive disease to manage with lifetime cost of care estimated for CD to be approximately $125,000 per patient in the United States and for IBD in general to be 1871 Euro (currently $2723 USD) per patient year in 8 European countries and Israel.[18,20] Hospitalizations and surgery account for the majority of the expenses in both the United States and Europe and are typically much higher within the first year of diagnosis.[20]

What Is the Prognosis Specifically Relating to Surgery, Neoplasia, and Mortality?

SURGERY

Using surgical rates as a marker for prognosis, review of the available referral center and population-based data would suggest that pediatric-onset IBD has a similar prognosis as that of adult-onset disease. Surgical rates in patients with pediatric-onset CD have been described from retrospective analyses of referral-based practices to be 17%, 28%, and 69% at 5, 10, and 20 years, respectively.[21,22] Similarly, available population-based analyses describe 5- and 10-year surgical rates to be approximately 33% and 23%, respectively.[9,12] These figures of approximately one-third of pediatric-onset CD patients requiring surgery at 10 years and two-thirds by 20 years are very similar to population-based studies of primarily adult-onset patients. Population-based data of adult patients with CD indicate a 60% to 70% rate of surgery over 20 years.[23-25] Depending upon the type of operation performed, recurrent CD occurs in 25% to 60% of adult patients over 10 years. Total proctocolectomy with end ileostomy leads to the lowest recurrence rates while ileorectostomy leads to the highest.[26,27] Accepting the limitations of the pediatric-specific data (retrospective nature, tertiary referral center bias, and heterogeneity of operations performed), recurrence rates have also been established to be quite high (40% to 50% at 5 years).[28,29]

As pediatric-onset UC appears to present more frequently as extensive disease, one might expect the colectomy rate to be higher than that of the adult-onset population. Retrospective referral-based studies describe more frequent progression of proctosigmoiditis to pancolitis (38%, pediatric onset versus 10%, adult onset)[30,31] and a high rate of colectomy for those moderate to severely affected young-onset patients within 5 years of the diagnosis (26%).[32] Importantly, the population-based data for colectomy rates and UC do not demonstrate significant differences between adult- and pediatric-onset disease. In a study of a population of pediatric-onset UC patients, the 20-year colectomy rate was 29%, which was not significantly different from adult-onset patients.[11,19] Another population-based study, the most recent European assessment of colectomy rates, reported an 8.7% colectomy rate at 10 years, and age at diagnosis was not found to be predictive in this population of over 700 patients across 7 countries.[33] Thus, roughly two-thirds of patients with CD and one-third of patients with UC undergo surgery within 20 years, and the available data do not suggest a different prognosis for patients with pediatric-onset disease.

NEOPLASIA

The risk of colorectal cancer (CRC) is increased among populations of patients with either UC or CD. While CRC among IBD patients accounts for only a small percentage of all CRC cases in the general population, CRC accounts for 1 in 6 deaths among populations of patients with IBD and thus is an important consideration, even among pediatric practitioners.[34,35] Population-based studies from Canada, Israel, and Sweden document an increased relative risk of CRC in patients with UC ranging from 1.4 to 6,[36-39] while population-based data from North America and Denmark demonstrate no differences in CRC rates over the background population.[40,41] It has been suggested that a similar high usage of 5-ASA medication and an active surgical approach to UC in Olmsted County, Minnesota and Copenhagen County, Denmark may affect the low rate of CRC in these populations.

Similar to the data for UC presented previously, there is variation of risk of CRC in populations of patients with CD from no-risk populations in Denmark,[42] Israel,[43] and Sweden[44] to modestly increased (relative risk approximately 2.5) in populations from Canada,[37] Sweden,[45] and Olmsted County.[41] Notably, 2 studies reported an increased risk among patients <30 years at the time of diagnosis.[41,45] While extremely rare, the relative risk of small bowel adenocarcinoma is quite high among patients with CD.[41,42,44]

Additional risk factors for CRC among patients with IBD include a positive family history of CRC,[46] concomitant primary sclerosing cholangitis,[47] and duration of disease.[41] Thus, in the pediatric-onset population, extensive counseling of the risk of CRC should be offered to all patients, with special attention given to those with extensive colonic disease, concomitant primary sclerosing cholangitis, and a family history of CRC.

MORTALITY

Regarding mortality data, it is very difficult to glean from the available population-based studies information unique to pediatric-onset patients. Mortality data are generally presented as a standardized mortality ratio (SMR), which is the ratio of observed deaths in a population (ie, IBD patients) over expected deaths in the background population. A number greater than 1 (ie, 185 deaths/100 deaths = 1.85) means that there were 85% more deaths than expected in the population of interest. It is clear that CD but not UC[48-52] is associated with increased mortality in most populations studied, ranging from rates 20% to 30% higher[51,52] to 70% to 90% higher than the general population.[48,53] It is also clear that an older age at diagnosis rather than younger is significantly associated with mortality,[53] yet this is often the case in mortality studies of any disease. In fact, in the one study large enough to evaluate age of onset in detail, hazard ratios for death were greatest among younger age groups (hazard ratio for death 5.3 among CD patients under 20), yet because these deaths are so uncommon numerically, the absolute risk continues to be highest with advancing age.[48]

Is It Possible to Predict Which Patients Will Experience Aggressive Disease Leading to Complications?

CORTICOSTEROID USAGE

Population-based data demonstrate that the first course of corticosteroids predicts a high rate of surgery (approximately one-third of the patient population) over the subsequent year for both pediatric and adult patients with either CD or UC.[6,54] Corticosteroid usage at disease presentation was again found predictive of complicated CD in a recent study of adults (along with young onset and penetrating disease).[55] Thus, initial disease severity requiring corticosteroid usage should alert the clinician to the possibility of a complicated disease course.

SEROLOGIC MARKERS

Serologic markers to microbial antigen have also been associated with complicated pediatric CD. While cross-sectional, retrospective studies of adult patients with CD have demonstrated an association between serologic responsiveness to microbial antigens and complicated CD (internal penetrating/fibrostenosing),[56-60] the most compelling data are derived from a large prospective study of pediatric CD patients.[61] A study of 4 bacterially associated antigens (anti-I2, anti-outer membrane porin C of Escherichia coli [OmpC], anti-CBir1 flagellin [CBir1], and anti-Saccharomyces cerevisiae antibody [ASCA]) in 196 pediatric patients demonstrated a markedly increased odds ratio (OR,) for developing penetrating or fibrostenosing disease among those patients with serology reactive against 3 (OR, 5.3) and 4 (OR, 11) microbial antigens.[61]

Regarding UC, serologic reactivity to microbial antigens has not yet produced equally strong prognostic data, and indeed, a lack of key antimicrobial antibodies in association with perinuclear antineutrophil cytoplasmic antibodies (pANCA) predicts UC in those indeterminate cases of

IBD.[62-64] The capability of serologic markers to predict chronic pouchitis is the one current exception. In those patients that require colectomy and ileal pouch anal anastomosis (IPAA), high-titer pANCA has been associated with chronic pouchitis in an initial retrospective analysis[65] and then subsequently in a prospective analysis (serum collected prior to IPAA) of adult patients with UC.[66] Responsiveness to microbial antigen has likewise been associated with chronic pouchitis[67] and even fistulizing disease.[68] Discriminating CD of the pouch and chronic pouchitis can be difficult; thus whether pre-IPAA serologic responsiveness to ASCA, OmpC, CBir1,[69] and I2 predicts pouchitis or Crohn's recurrence in the pouch is unclear.

GENOTYPE

Patient genotype may be predictive of a complicated disease course. Variants of the *NOD2* gene have been associated with young-onset CD of the terminal ileum, frequently leading to stricture, surgery, and higher rates of reoperation.[70-74] Polymorphic variation in 2 additional CD susceptibility genes, *OCTN* and *DLG5*, has been associated with penetrating CD in pediatric patients.[75] While the genes involved in the aforementioned immunologic response to microbial antigens have yet to be discovered, a heritable immunophenotype of ASCA and anti-OmpC positivity has been described. Family members of patients with CD demonstrate a significant serologic responsiveness to ASCA and OmpC when compared to healthy controls or family members of patients with UC.[76-78] Of note, limited data suggest that a family history of IBD is not an important factor predictive of disease course.[79]

Thus, a clinical, serologic, and genotypic profile predictive of a pediatric patient at high risk for complicated IBD appears to be emerging. The patient with CD that requires corticosteroids upon presentation, has extensive serologic reactivity to microbial antigen, and is polymorphic for *NOD2* appears to be at highest risk for complicated disease. Accordingly, one may consider early intervention in such patients. The pediatric patient with UC and extensive moderate to severely active disease that requires corticosteroids at presentation likewise appears to be at risk for early surgery. Those patients with colitis and serologic responsiveness to microbial antigens may be at high risk of chronic pouchitis or overt CD of the pouch post-IPAA. Whether early, effective intervention can decrease the frequency of these expected outcomes is the final consideration of this chapter.

Can Early, Effective Therapy Alter an Anticipated Poor Prognosis?

With the advent of biologic therapy for IBD, 2 phrases have emerged in the lexicon of IBD specialists: mucosal healing and step-up versus top-down. "Mucosal healing" rather than symptom control is now the desired outcome of effective medical therapy, and "step-up versus top-down" is an allegorical phrase representing oppositional management strategies of patients with IBD. Step-up refers to a strategy of matching the severity of disease to the intensity of therapy, while top-down refers to the implementation of universal early intensive therapy under the belief that if one effectively heals the mucosa, disease-associated complications (stricture, perforation, neoplasia, etc) will wane, leading to improved function and quality of life. The next 2 sections will present data in support of the step-up strategy followed by those data supporting the top-down approach.

In support of the step-up strategy, clinical experience tells us that not every patient is doomed from diagnosis to suffer an intractable disabling course. Indeed, only 65% of pediatric-onset patients with CD and 44% of patients with UC required corticosteroids in a population-based analysis.[6] Furthermore, no therapy to date (with the exception of a post-hoc analysis of the Accent II data)[80] has been demonstrated to alter the natural history of CD.[81] In a direct comparison of step-up versus top-down therapy of 129 adult patients with CD, no difference in corticosteroid-free clinical remission rates was evident between the 2 groups at 24 months.[82] As not every patient will require thiopurine and/or biologic therapy and newer therapies carry certain definable risks,[83,84] further refinement of outcomes-related research in IBD is required to match the risk of disease progression to the risk of effective therapy.

On the other hand, there are several lines of evidence that the top-down strategy has the potential to alter the natural history of CD but only limited data specific to UC. Further analysis of the aforementioned direct comparison of the step-up versus top-down approach reveals a marked advantage in the frequency of mucosal healing attributable to the top-down approach (73% of patients with complete mucosal healing) when compared to the step-up approach (30%) at 24 months.[82] This finding may be very significant as mucosal healing is a therapeutic endpoint that correlates with reduced hospitalization,[80,85] reduced surgery,[80,85] and improved quality of life[85,86] in studies of adult patients with CD.

Until recently, little data are available with a specific focus on children with IBD, yet these young patients are potentially at highest risk of a disabling course of disease (young onset and frequent steroid use), and thus have the most to gain from a theoretical intervention that alters the predicted natural history. Several studies of pediatric patients indicate that aggressive treatment early in the disease course affects response and remission rates. Thiopurine therapy when instituted at the time of CD diagnosis along with corticosteroids was vastly superior to placebo in achieving long-term, corticosteroid-free remission.[87] Duration of disease was found to be inversely proportional to the length of remission in pediatric patients treated with infliximab.[88] Two recent studies of a prospective pediatric IBD registry depicted the course of IBD in pediatric patients within the first year of corticosteroid usage.[89,90] Upon comparing surgical rates of this newly diagnosed prospective cohort with established natural history data from retrospective population-based analyses, a marked difference in surgical rates is evident. While enrollment specifications and outcome parameter definitions differ, the rate of surgery within 1 year of steroid usage in the registry studies is strikingly low (8% CD, 5% UC)[89,90] when compared to the available adult and pediatric population-based natural history studies (20% to 38% CD, 29% UC).[6,54,91] A major difference between the more recent prospective registry studies[89,90] and the population-based natural history studies[6,54,91] is the infrequent use of immunomodulatory or biologic therapy in the former studies and frequent use in the latter ones. The impact of biologic therapy on disease outcome was addressed directly in the CD study.[89] Thirty of 109 (28%) pediatric patients received infliximab therapy within 1 year of beginning corticosteroids. Among these 30 children, 67% successfully discontinued corticosteroid therapy and only 2 (6.7%) required surgery.

Thus, early intensive therapy appears to result in more frequent mucosal healing, and mucosal healing correlates well with outcome variables commonly used in natural history studies (hospitalization and surgery). Early intensive therapy is associated with a reduction in short-term (1 year) rates of surgery in children. Whether there is long-term benefit to early intensive treatment of inflammatory disease is the crux of the "step-up" versus "top-down" debate and future clinical trial design. The cornerstone of such a clinical trial is to adequately predict those patients at high risk of IBD-related complications, therefore justifying attendant risks of long-term intensive immunotherapy.

Summary

Pediatric IBD is a common disease affecting approximately 50,000 to 100,000 children in the United States. Patients with IBD experience a relapsing and remitting disease course, with fewer than 10% of patients maintaining long-term remission. Those patients with CD that have required corticosteroids for active disease have evidence of immunoreactivity to microbial antigen, and genotypic variation of *NOD2* are more likely to experience an aggressive disease course. Those patients with UC that require corticosteroids are at higher risk of colectomy, and concurrent positive serology for pANCA or microbial antigen places these postcolectomy patients at high risk for chronic pouchitis. Recent data suggest that intensive medical therapy may alter short-term surgical rates, providing optimism that future studies of early immunotherapy will alter the natural history in those patients with poor prognoses.

References

1. Kugathasan S, Judd RH, Hoffmann RG, et al. Epidemiologic and clinical characteristics of children with newly diagnosed inflammatory bowel disease in Wisconsin: a statewide population-based study. *J Pediatr.* 2003;143:525-531.
2. Auvin S, Molinie F, Gower-Rousseau C, et al. Incidence, clinical presentation and location at diagnosis of pediatric inflammatory bowel disease: a prospective population-based study in northern France (1988-1999). *J Pediatr Gastroenterol Nutr.* 2005;41:49-55.
3. Turunen P, Kolho KL, Auvinen A, Iltanen S, Huhtala H, Ashorn M. Incidence of inflammatory bowel disease in Finnish children, 1987-2003. *Inflamm Bowel Dis.* 2006;12:677-683.
4. Hildebrand H, Finkel Y, Grahnquist L, Lindholm J, Ekbom A, Askling J. Changing pattern of paediatric inflammatory bowel disease in northern Stockholm 1990-2001. *Gut.* 2003;52:1432-1434.
5. Perminow G, Frigessi A, Rydning A, Nakstad B, Vatn MH. Incidence and clinical presentation of IBD in children: comparison between prospective and retrospective data in a selected Norwegian population. *Scand J Gastroenterol.* 2006;41:1433-1439.
6. Tung J, Loftus EV Jr, Freese DK, et al. A population-based study of the frequency of corticosteroid resistance and dependence in pediatric patients with Crohn's disease and ulcerative colitis. *Inflamm Bowel Dis.* 2006;12:1093-1100.
7. Loftus CG, Loftus EV Jr, Harmsen WS, et al. Update on the incidence and prevalence of Crohn's disease and ulcerative colitis in Olmsted County, Minnesota, 1940-2000. *Inflamm Bowel Dis.* 2007;13:254-261.
8. Heyman MB, Kirschner BS, Gold BD, et al. Children with early-onset inflammatory bowel disease (IBD): analysis of a pediatric IBD consortium registry. *J Pediatr.* 2005;146:35-40.
9. Lindberg E, Lindquist B, Holmquist L, Hildebrand H. Inflammatory bowel disease in children and adolescents in Sweden, 1984-1995. *J Pediatr Gastroenterol Nutr.* 2000;30:259-264.
10. Faybush EM, Blanchard JF, Rawsthorne P, Bernstein CN. Generational differences in the age at diagnosis with IBD: genetic anticipation, bias, or temporal effects. *Am J Gastroenterol.* 2002;97:636-640.
11. Langholz E, Munkholm P, Krasilnikoff PA, Binder V. Inflammatory bowel diseases with onset in childhood: clinical features, morbidity, and mortality in a regional cohort. *Scand J Gastroenterol.* 1997;32:139-147.
12. Stordal K, Jahnsen J, Bentsen BS, Moum B. Pediatric inflammatory bowel disease in southeastern Norway: a five-year follow-up study. *Digestion.* 2004;70:226-230.
13. Mamula P, Telega GW, Markowitz JE, et al. Inflammatory bowel disease in children 5 years of age and younger. *Am J Gastroenterol.* 2002;97:2005-2010.
14. Carvalho RS, Abadom V, Dilworth HP, Thompson R, Oliva-Hemker M, Cuffari C. Indeterminate colitis: a significant subgroup of pediatric IBD. *Inflamm Bowel Dis.* 2006;12:258-262.
15. Markowitz J, Grancher K, Rosa J, Aiges H, Daum F. Growth failure in pediatric inflammatory bowel disease. *J Pediatr Gastroenterol Nutr.* 1993;16:373-380.
16. Griffiths AM, Nguyen P, Smith C, MacMillan JH, Sherman PM. Growth and clinical course of children with Crohn's disease. *Gut.* 1993;34:939-943.
17. Munkholm P, Langholz E, Davidsen M, Binder V. Disease activity courses in a regional cohort of Crohn's disease patients. *Scand J Gastroenterol.* 1995;30:699-706.
18. Silverstein MD, Loftus EV, Sandborn WJ, et al. Clinical course and costs of care for Crohn's disease: Markov model analysis of a population-based cohort. *Gastroenterology.* 1999;117:49-57.
19. Langholz E, Munkholm P, Davidsen M, Binder V. Course of ulcerative colitis: analysis of changes in disease activity over years. *Gastroenterology.* 1994;107:3-11.
20. Odes S, Vardi H, Friger M, et al. Cost analysis and cost determinants in a European inflammatory bowel disease inception cohort with 10 years of follow-up evaluation. *Gastroenterology.* 2006;131:719-728.
21. Farmer RG, Michener WM. Prognosis of Crohn's disease with onset in childhood or adolescence. *Dig Dis Sci.* 1979;24:752-757.
22. Gupta N, Cohen SA, Bostrom AG, et al. Risk factors for initial surgery in pediatric patients with Crohn's disease. *Gastroenterology.* 2006;130:1069-1077.
23. Dhillon S, Loftus Jr EV, Tremaine W, et al. The natural history of surgery for Crohn's disease in a population-based cohort from Olmsted County, Minnesota. *Am J Gastroenterol.* 2005;100:S305.
24. Binder V, Hendriksen C, Kreiner S. Prognosis in Crohn's disease—based on results from a regional patient group from the county of Copenhagen. *Gut.* 1985;26:146-150.

25. Munkholm P, Langholz E, Davidsen M, Binder V. Intestinal cancer risk and mortality in patients with Crohn's disease. *Gastroenterology.* 1993;105:1716-1723.

26. Bernell O, Lapidus A, Hellers G. Risk factors for surgery and postoperative recurrence in Crohn's disease. *Ann Surg.* 2000;231:38-45.

27. Bernell O, Lapidus A, Hellers G. Recurrence after colectomy in Crohn's colitis. *Dis Colon Rectum.* 2001;44:647-654.

28. Hyams JS, Grand RJ, Colodny AH, Schuster SR, Eraklis A. Course and prognosis after colectomy and ileostomy for inflammatory bowel disease in childhood and adolescence. *J Pediatr Surg.* 1982;17:400-405.

29. Griffiths AM, Wesson DE, Shandling B, Corey M, Sherman PM. Factors influencing postoperative recurrence of Crohn's disease in childhood. *Gut.* 1991;32:491-495.

30. Mir-Madjlessi SH, Michener WM, Farmer RG. Course and prognosis of idiopathic ulcerative proctosigmoiditis in young patients. *J Pediatr Gastroenterol Nutr.* 1986;5:571-575.

31. Henriksen M, Jahnsen J, Lygren I, et al. Ulcerative colitis and clinical course: results of a 5-year population-based follow-up study (the IBSEN study). *Inflamm Bowel Dis.* 2006;12:543-550.

32. Hyams JS, Davis P, Grancher K, Lerer T, Justinich CJ, Markowitz J. Clinical outcome of ulcerative colitis in children. *J Pediatr.* 1996;129:81-88.

33. Hoie O, Wolters FL, Riis L, et al. Low colectomy rates in ulcerative colitis in an unselected European cohort followed for 10 years. *Gastroenterology.* 2007;132:507-515.

34. Lennard-Jones JE. Cancer risk in ulcerative colitis: surveillance or surgery. *Br J Surg.* 1985;72:S84-S86.

35. Choi PM, Zelig MP. Similarity of colorectal cancer in Crohn's disease and ulcerative colitis: implications for carcinogenesis and prevention. *Gut.* 1994;35:950-954.

36. Karlen P, Lofberg R, Brostrom O, Leijonmarck CE, Hellers G, Persson PG. Increased risk of cancer in ulcerative colitis: a population-based cohort study. *Am J Gastroenterol.* 1999;94:1047-1052.

37. Bernstein CN, Blanchard JF, Kliewer E, Wajda A. Cancer risk in patients with inflammatory bowel disease: a population-based study. *Cancer.* 2001;91:854-862.

38. Gilat T, Fireman Z, Grossman A, et al. Colorectal cancer in patients with ulcerative colitis: a population study in central Israel. *Gastroenterology.* 1988;94:870-877.

39. Ekbom A, Helmick C, Zack M, Adami HO. Ulcerative colitis and colorectal cancer: a population-based study. *N Engl J Med.* 1990;323:1228-1233.

40. Winther KV, Jess T, Langholz E, Munkholm P, Binder V. Long-term risk of cancer in ulcerative colitis: a population-based cohort study from Copenhagen County. *Clin Gastroenterol Hepatol.* 2004;2:1088-1095.

41. Jess T, Loftus EV Jr, Velayos FS, et al. Risk of intestinal cancer in inflammatory bowel disease: a population-based study from olmsted county, Minnesota. *Gastroenterology.* 2006;130:1039-1046.

42. Jess T, Winther KV, Munkholm P, Langholz E, Binder V. Intestinal and extra-intestinal cancer in Crohn's disease: follow-up of a population-based cohort in Copenhagen County, Denmark. *Aliment Pharmacol Ther.* 2004;19:287-293.

43. Fireman Z, Grossman A, Lilos P, et al. Intestinal cancer in patients with Crohn's disease: a population study in central Israel. *Scand J Gastroenterol.* 1989;24:346-350.

44. Persson PG, Karlen P, Bernell O, et al. Crohn's disease and cancer: a population-based cohort study. *Gastroenterology.* 1994;107:1675-1679.

45. Ekbom A, Helmick C, Zack M, Adami HO. Increased risk of large-bowel cancer in Crohn's disease with colonic involvement. *Lancet.* 1990;336:357-359.

46. Askling J, Dickman PW, Karlen P, et al. Family history as a risk factor for colorectal cancer in inflammatory bowel disease. *Gastroenterology.* 2001;120:1356-1362.

47. Brentnall TA, Haggitt RC, Rabinovitch PS, et al. Risk and natural history of colonic neoplasia in patients with primary sclerosing cholangitis and ulcerative colitis. *Gastroenterology.* 1996;110:331-338.

48. Card T, Hubbard R, Logan RF. Mortality in inflammatory bowel disease: a population-based cohort study. *Gastroenterology.* 2003;125:1583-1590.

49. Hoie O, Schouten LJ, Wolters FL, et al. Ulcerative colitis: no rise in mortality in a European-wide population based cohort 10 years after diagnosis. *Gut.* 2007;56:497-503.

50. Winther KV, Jess T, Langholz E, Munkholm P, Binder V. Survival and cause-specific mortality in ulcerative colitis: follow-up of a population-based cohort in Copenhagen County. *Gastroenterology.* 2003;125:1576-1582.

51. Jess T, Loftus EV Jr, Velayos FS, et al. Risk factors for colorectal neoplasia in inflammatory bowel disease: a nested case-control study from Copenhagen county, Denmark and Olmsted county, Minnesota. *Am J Gastroenterol.* 2007;102:829-836.

52. Jess T, Loftus EV Jr, Harmsen WS, et al. Survival and cause-specific mortality in patients with inflammatory bowel disease: a long-term outcome study in Olmsted County, Minnesota, 1940-2004. *Gut.* 2006;55(9):1248-1254

53. Wolters FL, Russel MG, Sijbrandij J, et al. Crohn's disease: increased mortality 10 years after diagnosis in a Europe-wide population based cohort. *Gut.* 2006;55:510-518.

54. Faubion WA Jr, Loftus EV Jr, Harmsen WS, Zinsmeister AR, Sandborn WJ. The natural history of corticosteroid therapy for inflammatory bowel disease: a population-based study. *Gastroenterology.* 2001;121:255-260.

55. Beaugerie L, Seksik P, Nion-Larmurier I, Gendre JP, Cosnes J. Predictors of Crohn's disease. *Gastroenterology.* 2006;130:650-656.

56. Desir B, Amre DK, Lu SE, et al. Utility of serum antibodies in determining clinical course in pediatric Crohn's disease. *Clin Gastroenterol Hepatol.* 2004;2:139-146.

57. Arnott ID, Landers CJ, Nimmo EJ, et al. Sero-reactivity to microbial components in Crohn's disease is associated with disease severity and progression, but not NOD2/CARD15 genotype. *Am J Gastroenterol.* 2004;99:2376-2384.

58. Mow WS, Vasiliauskas EA, Lin YC, et al. Association of antibody responses to microbial antigens and complications of small bowel Crohn's disease. *Gastroenterology.* 2004;126:414-424.

59. Landers CJ, Cohavy O, Misra R, et al. Selected loss of tolerance evidenced by Crohn's disease-associated immune responses to auto- and microbial antigens. *Gastroenterology.* 2002;123:689-699.

60. Forcione DG, Rosen MJ, Kisiel JB, Sands BE. Anti-*Saccharomyces cerevisiae* antibody (ASCA) positivity is associated with increased risk for early surgery in Crohn's disease. *Gut.* 2004;53:1117-1122.

61. Dubinsky MC, Lin YC, Dutridge D, et al. Serum immune responses predict rapid disease progression among children with Crohn's disease: immune responses predict disease progression. *Am J Gastroenterol.* 2006;101:360-367.

62. Sandborn WJ, Loftus EV Jr, Colombel JF, et al. Evaluation of serologic disease markers in a population-based cohort of patients with ulcerative colitis and Crohn's disease. *Inflamm Bowel Dis.* 2001;7:192-201.

63. Joossens S, Reinisch W, Vermeire S, et al. The value of serologic markers in indeterminate colitis: a prospective follow-up study. *Gastroenterology.* 2002;122:1242-1247.

64. Zholudev A, Zurakowski D, Young W, Leichtner A, Bousvaros A. Serologic testing with ANCA, ASCA, and anti-OmpC in children and young adults with Crohn's disease and ulcerative colitis: diagnostic value and correlation with disease phenotype. *Am J Gastroenterol.* 2004;99:2235-2241.

65. Sandborn WJ, Landers CJ, Tremaine WJ, Targan SR. Antineutrophil cytoplasmic antibody correlates with chronic pouchitis after ileal pouch-anal anastomosis. *Am J Gastroenterol.* 1995;90:740-747.

66. Fleshner PR, Vasiliauskas EA, Kam LY, et al. High level perinuclear antineutrophil cytoplasmic antibody (pANCA) in ulcerative colitis patients before colectomy predicts the development of chronic pouchitis after ileal pouch-anal anastomosis. *Gut.* 2001;49:671-677.

67. Hui T, Landers C, Vasiliauskas E, et al. Serologic responses in indeterminate colitis patients before ileal pouch-anal anastomosis may determine those at risk for continuous pouch inflammation. *Dis Colon Rectum.* 2005;48:1254-1262.

68. Dendrinos KG, Becker JM, Stucchi AF, Saubermann LJ, LaMorte W, Farraye FA. Anti-*Saccharomyces cerevisiae* antibodies are associated with the development of postoperative fistulas following ileal pouch-anal anastomosis. *J Gastrointest Surg.* 2006;10:1060-1064.

69. Fleshner NE, Vasiliauskas E, Dubinsky M, et al. Both Preoperative pANCA and CBIR1 flagellin expression in ulcerative colitis (UC) patients influence pouchitis development after ileal pouch-anal anastomosis (IPAA). *Gastroenterology.* 2006;130:A130.

70. Abreu MT, Taylor KD, Lin YC, et al. Mutations in NOD2 are associated with fibrostenosing disease in patients with Crohn's disease. *Gastroenterology.* 2002;123:679-688.

71. Cuthbert AP, Fisher SA, Mirza MM, et al. The contribution of NOD2 gene mutations to the risk and site of disease in inflammatory bowel disease. *Gastroenterology.* 2002;122:867-874.

72. Annese V, Lombardi G, Perri F, et al. Variants of CARD15 are associated with an aggressive clinical course of Crohn's disease: an IG-IBD study. *Am J Gastroenterol.* 2005;100:84-92.

73. Helio T, Halme L, Lappalainen M, et al. CARD15/NOD2 gene variants are associated with familially occurring and complicated forms of Crohn's disease. *Gut.* 2003;52:558-562.

74. Buning C, Genschel J, Buhner S, et al. Mutations in the NOD2/CARD15 gene in Crohn's disease are associated with ileocecal resection and are a risk factor for reoperation. *Aliment Pharmacol Ther.* 2004;19:1073-1078.

75. Latiano A, Cucchiara S, Vieni G, et al. Genotype/phenotype analysis of a panel of genes in pediatric patients with IBD: a study of the Italian society for pediatric gastroenterology (SIGENP). *Gastroenterology.* 2006;130:A350.

76. Mei L, Targan SR, Landers CJ, et al. Familial expression of anti-*Escherichia coli* outer membrane porin C in relatives of patients with Crohn's disease. *Gastroenterology.* 2006;130:1078-1085.

77. Aisenberg J, Legnani PE, Nilubol N, et al. Are pANCA, ASCA, or cytokine gene polymorphisms associated with pouchitis? Long-term follow-up in 102 ulcerative colitis patients. *Am J Gastroenterol.* 2004;99:432-441.

78. Annese V, Andreoli A, Andriulli A, et al. Familial expression of anti-*Saccharomyces cerevisiae* Mannan antibodies in Crohn's disease and ulcerative colitis: a GISC study. *Am J Gastroenterol.* 2001;96:2407-2412.

79. Henriksen M, Jahnsen J, Lygren I, Vatn MH, Moum B. Are there any differences in phenotype or disease course between familial and sporadic cases of inflammatory bowel disease? Results of a population-based follow-up study. *Am J Gastroenterol.* 2007;102:1955-1963.

80. Lichtenstein GR, Yan S, Bala M, Blank M, Sands BE. Infliximab maintenance treatment reduces hospitalizations, surgeries, and procedures in fistulizing Crohn's disease. *Gastroenterology.* 2005;128:862-869.

81. Cosnes J, Cattan S, Blain A, et al. Long-term evolution of disease behavior of Crohn's disease. *Inflamm Bowel Dis.* 2002;8:244-250.

82. Hommes DW, Baert F, Van Assche G, et al. A randomized controlled trial evaluating the ideal medical management for Crohn's disease (CD): top-down versus step-up strategies. *Gastroenterology.* 2005;128:A577.

83. Sandborn WJ, Colombel JF, Enns R, et al. Natalizumab induction and maintenance therapy for Crohn's disease. *N Engl J Med.* 2005;353:1912-1925.

84. Ricart E, Panaccione R, Loftus EV, Tremaine WJ, Sandborn WJ. Infliximab for Crohn's disease in clinical practice at the Mayo Clinic: the first 100 patients. *Am J Gastroenterol.* 2001;96:722-729.

85. Lichtenstein GR, Yan S, Bala M, Hanauer S. Remission in patients with Crohn's disease is associated with improvement in employment and quality of life and a decrease in hospitalizations and surgeries. *Am J Gastroenterol.* 2004;99:91-96.

86. Feagan BG, Yan S, Bala M, Bao W, Lichtenstein GR. The effects of infliximab maintenance therapy on health-related quality of life. *Am J Gastroenterol.* 2003;98:2232-2238.

87. Markowitz J, Grancher K, Kohn N, Lesser M, Daum F. A multicenter trial of 6-mercaptopurine and prednisone in children with newly diagnosed Crohn's disease. *Gastroenterology.* 2000;119:895-902.

88. Kugathasan S, Werlin SL, Martinez A, Rivera MT, Heikenen JB, Binion DG. Prolonged duration of response to infliximab in early but not late pediatric Crohn's disease. *Am J Gastroenterol.* 2000;95:3189-3194.

89. Markowitz J, Hyams J, Mack D, et al. Corticosteroid therapy in the age of infliximab: acute and 1-year outcomes in newly diagnosed children with Crohn's disease. *Clin Gastroenterol Hepatol.* 2006;4:1124-1129.

90. Hyams J, Markowitz J, Lerer T, et al. The natural history of corticosteroid therapy for ulcerative colitis in children. *Clin Gastroenterol Hepatol.* 2006;4:1118-1123.

91. Munkholm P, Langholz E, Davidsen M, Binder V. Frequency of glucocorticoid resistance and dependency in Crohn's disease. *Gut.* 1994;35:360-362.

Financial disclosure: Dr. Faubion is principal investigator on active research protocols for Centocor and Abbott and serves as a consultant for Takeda Pharmaceuticals.

MEDICATION RESPONSIVENESS IN CHILDREN

Michael C. Stephens, MD, FAAP

The commonly uttered cliché that "children are not little adults" is perhaps most relevant when considering drug therapy. A tragic and striking example of this is the grey baby syndrome resulting from administration of chloramphenicol to infants.[1] Babies receiving this drug developed emesis, abdominal distention, cardiovascular collapse, and death. This outcome was the result of an immature conjugating system that reduced clearance and elimination. During growth and development, significant changes in body composition occur, which impact drug disposition. This includes changes in the relative size of fluid compartments, organs, and the expression of drug-metabolizing enzymes (DME) and other determinants of drug disposition. The results of these differences lead to differences in the pharmacokinetic and pharmacodynamic profiles of drugs in children. Because of the dynamic nature of these developmental changes, and the differences in substrate specificity of each factor, generalization across multiple drugs (even within the same class) is rarely possible. This illustrates the importance of conducting clinical drug trials in children and the pitfalls of attempting to apply adult experience to pediatric therapy. This chapter will outline key differences in disease behavior and responsiveness in children with inflammatory bowel disease (IBD). In most cases, the physiologic or pathophysiologic etiology of these differences is not well understood. A discussion of key concepts of the impact of human development on drug disposition will highlight the challenges in establishing safe and efficacious therapies for pediatric patients.

Differences in Disease Behavior and Corticosteroid Responsiveness

Differences exist in disease distribution, extent, and severity at diagnosis between adults and children with IBD. In Crohn's disease (CD), a higher rate of colonic involvement has been reported in children (two-thirds have colonic involvement with 20% to 30% of adults having only

Scherl EJ, Dubinsky MC.
*The Changing World of Inflammatory Bowel Disease:
Impact of Generation, Gender, and Global Trends (pp 91-100)*
© 2009 SLACK Incorporated.

colonic disease).[2] Younger patients with ulcerative colitis (UC) consistently have more extensive and severe disease. Eighty percent to 90% of pediatric patients have pancolitis at presentation.[2,3] Pancolitis is present in up to 60% of adults at diagnosis of UC.[4] Mucosal differences have also been demonstrated between adult and pediatric UC.[5-7] In contrast to the increased extent of involvement, these histologic differences include lesser degrees of inflammation, including architectural distortion and rectal sparing in pediatric UC.

Differences seen between adult- and childhood-onset disease behavior are reflected in corticosteroid (CS) responsiveness. An excellent point of reference for adult disease behavior is found in a study of 1-year outcomes in all patients with CD and UC in Olmsted County.[4] The short-term response rates to CS were 58% complete remission, 26% partial response, and 16% with no response in adults with CD. At 1 year, the rates were 32% sustained remission, 28% steroid dependence, and 38% required surgery. For UC, the short-term rates were 54% complete remission, 30% partial remission, and 16% nonresponders. At 1 year for UC, there was a prolonged response in 49%, CS dependence in 22%, and surgery was required in 29%. Importantly, the vast majority of patients did not receive immunomodulators (100% UC and 97% CD), and these data were collected in a prebiologic era.

Tung et al have published pediatric data from Olmsted County that included 50 patients with CD and 36 with UC.[8] A higher rate of CS use was seen in this cohort in comparison to adults. Sixty-five percent of patients with CD and 44% of patients with UC required CS in comparison to 43% and 34%, respectively, in the adult study. The short- and long-term CS response rates were similar to adults. In CD at 1 year, 46% had prolonged response, 31% were steroid dependent, and 27% had surgery. In UC at 1 year, 57% had prolonged response, 14% were CS dependent, and the surgery rate was 29%. Usage of immunomodulators was also low (7% in UC and 23% in CD). While increased requirement for CS suggests more severe disease in pediatric IBD, other explanations include differences in management practices between pediatric and adult gastroenterologists. Larger pediatric inception cohort studies have identified more significant differences in pediatric IBD.

A multi-center prospective inception cohort study of 97 children with UC demonstrated more severe disease in children.[3] As previously discussed, more extensive disease was noted at presentation, and a higher percentage of patients required CS therapy (79% versus 34% of adults in the Olmsted County study). The short-term response rate was similar to adults with 60% complete remission and 27% partial responders. However, 45% of children with UC were CS dependent at 1 year (versus 22% in adults). Important differences must be noted when comparing pediatric data to the adult data. A stricter definition was used for CS dependency and there was a lower rate of colectomy (4%). Conversely, 61% of the pediatric patients received immunomodulators and 12% received infliximab. Despite more aggressive therapy, there was a higher rate of CS dependency. This presents an overall picture of more extensive and refractory disease in childhood UC but also less need for surgery.

The same multi-center pediatric consortium has completed a similar inception to 1-year study in 109 children with moderate to severe CD.[9] The short-term response to steroids was nearly identical to the adult study; however, the long-term data identified key differences. A lower surgical rate was seen (8% versus 38% in adults). In an era with common use of immunomodulators and availability of infliximab, the 1-year response rate (sustained response off CS) was 61%. Infliximab use was a key factor in the higher response rate. One-fourth of these responders required infliximab, meaning only 46% of the overall group had a prolonged response and was not receiving CS or infliximab at 1 year. In comparison to the adult response rate of 32%, a modest improvement might be inferred from the use of immunomodulators. Eighty-one percent of the total cohort received immunomodulators (69% started within the first 4 months). Early use of immunomodulators is of well-known benefit in pediatric CD. In the landmark study by Markowitz et al, 27 patients received CS and 6-mercaptopurine at diagnosis and were compared with 28 patients who received CS and placebo.[10] After 18 months and a standardized protocol to withdraw CS,

91% of patients in the treatment group had sustained remission without CS. In the placebo group, only 50% had sustained remission and were independent of CS. The rate in the placebo group is higher than what is reported in adults, but the study was not designed and powered to address the question of CS responsiveness.

Infliximab

Infliximab is a monoclonal antibody to tumor necrosis factor alpha (TNF-α) and was the first biologic therapy approved for IBD. Consistently, a higher response rate has been seen in children versus adults. In the seminal adult study (Accent I), 48% of patients had response to infliximab at the end of 1 year of therapy for luminal CD.[11] In Accent II, which studied fistulizing disease in adults, the 54-week response rate was 46%.[12] The response rates have been much higher in pediatric studies. The REACH study, a prospective multi-center study of the efficacy and safety of infliximab in pediatric CD,[13] yielded response and remission rates of 64% and 56%, respectively, at week 54 for children on the same dosing schedule as Accent I and II. The initial response rates at week 10 were also higher for children: 88% responding and 59% in remission versus 69% responders in Accent II following the induction series of 3 doses. It should be noted that nearly all patients in REACH were on concomitant immunomodulators while only a minority of patients were in Accent I and II.

Early pediatric data suggest improved response with earlier use of infliximab. A prospective and smaller study (n = 15) by Kugathasan et al found improved response in children with early disease (within 2 years of diagnosis).[14] Specifically, patients with early disease were more likely to maintain remission with maintenance infusions following induction versus those with disease of longer duration. A retrospective study also found an improved rate of response in early CD (using a 1-year disease duration cut-off).[15] In contrast to this, the REACH data did not find a difference in response between early and late CD (1-year disease duration cut-off), suggesting that children in general have an improved response profile with infliximab. Adult data have also found improved response in early disease. For example, improved response and remission rates were seen in adults with early disease in the Precise 2 study of certolizumab (a humanized pegylated anti-TNF monoclonal antibody).[16] Response rates were 82% for patients with disease duration less than 2 years and 58.5% for greater than 2 years. Additionally, the response rate increased to 87% for patients younger than 36 years of age with early disease. Although improved response in children may be related to disease duration, the overall improved response rate may suggest differences between pediatric disease and adult disease. A clear pattern of immune senescence[17] is recognized in humans, which must be considered.

Understanding the mechanisms that impact response to therapy early in the course of IBD and in children can drive the development of improved therapeutic strategies. Many developmental and physiologic changes in human development can impact drug disposition and must be considered when treating pediatric patients.

Body Composition

Changes in body composition during human development can have an important impact on drug disposition and response. The relative amount and distribution of total body water (TBW) is a key factor in the volume of distribution of many drugs and varies through human development.[18,19] In infancy, TBW represents 75% of total body mass (and is even higher in preterm infants [92%]). This decreases to roughly 60% by 6 months of life and then remains stable. The distribution of TBW also varies with age and impacts compartment modeling for pharmacokinetics. The fraction of TBW that represents extracellular fluid (ECF) also decreases throughout

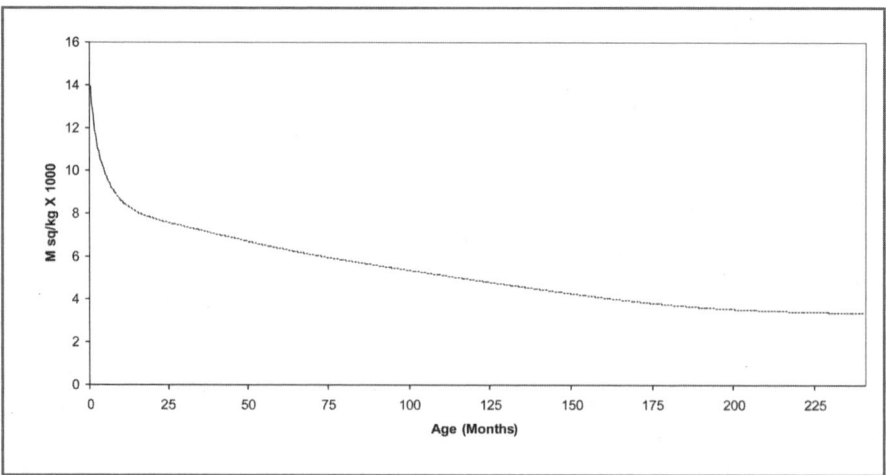

Figure 7-1. The ratio of BSA to weight (sq m/kg) is plotted versus age in months. Data taken from CDC 2000 growth charts (http://www.cdc.gov/growthcharts). The 50th percentile weight and height (Z = 0) were taken for each age and BSA calculated using the following formula: BSA = (Wt0.51456) x (Ht0.0235) x 0.0235.

development. Premature infants' ECF can represent as much as 50% TBW, is 45% at term, 28% at 1 year, and 20% in adults. Conversely, intracellular fluid increases throughout development. This leads to an increased volume of distribution for hydrophilic compounds.

Another important component of body composition that can impact drug distribution is the percentage of fat relative to total body mass. Fat content increases during the first year of life from 12% to 30%. This slowly decreases through adolescence. Puberty can also impact body fat composition differently between males and females.[20] Percent fat content significantly impacts the volume of distribution of lipophilic drugs, most notably many sedative hypnotics and inhalational anesthetics.

Body surface area (BSA) relative to weight is much higher in infancy than adulthood. Figure 7-1 demonstrates this trend. Because of this difference in proportion, extrapolation of adult doses to pediatric patients can yield very different results if BSA is used rather than mass, which increases in younger patients. This can become very significant when comparing BSA-based dosing versus weight-based dosing. In a 12 year old (assuming 50th percentile weight and height), a BSA-based dose extrapolated from adult dosing would be 20% higher versus weight-based dosing. This difference increases to 70% in a 2 year old. Most pediatric drugs used for IBD are dosed based on weight while BSA-based dosing is more commonly used in pediatric oncology. The rationale for using BSA-based dosing in children has included the increased volume of distribution often seen because of differences in TBW and its distribution (discussed previously), and increased clearance relative to body mass. As an example, early pediatric studies using high-dose busulfan chemotherapy utilized mg-per-kg doses extrapolated from adult standards. However, pharmacokinetic studies demonstrated increased clearance in children (8.4 mL/min/kg age less than 4 years, 4.4 mL/min/kg older children, and 2.5 mL/min/kg adults) and lower overall exposure to the drug.[21] When larger doses based on BSA were utilized, the total drug exposure increased and mirrored adult profiles.[22]

Liver and kidney sizes relative to total body mass also change during growth. The liver is relatively large in an infant (35 mL/kg body mass) and slowly becomes smaller during growth when normalized to patient weight.[23,24] Interestingly, this trend is not seen when liver size is normalized to BSA rather than weight. Differences in hepatic clearance with age may relate to the mechanism of hepatic clearance. A significant difference has been demonstrated with antipyrine (phase 2) but not indocyanine green (biliary secretion) and lorazepam (phase 1).[23] Other factors that must be considered include the substrate specificity of DME, that substrates are frequently metabolized by multiple DME, and the ontogeny of DME (discussed below). Thus, changes in clearance with age must be considered for each individual substrate.

Relative renal size and function also vary with age (reviewed in detail by Alcorn and McNamara[25]). The majority of this development occurs during infancy. At birth, glomerular filtration rate (GFR), tubular function, and transport function are very low but increase rapidly. This approaches adult levels (normalized to BSA) by 6 to 8 months of life. GFR continues to increase and exceeds adult levels in the first 12 years of life.[26] Tubular clearance beyond the newborn period also exceeds relative adult levels, declining during adolescence and correlating with pubertal development.[27]

Absorption

Other physiological changes associated with human development can impact drug disposition. The skin serves as a barrier to xenobiotics and is an increasingly used route of administration. Development of the primary barrier (the stratum corneum) is complete by 34 weeks gestation; however, it does not reach mature thickness until 4 months of age.[28] The result is increased permeability and increased insensible losses in younger (and especially preterm) infants.[29] Many examples of misadventure with either intentional or unintentional exposure to agents absorbed across the skin barrier exist from hospital nurseries. Increased theophylline absorption has been associated with increased skin permeability in infants.[30,31] Other examples include inadvertent exposure and toxicity from inactive ingredients in topical medication preparations (eg, propylene glycol[32]) or topical antiseptics (eg, hexachlorophene[33]).

Intestinal absorption can be altered by changes in gastric pH during development. Infants have a higher gastric pH, which can reduce the bioavailability of weakly acidic drugs. Other changes in gastrointestinal function include expression of phase 1 and 2 enzymes that impact first pass metabolism, bile acid secretion and absorption, motility, and secretion of digestive enzymes. These developmental differences are reviewed in detail by Kearns et al.[34] Much of this occurs during the first year of life, but gastric acid secretion can remain relatively low until 12 years of age. An example of the impact of gastric pH on absorption is the increased bioavailability of oral penicillin G in infants.[35]

Distribution

Protein binding is an important factor in the distribution of drugs. Infants have lower serum concentrations of key drug-binding proteins. At birth, albumin concentrations are 75% adult levels and alpha 1-acid glycoprotein is around 50%.[36] These concentrations slowly increase to adult levels by the early teens. This can be further compounded by the fact that neonates have lower blood pH since this impacts the fraction of protein-bound drug.[37,38] Other physiologic factors are important in younger patients. Bilirubin is frequently elevated in infancy and can compete with drugs for binding sites on albumin. As an example, sulfonamides administered to infants can displace albumin-bound bilirubin, leading to kernicterus.[39] Changes in protein binding of drugs as a result of physiological changes during human development affect a wide range of agents, many of which have significant side effects. For example, the free fraction of circulating fentanyl in an infant is double that of an adult (30% versus 16%).[36]

Metabolism and Elimination

Ontogeny refers to the study of the development of an organism. Changes in the expression of determinants of drug disposition (eg, DME, drug transporters, receptors) through human development play an important role in explaining differences in drug response in children. Although much of the early work in this field has focused on DME, all components of drug disposition must be considered. Several common patterns of expression have been noted.

Many DME are expressed at low levels during fetal development, begin to be expressed in the neonatal period, and reach adult levels within 1 to 2 years. The example of grey baby syndrome follows this pattern and is the result of immature uridine 5'-diphospho (UDP)-glucuronosyltransferase activity.[1] Another example is flavin-containing monooxygenase 3 (FMO3), which is the only known DME of ranitidine. Fetal expression is extremely low, begins to rise after birth, and does not reach adult levels until after 11 years of age.[40]

Another pattern in the developmental expression of DME involves transitioning from one predominant form during fetal development to another following parturition. Cytochrome P450 3A7 (CYP3A7) is the predominant CYP3A enzyme expressed in the fetal liver. This expression falls following delivery and there is an increase in CYP3A4 with CYP3A7 remaining the predominant enzyme until after the first year of life when CYP3A4 approaches adult levels (reviewed in detail by Hines[41]). The clinical significance of this transition is illustrated in the experience with cisapride. Cisapride is metabolized by CYP3A4 but not CYP3A7.[42] In vitro and in vivo kinetic studies have demonstrated a deficient metabolic activity in infants.[43,44] Reduced metabolism was also associated with increased side effects (prolongation of the QTc interval) in infants and was more pronounced in premature infants.[45] Marketing of cisapride in the United States was ultimately suspended primarily related to issues of cardiac toxicity.

Increased expression is also seen in children. Pediatric patients have an increased rate of sulfate conjugation early in life, which provides protection from acetaminophen toxicity.[46] Another example is thiopurine methyltransferase, which is a key enzyme in mercaptopurine and azathioprine metabolism. Activity in neonates exceeds adult levels by 1.5 fold.[47,48]

Currently, more is understood about the ontogeny of DME than most other determinants of drug distribution. Drug transporters such as P-glycoprotein (PGP) can impact elimination at the level of the renal tubule and bile duct and also distribution since it is expressed in the blood brain barrier.[49] PGP substrates include CSs, cyclosporine, tacrolimus, ondansetron, ranitidine, digoxin, erythromycin, and many other drugs. There are limited data regarding the ontogeny of PGP available.[50] Functional data suggest a direct relationship between age and function in human T lymphocytes but not B lymphocytes.[51] Whether other differences in expression related to age and location exist remains to be seen, as does any clinical significance.

Response/Pharmacodynamics

Changes in human development may also alter the pharmacodynamics of therapies. An important example of differences in drug effect in younger patients is warfarin. Takahashi et al have demonstrated that prepubertal and pubertal patients are 25% and 19% more sensitive than adult patients using mean international normalized ratio normalized to plasma drug concentrations.[52] Marshall and Kearns have demonstrated that the cyclosporine concentration at which 50% maximal effect and 90% maximal effect occur is 2 and 7 fold lower in infants, respectively, versus older age groups.[53] Increased responsiveness is not the only trend for age-related effects on cyclosporine. Differences are also seen in bioavailability and clearance, which impact cyclosporine dosing in children.[54] This highlights the fact that multiple developmental factors impact pediatric drug disposition, making extrapolation from adult data inadequate and often inappropriate.

Summary

The impact of developmental changes during growth (including body composition, physiological changes, and differences in expression of various proteins) creates significant differences in response to drugs in pediatric patients. Each factor can have substrate-specific impacts that make generalized inferences from adult experience inadequate in pediatric pharmacotherapy. Multiple models have attempted to incorporate what is known about these developmental factors to estimate pediatric dosing strategies.[36,55] However, a significant knowledge gap remains, and these models do not obviate the need for pediatric pharmacokinetic and pharmacodynamic studies. Historically, few drugs have received significant pediatric study before being used in infants and children. Recent legislative efforts in the United States (1997 FDA Modernization Act, 2002 Best Pharmaceuticals for Children Act, 2007 FDA Revitalization Act) and Europe (Regulation EC 1901/2006) have sought to improve this situation. Increased inclusion of pediatric patients in clinical trials, combined with further understanding of the ontogeny of all determinants of drug disposition, will help improve the efficacy and safety of the medications given to children.

References

1. Weiss CF, Glazko AJ, Weston JK. Chloramphenicol in the newborn infant: a physiologic explanation of its toxicity when given in excessive doses. *N Engl J Med.* 1960;262:787-794.
2. Kugathasan S, Judd RH, Hoffmann RG, et al. Epidemiologic and clinical characteristics of children with newly diagnosed inflammatory bowel disease in Wisconsin: a statewide population-based study. *J Pediatr.* 2003;143(4):525-531.
3. Hyams J, Markowitz J, Lerer T, et al. The natural history of corticosteroid therapy for ulcerative colitis in children. *Clin Gastroenterol Hepatol.* 2006;4(9):1118-1123.
4. Faubion WA Jr, Loftus EV Jr, Harmsen WS, Zinsmeister AR, Sandborn WJ. The natural history of corticosteroid therapy for inflammatory bowel disease: a population-based study. *Gastroenterology.* 2001;121(2):255-260.
5. Markowitz J, Kahn E, Grancher K, Hyams J, Treem W, Daum F. Atypical rectosigmoid histology in children with newly diagnosed ulcerative colitis. *Am J Gastroenterol.* 1993;88(12):2034-2037.
6. Robert ME, Tang L, Hao LM, Reyes-Mugica M. Patterns of inflammation in mucosal biopsies of ulcerative colitis: perceived differences in pediatric populations are limited to children younger than 10 years. *Am J Surg Pathol.* 2004;28(2):183-189.
7. Washington K, Greenson JK, Montgomery E, et al. Histopathology of ulcerative colitis in initial rectal biopsy in children. *Am J Surg Pathol.* 2002;26(11):1441-1449.
8. Tung J, Loftus EV Jr, Freese DK, et al. A population-based study of the frequency of corticosteroid resistance and dependence in pediatric patients with Crohn's disease and ulcerative colitis. *Inflamm Bowel Dis.* 2006;12(12):1093-1100.
9. Markowitz J, Hyams J, Mack D, et al. Corticosteroid therapy in the age of infliximab: acute and 1-year outcomes in newly diagnosed children with Crohn's disease. *Clin Gastroenterol Hepatol.* 2006;4(9):1124-1129.
10. Markowitz J, Grancher K, Kohn N, Lesser M, Daum F. A multicenter trial of 6-mercaptopurine and prednisone in children with newly diagnosed Crohn's disease. *Gastroenterology.* 2000;119(4):895-902.
11. Hanauer SB, Feagan BG, Lichtenstein GR, et al. Maintenance infliximab for Crohn's disease: the Accent I randomised trial. *Lancet.* 2002;359(9317):1541-1549.
12. Sands BE, Anderson FH, Bernstein CN, et al. Infliximab maintenance therapy for fistulizing Crohn's disease. *N Engl J Med.* 2004;350(9):876-885.
13. Hyams J, Crandall W, Kugathasan S, et al. Induction and maintenance infliximab therapy for the treatment of moderate-to-severe Crohn's disease in children. *Gastroenterology.* 2007;132(3):863-873; quiz 1165-1166.
14. Kugathasan S, Werlin SL, Martinez A, Rivera MT, Heikenen JB, Binion DG. Prolonged duration of response to infliximab in early but not late pediatric Crohn's disease. *Am J Gastroenterol.* 2000;95(11):3189-3194.
15. Lionetti P, Bronzini F, Salvestrini C, et al. Response to infliximab is related to disease duration in paediatric Crohn's disease. *Aliment Pharmacol Ther.* 2003;18(4):425-431.
16. Hanauer SB, Schreiber S, Thomsen OO, Lichtenstein GR, Bloomfield R, Sandborn WJ. Predictors of response in patients with active Crohn's disease treated with certolizumab pegol: a multiple regression analysis of precise 2 data. *Gastroenterology.* 2008;134(4, Supplement 1):A-489.
17. Butcher S, Chahel H, Lord JM. Review article: ageing and the neutrophil: no appetite for killing? *Immunology.* 2000;100(4):411-416.

18. Friis-Hansen B. Body composition during growth: in vivo measurements and biochemical data correlated to differential anatomical growth. *Pediatrics*. 1971;47(1):Suppl 2:264.

19. Friis-Hansen B. Water distribution in the foetus and newborn infant. *Acta Paediatr Scand Suppl*. 1983;305:7-11.

20. Lew KH, Ludwig EA, Milad MA, et al. Gender-based effects on methylprednisolone pharmacokinetics and pharmacodynamics. *Clin Pharmacol Ther*. 1993;54(4):402-414.

21. Grochow LB, Krivit W, Whitley CB, Blazar B. Busulfan disposition in children. *Blood*. 1990;75(8):1723-1727.

22. Vassal G, Deroussent A, Hartmann O, et al. Dose-dependent neurotoxicity of high-dose busulfan in children: a clinical and pharmacological study. *Cancer Res*. 1990;50(19):6203-6207.

23. Murry DJ, Crom WR, Reddick WE, Bhargava R, Evans WE. Liver volume as a determinant of drug clearance in children and adolescents. *Drug Metab Dispos*. 1995;23(10):1110-1116.

24. Noda T, Todani T, Watanabe Y, Yamamoto S. Liver volume in children measured by computed tomography. *Pediatr Radiol*. 1997;27(3):250-252.

25. Alcorn J, McNamara PJ. Pharmacokinetics in the newborn. *Adv Drug Deliv Rev*. 2003;55(5):667-686.

26. Schwartz GJ, Haycock GB, Edelmann CM Jr, Spitzer A. A simple estimate of glomerular filtration rate in children derived from body length and plasma creatinine. *Pediatrics*. 1976;58(2):259-263.

27. Linday LA, Drayer DE, Khan MA, Cicalese C, Reidenberg MM. Pubertal changes in net renal tubular secretion of digoxin. *Clin Pharmacol Ther*. 1984;35(4):438-446.

28. Evans NJ, Rutter N. Development of the epidermis in the newborn. *Biol Neonate*. 1986;49(2):74-80.

29. Nachman RL, Esterly NB. Increased skin permeability in preterm infants. *J Pediatr*. 1971;79(4):628-632.

30. Cartwright RG, Cartlidge PH, Rutter N, Melia CD, Davis SS. Transdermal delivery of theophylline to premature infants using a hydrogel disc system. *Br J Clin Pharmacol*. 1990;29(5):533-539.

31. Evans NJ, Rutter N, Hadgraft J, Parr G. Percutaneous administration of theophylline in the preterm infant. *J Pediatr*. 1985;107(2):307-311.

32. Peleg O, Bar-Oz B, Arad I. Coma in a premature infant associated with the transdermal absorption of propylene glycol. *Acta Paediatr*. 1998;87(11):1195-1196.

33. Tyrala EE, Hillman LS, Hillman RE, Dodson WE. Clinical pharmacology of hexachlorophene in newborn infants. *J Pediatr*. 1977;91(3):481-486.

34. Kearns GL, Abdel-Rahman SM, Alander SW, Blowey DL, Leeder JS, Kauffman RE. Developmental pharmacology: drug disposition, action, and therapy in infants and children. *N Engl J Med*. 2003;349(12):1157-1167.

35. Huang NN, High RH. Comparison of serum levels following the administration of oral and parenteral preparations of penicillin to infants and children of various age. *J Pediatr*. 1953;42:657-668.

36. McNamara PJ, Alcorn J. Protein binding predictions in infants. *AAPS PharmSci*. 2002;4(1):E4.

37. Morselli PL. Clinical pharmacology of the perinatal period and early infancy. *Clin Pharmacokinet*. 1989;17(Suppl 1):13-28.

38. Notarianni LJ. Plasma protein binding of drugs in pregnancy and in neonates. *Clin Pharmacokinet*. 1990;18(1):20-36.

39. Brodersen R. Bilirubin transport in the newborn infant, reviewed with relation to kernicterus. *J Pediatr*. 1980;96(3 Pt 1):349-356.

40. Koukouritaki SB, Simpson P, Yeung CK, Rettie AE, Hines RN. Human hepatic flavin-containing monooxygenases 1 (FMO1) and 3 (FMO3) developmental expression. *Pediatr Res*. 2002;51(2):236-243.

41. Hines RN. Ontogeny of human hepatic cytochromes P450. *J Biochem Mol Toxicol*. 2007;21(4):169-175.

42. Pearce RE, Gotschall RR, Kearns GL, Leeder JS. Cytochrome P450 involvement in the biotransformation of cisapride and racemic norcisapride in vitro: differential activity of individual human CYP3A isoforms. *Drug Metab Dispos*. 2001;29(12):1548-1554.

43. Kearns GL, Robinson PK, Wilson JT, et al. Cisapride disposition in neonates and infants: in vivo reflection of cytochrome P450 3A4 ontogeny. *Clin Pharmacol Ther*. 2003;74(4):312-325.

44. Treluyer JM, Rey E, Sonnier M, Pons G, Cresteil T. Evidence of impaired cisapride metabolism in neonates. *Br J Clin Pharmacol*. 2001;52(4):419-425.

45. Bernardini S, Semama DS, Huet F, Sgro C, Gouyon JB. Effects of cisapride on QTc interval in neonates. *Arch Dis Child Fetal Neonatal Ed*. 1997;77(3):F241-F243.

46. Alam SN, Roberts RJ, Fischer LJ. Age-related differences in salicylamide and acetaminophen conjugation in man. *J Pediatr*. 1977;90(1):130-135.

47. McLeod HL, Krynetski EY, Wilimas JA, Evans WE. Higher activity of polymorphic thiopurine S-methyltransferase in erythrocytes from neonates compared to adults. *Pharmacogenetics*. 1995;5(5):281-286.

48. Pacifici GM, Romiti P, Giuliani L, Rane A. Thiopurine methyltransferase in humans: development and tissue distribution. *Dev Pharmacol Ther*. 1991;17(1-2):16-23.

49. Schinkel AH, Jonker JW. Mammalian drug efflux transporters of the ATP binding cassette (ABC) family: an overview. *Adv Drug Deliv Rev*. 2003;55(1):3-29.

50. van Kalken CK, Giaccone G, van der Valk P, et al. Multidrug resistance gene (P-glycoprotein) expression in the human fetus. *Am J Pathol*. 1992;141(5):1063-1072.

51. Machado CG, Calado RT, Garcia AB, Falcao RP. Age-related changes of the multidrug resistance P-glycoprotein function in normal human peripheral blood T lymphocytes. *Braz J Med Biol Res*. 2003;36(12):1653-1657.

52. Takahashi H, Ishikawa S, Nomoto S, et al. Developmental changes in pharmacokinetics and pharmacodynamics of warfarin enantiomers in Japanese children. *Clin Pharmacol Ther.* 2000;68(5):541-555.

53. Marshall JD, Kearns GL. Developmental pharmacodynamics of cyclosporine. *Clin Pharmacol Ther.* 1999;66(1):66-75.

54. Cooney GF, Habucky K, Hoppu K. Cyclosporin pharmacokinetics in paediatric transplant recipients. *Clin Pharmacokinet.* 1997;32(6):481-495.

55. Johnson TN, Rostami-Hodjegan A, Tucker GT. Prediction of the clearance of eleven drugs and associated variability in neonates, infants and children. *Clin Pharmacokinet.* 2006;45(9):931-956.

CHAPTER 8

BONE AND INFLAMMATORY BOWEL DISEASE

Francisco A. Sylvester, MD

The skeleton is often depicted as a static scaffold for soft tissues, but its function is much broader. Bone is metabolically active in both adults and children. In addition to serving as the largest reservoir for calcium in the body, it is an important source of buffer and it harbors and interacts with the hematopoietic bone marrow. The skeleton is sensitive to systemic and local regulatory signals, both normal and pathological. Therefore, inflammatory bowel diseases (IBD) may affect bone cell function and consequently bone mass by multiple mechanisms. In this chapter, we will briefly review normal bone physiology in adults and children and then focus on bone mass deficits associated with IBD, the mechanisms involved, and the treatment options to optimize skeletal health in these patients.

Normal Bone Physiology

BONE CELLS

Two main cell types are responsible for bone metabolic activity: osteoblasts and osteoclasts. In addition, the cartilaginous growth plate is responsible for the linear growth of long bones in children. These cells can be influenced by alterations in homeostasis that occur in IBD.

Osteoblasts are cells from mesenchymal origin that synthesize a collagenous bone matrix, which is then mineralized with calcium and phosphate crystals. Consequently, osteoblasts are responsible for bone formation. Bone morphogenetic (BMP), Wnt, calcium/calmodulin, and insulin-like growth factor-I (IGF-I) signals, as well as the transcription factors Runx2 and Osterix, are all key regulators of osteoblast differentiation and function. These pathways are susceptible to the effects of cytokines and medications (eg, corticosteroids, calcineurin inhibitors).[1-6]

Osteoclasts originate from pluripotent hematopoietic precursors and resorb bone in response to local and systemic signals. Like osteoblasts, their differentiation and function are tightly controlled by cytokines, key signaling pathways, and transcription factors. For osteoclasts,

Scherl EJ, Dubinsky MC.
*The Changing World of Inflammatory Bowel Disease:
Impact of Generation, Gender, and Global Trends (pp 101-118)*
© 2009 SLACK Incorporated.

receptor activator of nuclear factor κ B-ligand (RANKL) stimulation of its cellular receptor RANK in osteoclast precursors is essential for their maturation, activation, and survival.[7] Osteoprotegerin (OPG) is a soluble decoy receptor for RANKL that inhibits osteoclastogenesis.[8] In addition, the transcription factors NF-κB and nuclear factor of activated T cells (NFAT) are both important for osteoclast differentiation.[9] Among the cytokines upregulated in IBD, IL-6 and TNF-α both stimulate osteoclastogenesis via RANKL, and TNF-α[10] also independently of RANKL.[11]

The growth plate of long bones is constituted by columns of chondrocytes of distinct characteristics. The growth plate generates a cartilaginous model for new bone trabeculae, which is substituted by bone by the combined actions of osteoclasts and osteoblasts. The growth plate is responsive to anabolic growth factors such as IGF-I.[12] In children, active IBD is associated with reduced systemic and perhaps local IGF-I concentrations, resulting in growth arrest.[13] Since the acquisition of bone mass is highly dependent on linear growth, stunting will significantly affect gains in skeletal mass.

BONE MODELING AND REMODELING

In growing children, long bones are reshaped as they increase in length to maintain proper morphological characteristics. In addition, bones increase in width by an expansion of the periosteal surface, while at the same time increasing the medullary cavity. This process is called *bone modeling* and occurs almost exclusively in children. In bone modeling, both osteoblasts and osteoclasts are active at the same time on different surfaces. Bone modeling affects primarily cortical bone and produces relatively large amounts of bone material.[14,15]

In both children and adults, the bone microarchitectural integrity is maintained by bone remodeling. Remodeling occurs in both trabecular and cortical bone. In this process, osteoclasts remove damaged or stressed bone by resorption and create a divot. A second wave of bone-forming osteoblasts then fills in the defect with bone matrix. In consequence, the activities of osteoclasts and osteoblasts are coupled and occur in sequence. In addition, the amount of bone generated in each remodeling cycle is small, over a period of 3 to 4 months. Therefore, this process is comparatively slower than bone modeling.[16]

PEAK BONE MASS AND AGE-RELATED BONE LOSS

Bone mass accumulates during growth and reaches a peak early in the third decade of life. Peak bone mass is largely determined genetically. After a period of stability, bone mass is steadily lost, beginning usually in the fifth decade of life.[17] Menopause accelerates bone loss. In addition to the reduction of bone mass, bone microarchitecture is compromised over time due to bone resorption and inadequate bone formation. This results in thinning and loss of trabecular bone and increases the risk of mechanical fragility and fractures.[18]

EVALUATION OF BONE MASS

There are a number of methods that can be used to estimate bone mass, including dual x-ray absorptiometry (DXA),[19] peripheral quantitative computed tomography (pQCT),[20] magnetic resonance imagining (MRI),[21] and quantitative broadband ultrasound (QUS).[22] The most widely available method is DXA, which is used in both children and adults, which will be discussed here in some detail. MRI is an experimental technology for the determination of bone mass and its use is limited to research at this time. QUS has the advantage of avoiding ionizing radiation, but there are technical issues that need to be resolved before it can be more widely used. pQCT is an emerging technology, mostly used in the research setting at this time, but with advantages over DXA in that it measures volumetric material density and provides measures of bone strength (see next).

In a DXA scan, 2 x-ray beams of different energies traverse the supine patient. The dose of radiation is minimal, comparable to background exposure from natural sources. As these 2 x-ray beams travel through soft tissue and bone, they are attenuated. The degree of tissue energy absorption is measured by an array of detectors facing the subject. This information is translated into bone mineral content, bone area, and fat and lean body mass. The instrument reports areal bone mineral density (BMD) (in g/cm^2). Consequently, DXA does not measure true volumetric bone density (in g/cm^3). For this reason, DXA tends to underestimate bone density in small individuals.[23,24] DXA can measure bone density of the whole body (minus the head) and of different regions of interest, including the lumbar spine, and hip. DXA also provides body composition data, including fat mass and lean body mass. These measurements can be helpful to follow the nutritional status of patients with IBD.

In adults, raw BMD data are compared to those of healthy, young individuals, and a *t* score is generated (observed BMD–mean BMD/standard deviation of the mean). According to the World Health Organization, a *t* score of >-1 is normal, <-2.5 is defined as osteoporosis, and >-1 but ≤-2.5 is osteopenia.[25] Importantly, correlations between *t* score and fracture risk have only been adequately studied in postmenopausal women and not yet in IBD. In addition, *t* score by itself does not predict the risk of fracture in a given individual. For example, a 50-year-old postmenopausal woman has a much lesser fracture risk than a 75-year-old woman with identical *t* scores.[18] This is probably due to changes in bone microarchitecture, impairments in vision and coordination, decreased muscle and fat mass (which cushion falls), and delayed reaction time to falls associated with aging.

In growing children, BMD data should be compared to individuals of the same age and sex to calculate a *z* score.[26] Since DXA can underestimate BMD in small individuals, *z* score calculations may need adjustments for height and bone age in patients with growth retardation or with pubertal delay. DXA reports for pediatric patients should never include *t* scores, as these will routinely underestimate their bone mass. The diagnosis of pediatric osteoporosis should not be made based on a low *z* score alone; instead a *z* score <-2 should be reported as significant deficit in bone mass. The terms *osteopenia* and *osteoporosis* should not be used in children.

Repeated measurements of BMD should ideally be performed in the same instrument to ensure that data at different time points are directly comparable. For children, the availability of pediatric software in the DXA scanner is essential to measure BMD appropriately. In addition, meticulous quality control and instrument calibration, as well as adequate patient positioning for each examination are all indispensable.[26]

pQCT measures true bone density in g/cm^3 and provides information on the mechanical properties of bone and its relationship to muscle mass.[27] Peripheral devices use a minimal dose of x-ray energy and are considered safe. Clinically, they are used in a handful of centers at the present time, but with the emerging availability of pediatric reference data, it is likely that their use will increase.

Bone Mass Deficits in Inflammatory Bowel Disease—Clinical Studies

Multiple studies in both adults and children with IBD document that reduced BMD is common. Most of these studies were cross-sectional studies in patients with long-standing disease.[28] However, some were performed at the time of diagnosis.[29-32] Longitudinal studies have also been conducted in both adults[33,34] and children.[32] The majority of studies used DXA to evaluate BMD in regions of interest such as the total body, lumbar spine, hip, or forearm.

Several lessons can be obtained from these papers. Firstly, the prevalence of low bone mass in patients with IBD ranges from 0% to 60% depending on the population studied.[29,35] This wide variation suggests that normal bone mass is attainable in patients with IBD and certain patient characteristics may increase the risk of bone mass deficits. In children, for example, indirect indicators of disease severity such as hypoalbuminemia, need for nasogastric tube feeds, total parenteral nutrition, use of 6-mercaptopurine,[36] and elevated serum IL-6[32,37] correlate with impaired bone mineral status. In addition, decreased body mass index (BMI) and lean body mass are powerful predictors of reduced BMD in both adults and children.[32,34,38-41] The use of corticosteroids has been inconsistently associated with low BMD in children with IBD,[32,36-38,42,43] but this correlation appears to be more robust in adults.[34,44-49] This may be explained by physiological differences between the pediatric and adult skeleton (bone in children may be able to recover faster upon corticosteroid withdrawal). Also the beneficial anti-inflammatory effects of short-term corticosteroid use may supersede their negative effects on bone.[50] It is likely, however, that steroid dependency may have deleterious effects on the skeleton in both adults and children.

Secondly, several studies have reported that patients with Crohn's disease have more significant bone deficits than those with ulcerative colitis.[32,38,42,51,52] It is important to evaluate specific features of the reports, including sample size (which may affect the ability to detect differences in BMD z and t scores between individuals with Crohn's disease and ulcerative colitis), patient characteristics (such as their age and sex [children versus adults, number of postmenopausal women]), the activity of disease, and the inclusion of patients with ulcerative proctitis, who may be less likely to lose bone mass because of minimal impact on overall health.[53] Although it is possible that patients with Crohn's disease may have decreased skeletal mass compared to those with ulcerative colitis, there are no sufficiently large studies to date to draw firm conclusions about differential effect of these 2 diseases on bone mass.

Thirdly, longitudinal studies in adults reveal that some patients with IBD may lose bone mass over time at an accelerated rate. For example, single photon absorptiometry (which precedes DXA) revealed increased rates of cortical bone loss in the radius,[33] and quantitative computed tomography showed excessive mineral losses in the lumbar spine.[54] Moreover, serial measurements of total body calcium by prompt gamma-neutron activation analysis showed an average decrease of 7.8% (-12.0% to -3.7%) per year.[55] Longitudinal studies using DXA have reported a decline in lumbar spine and femoral neck BMD in patients with Crohn's disease and ulcerative colitis,[56,57] while others have observed that bone loss is restricted to patients with ulcerative colitis receiving corticosteroids.[58] These studies need to be interpreted with caution because in some cases patients with IBD were not compared to individuals of the same age and sex (in adults, some degree of bone loss is expected over time, especially after menopause). In addition, BMD may decrease but stay within the normal range, raising the question about the clinical significance of these losses.

However, the majority of adults with IBD probably do not lose excess bone compared to unaffected individuals of the same age and sex.[34,59] In fact, gains in bone mass have been reported in patients with ulcerative colitis gains after colectomy and ileal-pouch anastomosis[56,60] and in patients with Crohn's disease that improve with therapy.[61,62] In addition, children with IBD gain bone mass,[63] although the rate of bone mineral accrual appears to be slower than normal, at least 2 years after diagnosis.[32] Moreover, a population-based study of 70 postmenopausal women less than 45 years of age who were diagnosed with IBD before age 20 years showed that only 3 individuals had a BMD t score <-2.5 at any site.[64] This suggests that patients diagnosed with IBD as children in most cases do not have significant bone mass deficits when they become adults. Why some adults with IBD lose bone mineral more quickly than normal is not clear, but ongoing steroid use and low BMI may be contributing factors.[54,65] In children, inadequate linear growth may stunt the normal acquisition of bone mineral.[66]

Markers of Bone Turnover in Inflammatory Bowel Disease

Several surrogate markers of osteoclast and osteoblast activity are available. These indicators can be measured in blood and in some cases in urine. In adults treated for IBD, biomarkers of bone formation (eg, serum osteocalcin, bone alkaline phosphatase, collagen propeptides) can be normal,[67,68] low,[44,69,70] and occasionally elevated.[47] Bone resorption markers (eg, degradation products of type I collagen such as cross-linking telopeptides and deoxypyridinoline) are often increased.[30,47,57,67,68,71-75] In consequence, bone resorption is more active in adults with IBD without adequate compensatory bone formation. This imbalance may result in loss of bone mass and deterioration of bone microarchitecture. In contrast, children with IBD at diagnosis have reduced biomarkers of both bone formation and resorption to levels that are ~30% normal.[32,76] This indicates a state of low bone turnover, which probably is mainly due to the stunting of growth commonly seen in children with IBD. With treatment and favorable clinical response, these markers of bone turnover increase to concentrations comparable to healthy children.[32]

Bone Biopsy Data

There are a handful of reports of transiliac bone biopsies in patients with IBD. The analysis of these biopsies provides direct insight into bone cell activity and bone structure. Hessov et al observed marked decreases in trabecular bone mass in patients with Crohn's disease after small bowel resection.[77] Croucher et al analyzed biopsies in 19 patients with IBD with decreased BMD, of which 11 were receiving prednisolone at the time of their biopsy. They found significant reductions in trabecular bone area and wall width and significant reductions in histological parameters of bone formation.[78] In patients with IBD with severe vitamin D deficiency, transiliac bone biopsies demonstrate osteomalacia, which improved after vitamin D therapy.[79] These studies were conducted in adult patients with long-standing disease, making it difficult to differentiate between disease and treatment effects on bone microarchitecture. More recently, Ward et al reported bone biopsy data in children with Crohn's disease at diagnosis before treatment was initiated. These data provide direct evidence that osteoblast function is decreased, while osteoclast function is not augmented in these patients (Ward L, oral communication, May 2007), confirming earlier bone biomarker data.[32] Consequently, in contrast to the high bone resorption state observed in adults affected by IBD evidenced by bone biomarker and biopsy data, children with IBD have decreased bone formation at diagnosis. Therefore, IBD affects the adult and pediatric skeleton differently, which needs to be considered when designing interventions to promote optimal bone health in these patients.

Fracture Risk in Inflammatory Bowel Disease

Patients with IBD often exhibit bone mass deficits, and their bone biomechanical properties may be compromised.[80] However, the central question of whether these changes are clinically significant, resulting in bone fracture, has not been conclusively answered. To date, there has not been a prospective study of fracture incidence as a primary endpoint in patients with IBD. There are several population-based studies in adults affected with IBD showing conflicting results. A study in Manitoba, Canada showed an increase in fracture risk of 40% greater than the general population.[81] In another population-based study in Denmark, fracture risk was increased in adults with Crohn's disease (from an incidence rate ratio of 1.15, 95% CI, 1.00 to 1.32 before diagnosis to 1.19, 95% CI, 1.06 to 1.33 after diagnosis) but not ulcerative colitis.[82] In addition, a primary care-based nested case-control study observed an increased risk of vertebral fracture (OR, 1.72; 95% CI, 1.13 to 2.61) and hip fracture (OR, 1.59; 95% CI, 1.14 to 2.23). The risk of hip fracture was greater in patients with Crohn's disease (OR, 1.86; 95% CI, 1.08 to 3.21) compared with ulcerative colitis (OR, 1.40; 95% CI, 0.92 to 2.13). Corticosteroid use and severe disease activity were risk factors for fractures.[83] However, population-based studies in Olmsted County, Minnesota did not detect increased fracture prevalence in adults with ulcerative colitis[84] or Crohn's disease.[85] Consequently, based on these data, fracture risk in adults with IBD may be modestly increased.

Fracture risk data for children with IBD are much more limited. A recent report did not find an increase in the number of long bone fractures in children with IBD compared to their unaffected siblings.[86] This was a retrospective, questionnaire-based study that was the first to address fracture risk in children with IBD. However, it has several methodological limitations, including not reporting the age when the fracture occurred, not performing DXA close to the time of fracture in children with IBD or their siblings, and not considering the time between the diagnosis of IBD and the occurrence of fracture. In addition, the sample size may not have been large enough to detect group differences due to the high frequency of fractures in growing children.[87] Consequently, additional prospective studies of fracture risk are needed in IBD.

The studies mentioned above were performed in subjects who sought medical treatment for their fractures. However, it is well known that vertebral compression fractures may be clinically silent, and consequently they may have been missed in population-based studies. Irrespective of symptoms, their occurrence is an important risk factor for future fractures.[88] In consequence, the occurrence of vertebral fractures is of interest for patients with IBD. There are several case reports of vertebral fractures in both adults and children affected by IBD.[44,89-93] In adults with IBD with low BMD (t score <-1 of the lumbar spine), the frequency of unsuspected vertebral fractures or deformities detected by conventional spine films was 22%.[94] However, vertebral fractures may occur in patients with IBD with normal BMD and in the absence of steroid use.[95,96] In consequence, asymptomatic vertebral fractures may occur in patients with IBD. Their prevalence in unselected populations of patients with IBD requires further study.

Bone Mass Deficits in Inflammatory Bowel Disease: Animal Studies

Bone formation and bone strength have been studied in animal models of IBD. Bone formation is reduced in rats with acute 2,4,6-trinitrobenzenesulfonic acid (TNBS) colitis. Bone mass improves as the colitis resolves. This effect is independent of food intake and likely reflects the effect of the underlying intestinal inflammation.[97] In the IL-10 knockout mice (IL-10$^{-/-}$; 129 Sv/Ev background), at 3-months of age femur and vertebral bone mineral content (BMC) and BMD are both decreased and biomechanical strength is reduced compared to wild-type mice.[98] This was confirmed in 8- to 12-week-old IL-10$^{-/-}$ (C57/BL6J background) mice, with evidence of trabecular and cortical bone loss and decreased bone formation.[99] In consequence, these models mimic the bone phenotype of growing children with IBD.

Changes in bone mass have also been investigated in adoptive transfer mouse models of colitis. These models are T-cell dependent and offer insight into the role of T cells in bone loss in IBD. In one such model, CD4+CD45RB^{Hi} T cells injected into scid/scid mice induce colitis, while mice injected with CD4+CD45RB^{Lo} remain disease free and serve as controls. Mice that received CD4+CD45RB^{Hi} showed decreased BMD, with decreased osteoblasts and increased osteoclasts. Treatment with an Fc-osteoprotegerin (OPG) fusion protein increased BMD in both RB^{Hi}- and RB^{Lo}-treated mice, probably due to a decrease in osteoclast differentiation and activity. Although this study does not answer whether colitogenic T cells are directly responsible for bone loss in this model, it is interesting that CD4+CD45RB^{Hi} recipients had a bone marrow inflammatory infiltrate expressing TNF-α, which suggests that intestinal inflammation may directly alter the bone microenvironment.[100] In a second study, IL-2$^{-/-}$ mice (which develop colitis and other signs of systemic inflammation) and C57BL/6-$Rag1^{-/-}$ mice that received splenic T cells from IL-2$^{-/-}$ showed decreased bone mass.[101] In this model, systemic OPG improved bone mass and also ameliorated the colitis, suggesting a potential therapeutic role for OPG in IBD.

Mechanisms of Bone Loss in Inflammatory Bowel Disease

Multiple factors are probably responsible for decreasing bone mass in IBD. These include nutritional deficits (produced by inadequate intake and/or intestinal losses), reduced physical activity, pubertal delay in children, exposure to corticosteroids, decreased muscle mass, and inflammatory cells and factors.

MALNUTRITION

IBD, especially Crohn's disease, is commonly associated with malnutrition, which is caused by a combination of decreased intake of calories and micronutrients, enteral losses, and probably inappropriate nutrient utilization. In both adults and children, reduced BMI is associated with low BMD.[32,102] In addition, Jahnsen et al reported in adults with Crohn's disease followed for 2 years that gains in BMI were positively correlated with changes in the total body BMD.[34] Collectively, these data suggest that weight gain has an anabolic effect on bone mass in IBD. However, since BMI does not discriminate between muscle and fat compartments, it is not clear whether gains in muscle, fat mass, or both are responsible for this effect.

CALCIUM AND VITAMIN D

Low serum vitamin D concentration is common in both adults and children with IBD, especially in individuals living in northern latitudes due to limited exposure to unfiltered ultraviolet B (UVB) radiation from the sun.[103-107] Vitamin D insufficiency may impair calcium absorption from the intestine and may increase calcium mobilization from the bone.[108] This is aggravated by low calcium intake, which is prevalent in adults and children with IBD.[109] However, it is not clear if these deficits have clinical impact on BMD in patients with IBD.[110]

Vitamin D supplementation of 1000 IU/day for 1 year has been shown to prevent decreases in BMD in a cohort of adults affected by IBD, especially in those who attained normal serum 25-hydroxyvitamin D.[111] Calcium (1 g) and vitamin D (800 IU) daily given for 1 year increased lumbar BMD in patients with IBD who had a baseline BMD *t* score <-2 and normal serum 25-hydroxyvitamin D.[112] However, in patients receiving corticosteroids and a baseline calcium intake that met the recommended daily allowance (RDA), calcium carbonate (1 g) and vitamin D (250 IU) did not improve spine BMD after 1 year.[113]

VITAMIN K

Vitamin K is required for the γ-carboxylation of glutamic acid residues in osteocalcin, a bone-active protein capable of binding hydroxyapatite that may have a role in bone matrix mineralization and is widely used as a biomarker of osteoblast activity.[114] In consequence, vitamin K deficiency results in decreased serum carboxylated osteocalcin, with a relative increase in the undercarboxylated fraction. Subclinical vitamin K deficiency may be present in patients with IBD[75,115-117] and may affect bone health in patients with Crohn's disease. For example, in a cohort of adults with Crohn's disease that affected the small bowel who were in remission, Schoon et al observed an inverse correlation between undercarboxylated osteocalcin and BMD of the spine.[115] However, this relationship was not present for proximal femur or total body BMD or between serum vitamin K and BMD at any measured site. Duggan et al observed that resorptive markers were increased in adults with Crohn's disease who had increased serum undercarboxylated osteocalcin.[116] Consequently, subclinical vitamin K deficiency may play a role in bone health in IBD, but its significance is unclear at this time. Future studies should include larger cohorts of patients and test whether vitamin K supplementation increases BMD in patients with IBD.

CORTICOSTEROIDS

Glucocorticoids have marked effects on bone metabolism. While in vivo they have indirect actions on bone metabolism, their primary effect is to suppress osteoblast function and bone formation through multiple mechanisms. In consequence, glucocorticoid excess in adults can lead to bone loss due to the unopposed bone resorption by osteoclasts.[118] Clinically, up to 50% of adults on chronic (>1 year) glucocorticoid therapy lose significant bone mass.[119] In addition, fracture risk also rises, both in adults and children.[120,121] However, in patients with IBD, it may be difficult to separate the effects of the underlying disease from those of corticosteroids on bone.[50] In addition, by controlling inflammation and improving general health, corticosteroids may potentially have beneficial effects on bone health. Therefore, it is not surprising that the relationship between corticosteroid use and bone mass deficits in IBD is inconsistent in the published literature.[46,65,122-125] It seems prudent, however, to monitor cumulative corticosteroid use, minimize corticosteroid use in patients with IBD when possible, to measure BMD periodically in patients who are steroid dependent, and to institute bone-active therapy in those patients with significant BMD deficits.[83]

DECREASED MUSCLE MASS

The skeleton continuously adapts its strength to physiological loads, primarily muscle contractions.[126] In consequence, decreased muscle force and mass is expected to reduce bone mass and strength. This is relevant to patients with IBD, who often have significant, persistent deficits in lean body mass, a surrogate indicator of muscle mass.[41,127] Mauro et al reported that total lean body mass was independently associated with BMC in adults with Crohn's disease.[128] These deficits in muscle mass occur despite adequate weight gain and seemingly adequate symptom control in both adults and children with IBD. Therefore, interventions to improve muscle mass and force may be anabolic to bone in IBD.

EXERCISE

Physical exercise increases BMD in healthy young adults and slows the rate of bone loss in later life. In a cohort of adults with Crohn's disease, however, a progressive low-impact exercise program had insignificant BMD increases at the femoral neck and spine compared to a control group.[129] Nonetheless, exercise may have several health benefits and should be encouraged in patients with IBD.[130]

INFLAMMATION

IBD is characterized by T-cell activation and cytokine production in the intestinal mucosa, with spillover into the circulation. In addition, circulating T cells also produce higher concentrations of cytokines in patients with active disease.[76] Genetic studies suggest that cytokines are involved in the pathogenesis of bone loss in IBD. For example, polymorphisms associated with increased production of the proinflammatory IL-6[131,132] and IL-1β are associated with reduced BMD,[133] while decreased production of the anti-inflammatory IL-1ra is associated with low bone mass.[131] This may be due to the direct effects of overproduced specific cytokines on bone or due to more severe IBD in individuals with these polymorphisms. However, a polymorphism associated with low IL-6 synthesis does not protect from low BMD in IBD patients.[134] In addition, and somewhat surprisingly, IBD patients with the high-producing -857 CC TNF-α genotype had normal overall BMD.[135] The effects of these genetic variants on overall bone mass, independently of IBD, may explain these discrepant results.

Excess proinflammatory cytokines or anti-inflammatory cytokine deficiencies may have direct effects on bone cells. There is extensive cross-talk between immune cells and bone cells via cytokines. Inflammatory cytokines such as IL-6 and TNF-α, both upregulated in IBD, can increase osteoclast formation, activity, and survival via RANKL-dependent and independent mechanisms.[10,136-138] INF-α on the other hand inhibits osteoclastogenesis by inhibiting RANKL signaling and decreases osteoblast function.[139,140] Serum from children with active Crohn's disease inhibits bone formation in vitro, an effect that is at least partially mediated by IL-6.[141] TNF-α inhibits osteoblast differentiation and function in vitro.[142-145] In the TNBS mouse model of colitis, TNF-α inhibits Phex expression, a gene that plays a role in bone matrix mineralization in calvariae. Treatment of mice with colitis with an anti-TNF-α antibody and with curcumin, which ameliorates that severity of TNBS colitis, restored *Phex* expression.[146] This work suggests that systemic TNF-α affects osteoblast function in the context of intestinal inflammation. In consequence, soluble inflammatory factors generated by the gut in IBD may affect bone cell differentiation and function.

It is also possible that the bone microenvironment itself may be altered in IBD. For example, Byrne et al[100] observed that in the CD4+CD45RB^Hi transfer model of colitis, there is an inflammatory infiltrate in the bone marrow containing cells that produce TNF-α. It is not clear whether these are endogenous bone marrow cells activated by intestinal inflammation or if they originated in the gut and migrated into the bone marrow.

T CELLS AND BONE LOSS

T cells are emerging as important regulators of bone cell function in the context of postmenopausal osteoporosis and inflammation. Activated T cells generate RANKL-dependent and independent signals that can regulate osteoclast formation, activity, and survival. T-cell–induced bone resorption has been implicated in tissue injury in animal models of arthritis and periodontal disease.[147,148] In ovariectomized mice, an animal model of menopause, T cells play an important role in bone loss, but these observations await replication in humans.[149] In this model, it is intriguing that TNF-α–producing T cells are expanded, presumably due to exposure to microbial antigens from the gut or genital tract, or to putative self-antigens.[150] In IBD, circulating T cells that produce cytokines that regulate bone cell function may reach the bone marrow, or activated T cells or other immune cells may be generated in the bone marrow and influence bone cell function more directly.[76] These hypotheses await further research.

RANKL–OPG

RANKL is indispensable to induce osteoclast differentiation. OPG, a soluble decoy receptor for RANKL, is a potent inhibitor of osteoclast development. In bone, OPG is produced by osteoblasts. Both cytokines have important functions in the immune system as well.[151] Serum OPG concentration is modestly elevated in both adults and children with IBD. In addition, the inflamed intestine in adults with IBD produces increased OPG and RANKL.[152,153] Therefore, elevated serum OPG may originate from osteoblasts and intestinal inflammatory cells in IBD. In addition, in animal models of IBD in which osteoclast activity is increased, exogenous OPG improves bone mass and in one case also decreased gut inflammation, suggesting a potential role for OPG as a therapeutic agent in human IBD.[101]

THERAPEUTIC STRATEGIES

Several therapies are available to increase bone mass, including bisphosphonates, hormone replacement therapy, raloxifene, teriparatide, strontium ranelate, and combined vitamin D and calcium. Before deciding on a specific therapeutic regimen, the practitioner should consider that these have been studied primarily in postmenopausal women, and studies in patients with IBD are sparse. As stated above, IBD affects the skeletal health of growing children (typically not included in trials with these agents) and adults differently. Moreover, the effects of IBD and menopause on bone are likely to be distinct. Furthermore, orally administered agents may not be well absorbed in IBD, and patients with IBD have not been well represented in studies of glucocorticoid-induced osteoporosis.[154] Lastly, low BMD is associated with increased fracture risk in menopause.[155] In IBD, it is still yet unclear whether fracture risk is significantly increased.

To optimize skeletal health in patients with IBD, it probably makes good sense to control inflammation and minimize steroid exposure, as this has been shown to increase BMD.[62,125,156,157] Infliximab may be considered in patients with significant deficits in bone mass, as its use is associated in the short term with a rise in biomarkers of bone formation in both adults and children and increases in bone mass.[158-161] This probably reflects decreases in inflammation, improvement in general health, and reduction in corticosteroid use associated with the use of infliximab.[162-165] It also is sensible to improve nutrition and promote physical activity[159,166] and optimize calcium and vitamin D supplementation.[167]

Other bone-active agents may be considered in patients with documented fractures and those with significant bone mass deficits.[168] Bisphosphonates, which are stable derivatives of pyrophosphate, increase BMD and reduce fracture risk in postmenopausal women. Studies involving patients with IBD have used changes in BMD as their primary outcome and have involved a small number of patients. For example, Haderslev et al conducted a 12-month double-blind placebo-controlled study of 10 mg of daily oral alendronate (sponsored by the manufacturer) in 32 patients with t score <-1 at the lumbar spine or hip. They observed an increase in BMD of the lumbar spine of 4.6%±1.2% (mean±SEM) in the alendronate group compared with a decrease of 0.9%±1.0% in patients receiving placebo (P<0.01). BMD of the hip was unaffected. Treatment with alendronate significantly decreased biochemical markers of bone turnover.[169] Although in this trial no significant adverse events were reported, oral bisphosphonates can have gastrointestinal side effects, so the intravenous bisphosphonates have been used as alternatives. Stokkers et al treated 49 adult IBD patients (mean age, 40 years) with decreased BMD t scores and who received calcium and vitamin D supplementation with 30 mg of pamidronate administered every 3 months. After 1 year, mean t score of the lumbar spine increased by 0.51 (95% CI, 0.35 to 0.67; p<0.0004) and 0.39 in the femoral neck (95% CI, 0.24 to 0.53; p<0.0004). One patient developed fever with the infusion but otherwise the drug was well tolerated.[170] In another study, von Tirpitz et al infused ibandronate IV (1 mg every 3 months) in addition to daily calcium/vitamin D in 68 patients. The infusion was well tolerated and spine BMD increased by 5.4% after 27 months (p = 0.003). Treatment significantly reduced biomarkers of bone resorption.[171]

Summary

These data collectively show that oral and intravenous bisphosphonates can increase BMD, especially in the lumbar spine, in adults with IBD.

References

1. Nakashima K, Zhou X, Kunkel G, et al. The novel zinc finger-containing transcription factor Osterix is required for osteoblast differentiation and bone formation. Cell. 2002;108:17-29.

2. Zhang M, Xuan S, Bouxsein ML, et al. Osteoblast-specific knockout of the insulin-like growth factor (IGF) receptor gene reveals an essential role of IGF signaling in bone matrix mineralization. J Biol Chem. 2002;277(46):44005-44012.

3. Lian JB, Stein GS. Runx2/Cbfa1: a multifunctional regulator of bone formation. Curr Pharm Des. 2003;9(32):2677-2685.

4. Krishnan V, Bryant HU, MacDougald OA. Regulation of bone mass by Wnt signaling. J Clin Invest. 2006;116(5):1202-1209.

5. Winslow MM, Pan M, Starbuck M, et al. Calcineurin/NFAT signaling in osteoblasts regulates bone mass. Dev Cell. 2006;10(6):771-782.

6. Zayzafoon M. Calcium/calmodulin signaling controls osteoblast growth and differentiation. J Cellular Biochem. 2006;97(1):56-70.

7. Fuller K, Wong B, Fox S, Choi Y, Chambers TJ. TRANCE is necessary and sufficient for osteoblast-mediated activation of bone resorption in osteoclasts. *J Exp Med.* 1998;188(5):997-1001.

8. Udagawa N, Takahashi N, Yasuda H, et al. Osteoprotegerin produced by osteoblasts is an important regulator in osteoclast development and function. *Endocrinology.* 2000;141(9):3478-3484.

9. Takayanagi H, Kim S, Koga T, et al. Induction and activation of the transcription factor NFATc1 (NFAT2) integrate RANKL signaling in terminal differentiation of osteoclasts. *Dev Cell.* 2002;3(6):889-901.

10. Zhang YH, Heulsmann A, Tondravi MM, Mukherjee A, Abu-Amer Y. Tumor necrosis factor-alpha (TNF) stimulates RANKL-induced osteoclastogenesis via coupling of TNF type 1 receptor and RANK signaling pathways. *J Biol Chem.* 2001;276(1):563-568.

11. Kudo O, Fujikawa Y, Itonaga I, Sabokbar A, Torisu T, Athanasou NA. Proinflammatory cytokine (TNFalpha/IL-1alpha) induction of human osteoclast formation. *J Pathol.* 2002;198(2):220-227.

12. Yakar S, Rosen CJ, Beamer WG, et al. Circulating levels of IGF-1 directly regulate bone growth and density. *J Clin Invest.* 2002;110(6):771-781.

13. Kirschner BS, Sutton MM. Somatomedin-C levels in growth-impaired children and adolescents with chronic inflammatory bowel disease. *Gastroenterology.* 1986;91(4):830-836.

14. Schoenau E, Saggese G, Peter F, et al. From bone biology to bone analysis. *Horm Res.* 2004;61(6):257-269.

15. Canalis E. The fate of circulating osteoblasts. *N Engl J Med.* 2005;352(19):2014-2016.

16. Stains JP, Civitelli R. Cell-to-cell interactions in bone. *Biochem Biophys Res Commun.* 2005;328(3):721-727.

17. Soyka LA, Fairfield WP, Klibanski A. Clinical review 117: hormonal determinants and disorders of peak bone mass in children. *J Clin Endocrinol Metab.* 2000;85(11):3951-3963.

18. Raisz LG. Pathogenesis of osteoporosis: concepts, conflicts, and prospects. *J Clin Invest.* 2005;115(12):3318-3325.

19. Sanchez MM, Gilsanz V. Pediatric DXA bone measurements. *Pediatr Endocrinol Rev.* 2005;2(Suppl 3):337-341.

20. Schoenau E, Neu CM, Beck B, Manz F, Rauch F. Bone mineral content per muscle cross-sectional area as an index of the functional muscle-bone unit. *J Bone Miner Res.* 2002;17(6):1095-1101.

21. Wehrli FW, Song HK, Saha PK, Wright AC. Quantitative MRI for the assessment of bone structure and function. *NMR Biomed.* 2006;19(7):731-764.

22. Wren TA, Gilsanz V. Assessing bone mass in children and adolescents. *Curr Osteoporos Rep.* 2006;4(4):153-158.

23. Herzog D, Bishop N, Glorieux F, Seidman EG. Interpretation of bone mineral density values in pediatric Crohn's disease. *Inflamm Bowel Dis.* 1998;4(4):261-267.

24. Ahmed SF, Horrocks IA, Patterson T, et al. Bone mineral assessment by dual energy x-ray absorptiometry in children with inflammatory bowel disease: evaluation by age or bone area. *J Pediatr Gastroenterol Nutr.* 2004;38(3):276-280.

25. Assessment of fracture risk and its application to screening for postmenopausal osteoporosis: report of a WHO Study Group. *World Health Organ Tech Rep Ser.* 1994;843:1-129.

26. Writing Group for the ISCD Position Development Conference. Diagnosis of osteoporosis in men, premenopausal women, and children. *J Clin Densitom.* 2004;7(1):17-26.

27. Schoenau E, Neu MC, Manz F. Muscle mass during childhood: relationship to skeletal development. *J Musculoskelet Neuronal Interact.* 2004;4(1):105-108.

28. Semeao EJ, Jawad AF, Zemel BS, Neiswender KM, Piccoli DA, Stallings VA. Bone mineral density in children and young adults with Crohn's disease. *Inflamm Bowel Dis.* 1999;5(3):161-166.

29. Schoon EJ, Blok BM, Geerling BJ, Russel MG, Stockbrugger RW, Brummer RJ. Bone mineral density in patients with recently diagnosed inflammatory bowel disease. *Gastroenterology.* 2000;119(5):1203-1208.

30. Lamb EJ, Wong T, Smith DJ, et al. Metabolic bone disease is present at diagnosis in patients with inflammatory bowel disease. *Aliment Pharmacol Ther.* 2002;16(11):1895-1902.

31. Harpavat M, Keljo DJ, Regueiro MD. Metabolic bone disease in inflammatory bowel disease. *J Clin Gastroenterol.* 2004;38(3):218-224.

32. Sylvester FA, Wyzga N, Hyams JS, et al. Natural history of bone metabolism and bone mineral density in children with inflammatory bowel disease. *Inflamm Bowel Dis.* 2007;13(1):42-50.

33. Clements D, Motley RJ, Evans WD, et al. Longitudinal study of cortical bone loss in patients with inflammatory bowel disease. *Scand J Gastroenterol.* 1992;27(12):1055-1060.

34. Jahnsen J, Falch JA, Mowinckel P, Aadland E. Bone mineral density in patients with inflammatory bowel disease: a population-based prospective two-year follow-up study. *Scand J Gastroenterol.* 2004;39(2):145-153.

35. Schoon EJ, van Nunen AB, Wouters RS, Stockbrugger RW, Russel MG. Osteopenia and osteoporosis in Crohn's disease: prevalence in a Dutch population-based cohort. *Scand J Gastroenterol.* 2000;232:43-47.

36. Semeao EJ, Jawad AF, Stouffer NO, Zemel BS, Piccoli DA, Stallings VA. Risk factors for low bone mineral density in children and young adults with Crohn's disease. *J Pediatr.* 1999;135(5):593-600.

37. Paganelli M, Albanese C, Borrelli O, et al. Inflammation is the main determinant of low bone mineral density in pediatric inflammatory bowel disease. *Inflamm Bowel Dis.* 2007;13(4):416-423.

38. Boot AM, Bouquet J, Krenning EP, de Muinck Keizer-Schrama SM. Bone mineral density and nutritional status in children with chronic inflammatory bowel disease. *Gut.* 1998;42(2):188-194.

39. Andreassen H, Hylander E, Rix M. Gender, age, and body weight are the major predictive factors for bone mineral density in Crohn's disease: a case-control cross-sectional study of 113 patients. *Am J Gastroenterol.* 1999;94(3):824-828.

40. Burnham JM, Shults J, Semeao E, et al. Whole body BMC in pediatric Crohn disease: independent effects of altered growth, maturation, and body composition. *J Bone Miner Res.* 2004;19(12):1961-1968.

41. Burnham JM, Shults J, Semeao E, et al. Body-composition alterations consistent with cachexia in children and young adults with Crohn disease. *Am J Clin Nutr.* 2005;82(2):413-420.

42. Cowan FJ, Warner JT, Dunstan FD, Evans WD, Gregory JW, Jenkins HR. Inflammatory bowel disease and predisposition to osteopenia. *Arch Dis Child.* 1997;76(4):325-329.

43. von Scheven E, Gordon CM, Wypij D, Wertz M, Gallagher KT, Bachrach L. Variable deficits of bone mineral despite chronic glucocorticoid therapy in pediatric patients with inflammatory diseases: a Glaser Pediatric Research Network study. *J Pediatr Endocrinol Metab.* 2006;19(6):821-830.

44. Abitbol V, Roux C, Chaussade S, et al. Metabolic bone assessment in patients with inflammatory bowel disease. *Gastroenterology.* 1995;108(2):417-422.

45. Bernstein CN, Seeger LL, Sayre JW, Anton PA, Artinian L, Shanahan F. Decreased bone density in inflammatory bowel disease is related to corticosteroid use and not disease diagnosis. *J Bone Miner Res.* 1995;10(2):250-256.

46. Silvennoinen JA, Karttunen TJ, Niemela SE, Manelius JJ, Lehtola JK. A controlled study of bone mineral density in patients with inflammatory bowel disease. *Gut.* 1995;37(1):71-76.

47. Ardizzone S, Bollani S, Bettica P, Bevilacqua M, Molteni P, Bianchi Porro G. Altered bone metabolism in inflammatory bowel disease: there is a difference between Crohn's disease and ulcerative colitis. *J Intern Med.* 2000;247(1):63-70.

48. Siffiledeen JS, Fedorak RN, Siminoski K, et al. Bones and Crohn's: risk factors associated with low bone mineral density in patients with Crohn's disease. *Inflamm Bowel Dis.* 2004;10(3):220-228.

49. Frei P, Fried M, Hungerbuhler V, Rammert C, Rousson V, Kullak-Ublick GA. Analysis of risk factors for low bone mineral density in inflammatory bowel disease. *Digestion.* 2006;73(1):40-46.

50. Leonard MB. Glucocorticoid-induced osteoporosis in children: impact of the underlying disease. *Pediatrics.* 2007;119(Suppl 2):S166-S174.

51. Ghosh S, Cowen S, Hannan WJ, Ferguson A. Low bone mineral density in Crohn's disease, but not in ulcerative colitis, at diagnosis. *Gastroenterology.* 1994;107(4):1031-1039.

52. Gokhale R, Favus MJ, Karrison T, Sutton MM, Rich B, Kirschner BS. Bone mineral density assessment in children with inflammatory bowel disease. *Gastroenterology.* 1998;114(5):902-911.

53. Bernstein CN. Determinants of bone density in inflammatory bowel disease. *Gastroenterology.* 1995;108(5):1607-1609.

54. Motley RJ, Crawley EO, Evans C, Rhodes J, Compston JE. Increased rate of spinal trabecular bone loss in patients with inflammatory bowel disease. *Gut.* 1988;29(10):1332-1336.

55. Ryde SJ, Clements D, Evans WD, et al. Total body calcium in patients with inflammatory bowel disease: a longitudinal study. *Clin Sci (Lond).* 1991;80(4):319-324.

56. Roux C, Abitbol V, Chaussade S, Kolta S, Guillemant S, Dougados M, et al. Bone loss in patients with inflammatory bowel disease: a prospective study. *Osteoporos Int.* 1995;5(3):156-160.

57. Dresner-Pollak R, Karmeli F, Eliakim R, Ackerman Z, Rachmilewitz D. Increased urinary N-telopeptide cross-linked type 1 collagen predicts bone loss in patients with inflammatory bowel disease. *Am J Gastroenterol.* 2000;95(3):699-704.

58. Dinca M, Fries W, Luisetto G, et al. Evolution of osteopenia in inflammatory bowel disease. *Am J Gastroenterol.* 1999;94(5):1292-1297.

59. Motley RJ, Clements D, Evans WD, et al. A four-year longitudinal study of bone loss in patients with inflammatory bowel disease. *Bone Miner.* 1993;23(2):95-104.

60. Abitbol V, Roux C, Guillemant S, et al. Bone assessment in patients with ileal pouch-anal anastomosis for inflammatory bowel disease. *Br J Surg.* 1997;84(11):1551-1554.

61. de Jong DJ, Mannaerts L, van Rossum LG, Corstens FH, Naber AH. Longitudinal study of bone mineral density in patients with Crohn's disease. *Dig Dis Sci.* 2003;48(7):1355-1359.

62. Reffitt DM, Meenan J, Sanderson JD, Jugdaohsingh R, Powell JJ, Thompson RP. Bone density improves with disease remission in patients with inflammatory bowel disease. *Eur J Gastroenterol Hepatol.* 2003;15(12):1267-1273.

63. Issenman RM, Atkinson SA, Radoja C, Fraher L. Longitudinal assessment of growth, mineral metabolism, and bone mass in pediatric Crohn's disease. *J Pediatr Gastroenterol Nutr.* 1993;17(4):401-406.

64. Bernstein CN, Leslie WD, Taback SP. Bone density in a population-based cohort of premenopausal adult women with early onset inflammatory bowel disease. *Am J Gastroenterol.* 2003;98(5):1094-1100.

65. Haugeberg G, Vetvik K, Stallemo A, Bitter H, Mikkelsen B, Stokkeland M. Bone density reduction in patients with Crohn disease and associations with demographic and disease variables: cross-sectional data from a population-based study. *Scand J Gastroenterol.* 2001;36(7):759-765.

66. Gupta A, Paski S, Issenman R, Webber C. Lumbar spine bone mineral density at diagnosis and during follow-up in children with IBD. *J Clin Densitom.* 2004;7(3):290-295.

67. Silvennoinen J, Risteli L, Karttunen T, Risteli J. Increased degradation of type I collagen in patients with inflammatory bowel disease. *Gut.* 1996;38(2):223-228.

68. Robinson RJ, Iqbal SJ, Abrams K, Al-Azzawi F, Mayberry JF. Increased bone resorption in patients with Crohn's disease. *Aliment Pharmacol Ther.* 1998;12(8):699-705.

69. Bischoff SC, Herrmann A, Goke M, Manns MP, von zur Muhlen A, Brabant G. Altered bone metabolism in inflammatory bowel disease. *Am J Gastroenterol.* 1997;92(7):1157-1163.

70. Schoon EJ, Geerling BG, Van Dooren IM, et al. Abnormal bone turnover in long-standing Crohn's disease in remission. *Aliment Pharmacol Ther.* 2001;15(6):783-792.

71. Bjarnason I, Macpherson A, Mackintosh C, Buxton-Thomas M, Forgacs I, Moniz C. Reduced bone density in patients with inflammatory bowel disease. *Gut.* 1997;40(2):228-233.

72. Schulte C, Dignass AU, Mann K, Goebell H. Reduced bone mineral density and unbalanced bone metabolism in patients with inflammatory bowel disease. *Inflamm Bowel Dis.* 1998;4(4):268-275.

73. Bregenzer N, Erban P, Albrich H, et al. Screening for osteoporosis in patients with inflammatory bowel disease by using urinary N-telopeptides. *Eur J Gastroenterol Hepatol.* 2002;14(6):599-605.

74. Bartram SA, Peaston RT, Rawlings DJ, Walshaw D, Francis RM, Thompson NP. Mutifactorial analysis of risk factors for reduced bone mineral density in patients with Crohn's disease. *World J Gastroenterol.* 2006;12(35):5680-5686.

75. Gilman J, Shanahan F, Cashman KD. Altered levels of biochemical indices of bone turnover and bone-related vitamins in patients with Crohn's disease and ulcerative colitis. *Aliment Pharmacol Ther.* 2006;23(7):1007-1016.

76. Sylvester FA, Davis PM, Wyzga N, Hyams JS, Lerer T. Are activated T cells regulators of bone metabolism in children with Crohn disease? *J Pediatr.* 2006;148(4):461-466.

77. Hessov I, Mosekilde L, Melsen F, et al. Osteopenia with normal vitamin D metabolites after small-bowel resection for Crohn's disease. *Scand J Gastroenterol.* 1984;19(5):691-696.

78. Croucher PI, Vedi S, Motley RJ, Garrahan NJ, Stanton MR, Compston JE. Reduced bone formation in patients with osteoporosis associated with inflammatory bowel disease. *Osteoporos Int.* 1993;3(5):236-241.

79. Driscoll RH, Jr., Meredith SC, Sitrin M, Rosenberg IH. Vitamin D deficiency and bone disease in patients with Crohn's disease. *Gastroenterology.* 1982;83(6):1252-1258.

80. Burnham JM, Shults J, Petit MA, et al. Alterations in proximal femur geometry in children treated with glucocorticoids for Crohn disease or nephrotic syndrome: impact of the underlying disease. *J Bone Miner Res.* 2007;22(4):551-559.

81. Bernstein CN, Blanchard JF, Leslie W, Wajda A, Yu BN. The incidence of fracture among patients with inflammatory bowel disease: a population-based cohort study. *Ann Intern Med.* 2000;133(10):795-799.

82. Vestergaard P, Mosekilde L. Fracture risk in patients with celiac disease, Crohn's disease, and ulcerative colitis: a nationwide follow-up study of 16,416 patients in Denmark. *Am J Epidemiol.* 2002;156(1):1-10.

83. van Staa TP, Cooper C, Brusse LS, Leufkens H, Javaid MK, Arden NK. Inflammatory bowel disease and the risk of fracture. *Gastroenterology.* 2003;125(6):1591-1597.

84. Loftus EV Jr, Achenbach SJ, Sandborn WJ, Tremaine WJ, Oberg AL, Melton LJ, 3rd. Risk of fracture in ulcerative colitis: a population-based study from Olmsted County, Minnesota. *Clin Gastroenterol Hepatol.* 2003;1(6):465-473.

85. Loftus EV Jr, Crowson CS, Sandborn WJ, Tremaine WJ, O'Fallon WM, Melton LJ, 3rd. Long-term fracture risk in patients with Crohn's disease: a population-based study in Olmsted County, Minnesota. *Gastroenterology.* 2002;123(2):468-475.

86. Persad R, Jaffer I, Issenman RM. The prevalence of long bone fractures in pediatric inflammatory bowel disease. *J Pediatr Gastroenterol Nutr.* 2006;43(5):597-602.

87. Sylvester FA. Do bones crack under the effects of inflammatory bowel disease in children? *J Pediatr Gastroenterol Nutr.* 2006;43(5):563-565.

88. Roux C, Fechtenbaum J, Kolta S, Briot K, Girard M. Mild prevalent and incident vertebral fractures are risk factors for new fractures. *Osteoporos Int.* 2007;18(12):1617-1624.

89. Compston JE, Judd D, Crawley EO, et al. Osteoporosis in patients with inflammatory bowel disease. *Gut.* 1987;28(4):410-415.

90. Pigot F, Roux C, Chaussade S, et al. Low bone mineral density in patients with inflammatory bowel disease. *Dig Dis Sci.* 1992;37(9):1396-1403.

91. Cowan FJ, Parker DR, Jenkins HR. Osteopenia in Crohn's disease. *Arch Dis Child.* 1995;73(3):255-256.

92. Semeao EJ, Stallings VA, Peck SN, Piccoli DA. Vertebral compression fractures in pediatric patients with Crohn's disease. *Gastroenterology.* 1997;112(5):1710-1713.

93. Thearle M, Horlick M, Bilezikian JP, et al. Osteoporosis: an unusual presentation of childhood Crohn's disease. *J Clin Endocrinol Metab.* 2000;85(6):2122-2126.

94. Klaus J, Armbrecht G, Steinkamp M, et al. High prevalence of osteoporotic vertebral fractures in patients with Crohn's disease. *Gut.* 2002;51(5):654-658.

95. Stockbrugger RW, Schoon EJ, Bollani S, et al. Discordance between the degree of osteopenia and the prevalence of spontaneous vertebral fractures in Crohn's disease. *Aliment Pharmacol Ther.* 2002;16(8):1519-1527.

96. Siffledeen JS, Siminoski K, Jen H, Fedorak RN. Vertebral fractures and role of low bone mineral density in Crohn's disease. *Clin Gastroenterol Hepatol.* 2007;5(6):721-728.

97. Lin CL, Moniz C, Chambers TJ, Chow JW. Colitis causes bone loss in rats through suppression of bone formation. *Gastroenterology.* 1996;111(5):1263-1271.

98. Cohen SL, Moore AM, Ward WE. Interleukin-10 knockout mouse: a model for studying bone metabolism during intestinal inflammation. *Inflamm Bowel Dis.* 2004;10(5):557-563.

99. Dresner-Pollak R, Gelb N, Rachmilewitz D, Karmeli F, Weinreb M. Interleukin 10-deficient mice develop osteopenia, decreased bone formation, and mechanical fragility of long bones. *Gastroenterology.* 2004;127(3):792-801.

100. Byrne FR, Morony S, Warmington K, et al. CD4+CD45RBHi T cell transfer induced colitis in mice is accompanied by osteopenia which is treatable with recombinant human osteoprotegerin. *Gut.* 2005;54(1):78-86.

101. Ashcroft AJ, Cruickshank SM, Croucher PI, et al. Colonic dendritic cells, intestinal inflammation, and T cell-mediated bone destruction are modulated by recombinant osteoprotegerin. *Immunity.* 2003;19(6):849-861.

102. Hela S, Nihel M, Faten L, et al. Osteoporosis and Crohn's disease. *Joint Bone Spine.* 2005;72(5):403-407.

103. Andreassen H, Rix M, Brot C, Eskildsen P. Regulators of calcium homeostasis and bone mineral density in patients with Crohn's disease. *Scand J Gastroenterol.* 1998;33(10):1087-1093.

104. Sentongo TA, Semaeo EJ, Stettler N, Piccoli DA, Stallings VA, Zemel BS. Vitamin D status in children, adolescents, and young adults with Crohn disease. *Am J Clin Nutr.* 2002;76(5):1077-1081.

105. Siffledeen JS, Siminoski K, Steinhart H, Greenberg G, Fedorak RN. The frequency of vitamin D deficiency in adults with Crohn's disease. *Can J Gastroenterol.* 2003;17(8):473-478.

106. McCarthy D, Duggan P, O'Brien M, et al. Seasonality of vitamin D status and bone turnover in patients with Crohn's disease. *Aliment Pharmacol Ther.* 2005;21(9):1073-1083.

107. Pappa HM, Gordon CM, Saslowsky TM, et al. Vitamin D status in children and young adults with inflammatory bowel disease. *Pediatrics.* 2006;118(5):1950-1961.

108. Haderslev KV, Jeppesen PB, Sorensen HA, Mortensen PB, Staun M. Vitamin D status and measurements of markers of bone metabolism in patients with small intestinal resection. *Gut.* 2003;52(5):653-658.

109. Silvennoinen J, Lamberg-Allardt C, Karkkainen M, Niemela S, Lehtola J. Dietary calcium intake and its relation to bone mineral density in patients with inflammatory bowel disease. *J Intern Med.* 1996;240(5):285-292.

110. Bernstein CN, Bector S, Leslie WD. Lack of relationship of calcium and vitamin D intake to bone mineral density in premenopausal women with inflammatory bowel disease. *Am J Gastroenterol.* 2003;98(11):2468-2473.

111. Vogelsang H, Ferenci P, Resch H, Kiss A, Gangl A. Prevention of bone mineral loss in patients with Crohn's disease by long-term oral vitamin D supplementation. *Eur J Gastroenterol Hepatol.* 1995;7(7):609-614.

112. Abitbol V, Mary JY, Roux C, et al. Osteoporosis in inflammatory bowel disease: effect of calcium and vitamin D with or without fluoride. *Aliment Pharmacol Ther.* 2002;16(5):919-927.

113. Bernstein CN, Seeger LL, Anton PA, et al. A randomized, placebo-controlled trial of calcium supplementation for decreased bone density in corticosteroid-using patients with inflammatory bowel disease: a pilot study. *Aliment Pharmacol Ther.* 1996;10(5):777-786.

114. Compston JE. Boning up on vitamin K. *Gut.* 2001;48(4):448-449.

115. Schoon EJ, Muller MCA, Vermeer C, Schurgers LJ, Brummer R-JM, Stockbrugger RW. Low serum and bone vitamin K status in patients with longstanding Crohn's disease: another pathogenetic factor of osteoporosis in Crohn's disease? *Gut.* 2001;48(4):473-477.

116. Duggan P, O'Brien M, Kiely M, McCarthy J, Shanahan F, Cashman KD. Vitamin K status in patients with Crohn's disease and relationship to bone turnover. *Am J Gastroenterol.* 2004;99(11):2178-2185.

117. Franchimont N, Reenaers C, Lambert C, et al. Increased expression of receptor activator of NF-kappa B ligand (RANKL), its receptor RANK and its decoy receptor osteoprotegerin in the colon of Crohn's disease patients. *Clin Exp Immunol.* 2004;138(3):491-498.

118. Canalis E. Clinical review 83: Mechanisms of glucocorticoid action in bone: implications to glucocorticoid-induced osteoporosis. *J Clin Endocrinol Metab.* 1996;81(10):3441-3447.

119. Reid IR. Glucocorticoid effects on bone. *J Clin Endocrinol Metab.* 1998;83(6):1860-1862.

120. van Staa TP, Cooper C, Leufkens HG, Bishop N. Children and the risk of fractures caused by oral corticosteroids. *J Bone Miner Res.* 2003;18(5):913-918.

121. van Staa TP, Leufkens HG, Abenhaim L, Zhang B, Cooper C. Oral corticosteroids and fracture risk: relationship to daily and cumulative doses. *Rheumatology (Oxford).* 2000;39(12):1383-1389.

122. Dear KL, Compston JE, Hunter JO. Treatments for Crohn's disease that minimise steroid doses are associated with a reduced risk of osteoporosis. *Clin Nutr.* 2001;20(6):541-546.

123. von Tirpitz C, Epp S, Klaus J, et al. Effect of systemic glucocorticoid therapy on bone metabolism and the osteoprotegerin system in patients with active Crohn's disease. *Eur J Gastroenterol Hepatol.* 2003;15(11):1165-1170.

124. Walther F, Fusch C, Radke M, Beckert S, Findeisen A. Osteoporosis in pediatric patients suffering from chronic inflammatory bowel disease with and without steroid treatment. *J Pediatr Gastroenterol Nutr.* 2006;43(1):42-51.

125. Schoon EJ, Bollani S, Mills PR, et al. Bone mineral density in relation to efficacy and side effects of budesonide and prednisolone in Crohn's disease. *Clin Gastroenterol Hepatol.* 2005;3(2):113-121.

126. Frost HM. Bone "mass" and the "mechanostat": a proposal. *Anat Rec.* 1987;219(1):1-9.

127. Jahnsen J, Falch JA, Mowinckel P, Aadland E. Body composition in patients with inflammatory bowel disease: a population-based study. *Am J Gastroenterol.* 2003;98(7):1556-1562.

128. Mauro M, Armstrong D. Evaluation of densitometric bone-muscle relationships in Crohn's disease. *Bone.* 2007;40(6):1610-1614.

129. Tjellesen L, Nielsen PK, Staun M. Body composition by dual-energy x-ray absorptiometry in patients with Crohn's disease. *Scand J Gastroenterol.* 1998;33(9):956-960.

130. Ng V, Millard W, Lebrun C, Howard J. Exercise and Crohn's disease: speculations on potential benefits. *Can J Gastroenterol.* 2006;20(10):657-660.

131. Schulte CM, Dignass AU, Goebell H, Roher HD, Schulte KM. Genetic factors determine extent of bone loss in inflammatory bowel disease. *Gastroenterology.* 2000;119(4):909-920.

132. Todhunter CE, Sutherland-Craggs A, Bartram SA, et al. The influence of IL6, COL1A1 and VDR gene polymorphisms on bone mineral density in Crohn's disease. *Gut.* 2005;54(11):1579-1584.

133. Nemetz A, Toth M, Garcia-Gonzalez MA, et al. Allelic variation at the interleukin 1beta gene is associated with decreased bone mass in patients with inflammatory bowel diseases. *Gut.* 2001;49(5):644-649.

134. Schulte C, Goebell H, Roher HD, Schulte KM. Genetic determinants of IL-6 expression levels do not influence bone loss in inflammatory bowel disease. *Dig Dis Sci.* 2001;46(11):2521-2528.

135. Lee N, Fowler E, Mason S, Lincoln D, Taaffe DR, Radford-Smith G. Tumor necrosis factor-alpha haplotype is strongly associated with bone mineral density in patients with Crohn's disease. *J Gastroenterol Hepatol.* 2007;22(6):913-919.

136. Kudo O, Sabokbar A, Pocock A, Itonaga I, Fujikawa Y, Athanasou NA. Interleukin-6 and interleukin-11 support human osteoclast formation by a RANKL-independent mechanism. *Bone.* 2003;32(1):1-7.

137. Udagawa N, Takahashi N, Katagiri T, et al. Interleukin (IL)-6 induction of osteoclast differentiation depends on IL-6 receptors expressed on osteoblastic cells but not on osteoclast progenitors. *J Exp Med.* 1995;182(5):1461-1468.

138. Zou W, Hakim I, Tschoep K, Endres S, Bar-Shavit Z. Tumor necrosis factor-alpha mediates RANK ligand stimulation of osteoclast differentiation by an autocrine mechanism. *J Cell Biochem.* 2001;83(1):70-83.

139. Gowen M, MacDonald BR, Russell RG. Actions of recombinant human gamma-interferon and tumor necrosis factor alpha on the proliferation and osteoblastic characteristics of human trabecular bone cells in vitro. *Arthritis Rheum.* 1988;31(12):1500-1507.

140. Takayanagi H, Ogasawara K, Hida S, et al. T-cell-mediated regulation of osteoclastogenesis by signaling cross-talk between RANKL and IFN-gamma. *Nature.* 2000;408(6812):600-605.

141. Sylvester FA, Wyzga N, Hyams JS, Gronowicz GA. Effect of Crohn's disease on bone metabolism in vitro: a role for interleukin-6. *J Bone Miner Res.* 2002;17(4):695-702.

142. Gilbert L, He X, Farmer P, et al. Inhibition of osteoblast differentiation by tumor necrosis factor-alpha. *Endocrinology.* 2000;141(11):3956-3964.

143. Gilbert L, He X, Farmer P, et al. Expression of the osteoblast differentiation factor RUNX2 (Cbfa1/AML3/Pebp2alpha A) is inhibited by tumor necrosis factor-alpha. *J Biol Chem.* 2002;277(4):2695-2701.

144. Kaneki H, Guo R, Chen D, et al. Tumor necrosis factor promotes Runx2 degradation through up-regulation of Smurf1 and Smurf2 in osteoblasts. *J Biol Chem.* 2006;281(7):4326-4333.

145. Lu X, Gilbert L, He X, Rubin J, Nanes MS. Transcriptional regulation of the Osterix (Osx, Sp7) promoter by tumor necrosis factor identifies disparate effects of mitogen-activated protein kinase and NF kappa B pathways. *J Biol Chem.* 2006;281(10):6297-6306.

146. Uno JK, Kolek OI, Hines ER, et al. The role of tumor necrosis factor-α in down-regulation of osteoblast Phex gene expression in experimental murine colitis. *Gastroenterology.* 2006;131(2):497-509.

147. Teng Y-TA, Nguyen H, Gao X, et al. Functional human T-cell immunity and osteoprotegerin ligand control alveolar bone destruction in periodontal infection. *J Clin Invest.* 2000;106(6):R59-R67.

148. Kotake S, Udagawa N, Hakoda M, et al. Activated human T cells directly induce osteoclastogenesis from human monocytes: possible role of T cells in bone destruction in rheumatoid arthritis patients. *Arthritis Rheum.* 2001;44(5):1003-1012.

149. Pacifici R. T cells and post menopausal osteoporosis in murine models. *Arthritis Res Ther.* 2007;9(2):102.

150. Roggia C, Tamone C, Cenci S, Pacifici R, Isaia GC. Role of TNF-alpha producing T-cells in bone loss induced by estrogen deficiency. *Minerva Med.* 2004;95(2):125-132.

151. Ashcroft AJ, Carding SR. RANK ligand and osteoprotegerin: emerging roles in mucosal inflammation. *Gut.* 2005;54(9):1345-1346.

152. Bernstein CN, Sargent M, Leslie WD. Serum osteoprotegerin is increased in Crohn's disease: a population-based case control study. *Inflamm Bowel Dis.* 2005;11(4):325-330.

153. Moschen AR, Kaser A, Enrich B, et al. The RANKL/OPG system is activated in inflammatory bowel disease and relates to the state of bone loss. *Gut.* 2005;54(4):479-487.

154. Compston J. Osteoporosis in inflammatory bowel disease. *Gut.* 2003;52(1):63-64.

155. Recommendations for the prevention and treatment of glucocorticoid-induced osteoporosis: 2001 update. American College of Rheumatology Ad Hoc Committee on Glucocorticoid-Induced Osteoporosis. *Arthritis Rheum.* 2001;44(7):1496-1503.

156. D'Haens G, Verstraete A, Cheyns K, Aerden I, Bouillon R, Rutgeerts P. Bone turnover during short-term therapy with methylprednisolone or budesonide in Crohn's disease. *Aliment Pharmacol Ther.* 1998;12(5):419-424.

157. Floren CH, Ahren B, Bengtsson M, Bartosik J, Obrant K. Bone mineral density in patients with Crohn's disease during long-term treatment with azathioprine. *J Intern Med.* 1998;243(2):123-126.

158. Bernstein M, Irwin S, Greenberg GR. Maintenance infliximab treatment is associated with improved bone mineral density in Crohn's disease. *Am J Gastroenterol.* 2005;100(9):2031-2035.

159. Lee N, Radford-Smith G, Taaffe DR. Bone loss in Crohn's disease: exercise as a potential countermeasure. *Inflamm Bowel Dis.* 2005;11(12):1108-1118.

160. Pazianas M, Rhim AD, Weinberg AM, Su C, Lichtenstein GR. The effect of anti-TNF-alpha therapy on spinal bone mineral density in patients with Crohn's disease. *Ann N Y Acad Sci.* 2006;1068:543-556.

161. Thayu M, Leonard MB, Hyams J. Improvement in a biomarker of bone formation during infliximab therapy in pediatric Crohn Disease: results of the REACH study. In: First International Symposium on Pediatric Inflammatory Bowel Disease; Rome, Italy; 2006.

162. Franchimont N, Putzeys V, Collette J, et al. Rapid improvement of bone metabolism after infliximab treatment in Crohn's disease. *Aliment Pharmacol Ther.* 2004;20(6):607-614.

163. Ryan BM, Russel MG, Schurgers L, et al. Effect of antitumor necrosis factor-alpha therapy on bone turnover in patients with active Crohn's disease: a prospective study. *Aliment Pharmacol Ther.* 2004;20(8):851-857.

164. Abreu MT, Geller JL, Vasiliauskas EA, et al. Treatment with infliximab is associated with increased markers of bone formation in patients with Crohn's disease. *J Clin Gastroenterol.* 2006;40(1):55-63.

165. Miheller P, Muzes G, Zagoni T, Toth M, Racz K, Tulassay Z. Infliximab therapy improves the bone metabolism in fistulizing Crohn's disease. *Dig Dis.* 2006;24(1-2):201-206.

166. Robinson RJ, Krzywicki T, Almond L, et al. Effect of a low-impact exercise program on bone mineral density in Crohn's disease: a randomized controlled trial. *Gastroenterology.* 1998;115(1):36-41.

167. Siffledeen JS, Fedorak RN, Siminoski K, et al. Randomized trial of etidronate plus calcium and vitamin D for treatment of low bone mineral density in Crohn's disease. *Clin Gastroenterol Hepatol.* 2005;3(2):122-132.

168. Bartram SA, Peaston RT, Rawlings DJ, Francis RM, Thompson NP. A randomized controlled trial of calcium with vitamin D, alone or in combination with intravenous pamidronate, for the treatment of low bone mineral density associated with Crohn's disease. *Aliment Pharmacol Ther.* 2003;18(11-12):1121-1127.

169. Haderslev KV, Tjellesen L, Sorensen HA, Staun M. Alendronate increases lumbar spine bone mineral density in patients with Crohn's disease. *Gastroenterology.* 2000;119(3):639-646.

170. Stokkers PC, Deley M, Van Der Spek M, Verberne HJ, Van Deventer SJ, Hommes DW. Intravenous pamidronate in combination with calcium and vitamin D: highly effective in the treatment of low bone mineral density in inflammatory bowel disease. *Scand J Gastroenterol.* 2006;41(2):200-204.

171. von Tirpitz C, Klaus J, Steinkamp M, et al. Therapy of osteoporosis in patients with Crohn's disease: a randomized study comparing sodium fluoride and ibandronate. *Aliment Pharmacol Ther.* 2003;17(6):807-816.

INFLAMMATORY BOWEL DISEASE AND THE ADOLESCENT

*Robbyn E. Sockolow, MD; Aliza B. Solomon, DO;
and Oren L. Koslowe, MD*

Childhood-onset inflammatory bowel disease (IBD) poses unique clinical and psychosocial challenges for the pediatric gastroenterologist. It is during this time when a child with IBD transitions from adolescence to adulthood that situations arise that may not have been addressed previously. IBD is not unique, being a chronic illness affecting children and adults alike. The challenges in treating patients with IBD transitioning from childhood to adulthood have little to do with disease progression and a lot to do with individual progression.

Adolescence is a stage during which people are searching for their identities, struggling to maintain individuality, and dealing with their sexuality. The attention paid to a chronic illness often falls by the wayside during such a trying time. It is therefore the job of the health care team to provide an environment that allows for individual growth and maturity, separation from parents, and promotion of personal responsibility. This process begins with an open dialogue between the health care provider and the young IBD patient to discuss information about his or her disease and address questions and concerns he or she may have.

A hallmark of the adolescent period is the struggle to become independent and autonomous.[1] During early adolescence, there is a tendency to separate from family while spending more time with friends and peers. The onset of puberty poses an even greater strain on the relationship between adolescents and their families as hormones rage and defiance sets in. Chronic disease, IBD in particular, can be most difficult to handle during this period because of delayed growth or menarche, altered physical appearance due to disease or medications, and delayed intellectual maturity. With advancing age follows the desire for self-sufficiency and the increasing propensity for children to distance themselves from their parents both physically and socially. Finally, these children begin to think about their futures in concrete terms while in the past their futures were only hypothetical.[1]

This dynamic presents an interesting and complex situation for physicians working with children who have chronic medical conditions. During this time, teenage issues such as grades, gym, driving, and the search for independence give way to sexual intimacy, work and disability, starting a family, and additional disease processes.[2,3]

Scherl EJ, Dubinsky MC.
*The Changing World of Inflammatory Bowel Disease:
Impact of Generation, Gender, and Global Trends (pp 119-126)*
© 2009 SLACK Incorporated.

The issue of quality of life as it relates to adolescents with IBD involves several components. Not all components affect each adolescent equally, but most of those with IBD will be impacted in some way. There are several other factors, each important with respect to IBD in the adolescent, that when taken together may be seen to alter and impact on the daily activities of these young adults. Such factors include the physical signs associated with IBD, medication use, depression, anxiety, substance abuse, fatigue, hospitalization, and altered bowel habits.[4]

There is a wide range of physical stigmata that may be associated with IBD, any one of which may be particularly bothersome to an individual. Growth retardation and delayed menarche are not the subjects of this chapter, but their association with IBD plays a profound role in affecting adolescent self-image. Adolescence is a key period of physical and psychological development when fitting in is crucial, and in altering one's ability to assimilate, IBD can be devastating. Furthermore, adolescents who have undergone surgery are often left with large scars or ostomies. These marks may be easier to conceal than short stature or delayed development, but they may have a deep impact on self-esteem and willingness to partake in events and physical activities. Finally, anorectal disease may have significant consequences related to sexual intimacy. Fistulous tracts, abscesses, and enlarged skin tags may all contribute to decreased sexual activity. While the impact of IBD on sexual function has only been studied in adults,[5,6] there is no doubt that pediatric gastroenterologists care for a sizable sexually active community whose lives are also significantly affected.

Related to physical stigmata, as well as the notion of self-image, are eating disorders. IBD and Crohn's disease in particular have many overlapping features with eating disorders. The weight loss, decreased appetite, loss of energy, and depression seen with IBD may lead a practitioner in the appropriate setting to think of anorexia nervosa. The appropriate setting is precisely the topic of this chapter (ie, adolescence). Anorexia is most frequently diagnosed in teenage girls, and the shared features of the disease can make the correct diagnosis difficult. The main distinguishing feature that is present in anorexia and absent in Crohn's disease is an altered self-image, here referring specifically to the belief that he or she is overweight when he or she is not. While people with IBD may certainly have a poor self-image as described above, it is not usually that they are overweight. There are case reports of IBD and anorexia occurring simultaneously[7-10]; however, it is quite rare and there is no evidence that the incidence of eating disorders among those with IBD is greater than that in the general population. The current availability of laboratory tests, serology, and endoscopy should all but eliminate the number of individuals with eating disorders previously thought to have IBD. Conversely, the increasing awareness of IBD, especially within the adolescent population, and a wide array of diagnostic tools should prevent the prolonged misdiagnosis of eating disorders in patients with IBD.

Management of IBD involves the administration of medication, and often children are required to take numerous pills during the course of a single day. Early diagnosis often leads to the need to cope with the disease and inconvenience of medications for years. Some studies suggest that adolescents have low rates of adherence with their medication regimens.[11] Obstacles to medication use may include pill size, number of pills needed to be taken, and frequency of administration. Additionally, physicians may prescribe medications in the form of rectal preparations. Noncompliance with rectal medications is thought to be due to reluctance to use them because of perceived social stigmata, frustration, or inability to use them correctly.[12] Rectal medications often require specific instructions for proper use, which may not be routinely addressed by the physician. It is often inconvenient to administer them, as they may need to be given in the evening or multiple times during the day. This may cause embarrassment for the adolescent because the medications may need to be administered during school or when socializing with friends. Also, administration may cause local pain, leading to further noncompliance. Physicians must find creative methods for detecting noncompliance. In studies with children with HIV, useful methods for monitoring compliance include pill counts and therapeutic drug monitoring.[13] Thiopurine drug monitoring has been used to guide therapy as well as detect noncompliance in IBD.[14,15] It has been suggested that there is a higher level of family dysfunction in children with IBD compared to both healthy controls and other chronic illnesses.[15] Family dysfunction and inadequate coping strategies are issues that may contribute to noncompliance.[11]

Adolescence is a time during which there is an emphasis on peer relationship, and IBD often has its onset during this period. The symptoms of IBD, including abdominal bloating, diarrhea, delayed growth, or delayed puberty, may cause embarrassing and stressful situations for these teens. These symptoms may limit social interactions and isolate the adolescent. Adolescents with IBD have been reported to have more anxious or depressed symptoms and have more significant social problems than healthy controls.[16] They have also reported having fewer friends compared to healthy adolescents.[16]

This isolation and limited social interaction may contribute to the development of depressive symptoms. Patients with ulcerative colitis (UC) and Crohn's disease (CD) have been found to have a higher incidence of depression and anxiety.[17,18] Social support has been shown to have an inverse relationship with depression, and those who are single often report more depression than those who are married.[19] Adolescence is a time when there is a movement toward independence and a disconnection from families. As previously stated, the consequences of suffering from IBD may further limit social interactions and offer an insight into why adolescents with IBD suffer from depression.

The anxiety felt by adolescents with IBD stems a great deal from fear of relapse, which makes it difficult to enjoy life even while in remission. Everything from nights out with friends, to going to museums, to test taking is fraught with concern of relapse and fear that the closest bathroom may be too far away or occupied.[20] This baseline anxiety affects mood, character, and appetite and may promote symptoms of irritable bowel syndrome in those who are predisposed. Such anxiety may be all consuming and prevent participation in even the most mundane activities. Not only does it limit one's desire to participate, but its presence decreases the desire of his or her peers to include him or her in events.[21,22]

Substance abuse is a situation known to plague adolescents. In general, it is a frequent comorbid condition with anxiety and depression.[23] Screening for recreational drug use should be an element of a physician's history. Frequently, these questions are addressed to the adolescent independently from his or her parents. Cigarettes are a commonly abused substance during adolescence.[23] Smoking has been studied in IBD and affects UC and CD differently. Smoking may have a protective effect on UC, but often worsens CD.[24] Questioning about its use may aid the practitioner in tailoring therapy or understanding persistence of disease activity despite medication administration.

Fatigue is a very common complaint among adolescents with IBD and is often one of the first signs of an ensuing flare. It impacts peoples' lives in a more subtle way than anxiety but may be just as damaging to their enjoyment of daily activities. While the presence of anxiety is frequently volunteered by the patient or ascertained by an observant physician, fatigue is rarely noted unless specifically inquired about. Upon questioning, adolescents may acknowledge an inability to run as long as usual, climb as many steps, or stay awake in class. Fatigue may therefore impact some of the most important components of adolescents' lives, including academics and athletics. The element of fatigue is not limited to disruption of events during the school year but throughout the year. This includes participation, or even attendance, at camp, weekends with friends, and family vacations. The inability to participate in family events is of particular importance as it may focus feelings of disappointment from other family members onto the child with IBD. Such children often feel compelled to attend events or partake in activities that frequently result in further setbacks due to progression of disease activity.[21,22]

In a similar vein, recurrent hospitalizations upset the routine of life in high school.[21,22] Exams, proms, trips, and vacations are all crucial events during adolescence. Missing out on them due to hospitalization may lead to a sense of isolation and loss of camaraderie from friends and classmates.[25] Those who are frequently admitted come to look at the hospital as home, and its staff as friends. A series of cyclical events ensues through which hospitalization promotes isolation, leading to depression and anxiety, prolonging hospital stays. Adolescence is a time for participation—be it in class, extracurricular activities, the movies, or dating—and frequent hospitalization disrupts all of these activities.

The change in bowel habits associated with IBD may mean anywhere from 2 to 20 liquid stools per day, increased urgency, incontinence, and flatulence. Each of those could significantly alter one's daily activities, and in combination may make things quite unmanageable. Social norms being what they are and teenagers being who they are, it is not at all difficult to imagine why the thought of attending school with any of the above symptoms does not seem at all attractive. These issues may be of particular concern to adolescent girls for whom there is little acceptance among peers for someone who seems at all different. The issue of sexuality comes in to play here again as disease activity and increased urgency are likely to dissuade individuals from intimacy.[5,6]

As mentioned above, all the components of disease activity taken together significantly impact the quality of life for adolescents with IBD. As such, it is incumbent upon the pediatric gastroenterologist to address each issue. It may be clear during a visit that a child appears depressed, but the source of that depression must be addressed. Often the most important feature of disease to control from the physician standpoint is not the same as from the patient standpoint. Such incongruity may lead to frustration and a deepening sense of isolation due to the adolescent's feeling that he or she is misunderstood.[20] Social programs and camps for children and adolescents with IBD may be particularly helpful to such individuals and may help them learn to express their specific concerns more concretely to their physician, family, and friends. Camps in particular should be discussed as they are often short, 1 or 2 weeks, and may provide the first opportunity for adolescents to be open about their fears as well as hear how others have endured similar circumstances to their own.[26]

Outpatient and inpatient care must also be formatted uniquely for adolescents. Physicians must be aware of local laws that may impact when patients can be seen alone, until what ages they are covered by parental insurance, and what steps must be taken to ensure appropriate follow-up. They must also be aware of laws that impact their patients' education. Section 504 of the Rehabilitation Act of 1973, the Americans with Disabilities Act (ADA) of 1990, and the Individuals with Disabilities Education Act (IDEA)—amended in 2004—should all be familiar to the medical provider. Section 504 protects individuals such as those with physical impairments that limit major life activities from discrimination, including denial of equal education benefits. The ADA essentially extended the Civil Rights Act of 1964 to apply to those with disabilities as well. The IDEA mandates that any state or school district receiving federal funds provide a "free appropriate public education (FAPE)," identify those children in need of special services, and create an "individual education program (IEP)" outlining what is required for individuals that will receive services. This is common terminology in public schools, and parents will inquire about their child's ability to qualify for special considerations under those laws. Pediatric gastroenterologists must often author letters to school boards for extended time for exams, frequent restroom visits, and prolonged absences. More information related to education may be found at www.CCFA.org and www.ed.gov. As parents are often overwhelmed with the medical components of their child's illness, physicians should be forthcoming about information related to available services and programs in the event that the parent does not ask. In certain circumstances, such services may provide some relief of the significant financial burden that can accompany IBD, as well as alleviate some of the academic stress on the child.

The hospitalization of patients in their late teens and early twenties must be worked out with the adult and pediatric services as hospitals frequently have guidelines in place mandating that people above a certain age be placed on an adult floor and vice-versa. Such placement often impedes the ability of the primary physician to provide appropriate care. In such circumstances, an earlier move to an adult gastroenterologist may be warranted to avoid an awkward transition during a hospital stay. Steps for transitioning a patient from adolescent care to adult care will be discussed in Chapter 10.

There are several concerns beyond age that warrant special mention in this chapter and have been mentioned in position statements by the American Academy of Pediatrics, American Academy of Family Physicians, North American Society for Pediatric Gastroenterology, Hepatology and Nutrition, and others.[27-29] The American Academy of Pediatrics published a policy statement in 2002 that emphasized not only the need for developmentally appropriate care but also coordination of care and health care coverage for young adults with special needs.[27] A position paper from the Society for Adolescent Medicine (SAM) published in 2003 included recommendations for ensuring successful transition to adult care.[28] The SAM recommendations included designating a responsible primary physician to coordinate health care, ongoing patient and family education, increasing availability of services for adolescents, and encouraging further research in this area. As it is often the pediatric gastroenterologist that assumes the role of primary care provider for children with IBD, he or she becomes the focus of such position statements. Gastroenterologists must advocate for the patient in all areas, particularly those in which the patient and family are not well versed. In the area of chronic illness, it is often in the physician's capacity to address the questions not asked and assess the fears not mentioned that determines how successfully the disease is managed.

References

1. Behrman RE, Kliegman R, Jenson HB. *Nelson Textbook of Pediatrics.* 17th ed. Philadelphia, PA: Saunders; 2004:53-58.
2. Rettig P, Athreya BH. Adolescents with chronic disease: transition to adult health care. *Arthritis Care Res.* 1991;4(4):174-180.
3. Wallis C. Transition of care in children with chronic disease. *BMJ.* 2007;334(7606):1231-1232.
4. Calsbeek H, Rijken M, Bekkers MJ, Dekker J, van Berge Henegouwen GP. School and leisure activities in adolescents and young adults with chronic digestive disorders: impact of burden of disease. *Int J Behav Med.* 2006;13(2):121-130.
5. Trachter AB, Rogers AI, Leiblum SR. Inflammatory bowel disease in women: impact on relationship and sexual health. *Inflamm Bowel Dis.* 2002;8(6):413-421.
6. Timmer A, Bauer A, Dignass A, Rogler G. Sexual function in persons with inflammatory bowel disease: a survey with matched controls. *Clin Gastroenterol Hepatol.* 2007;5(1):87-94.
7. Holaday M, Smith KE, Robertson S, Dallas J. An atypical eating disorder with Crohn's disease in a fifteen-year-old male: a case study. *Adolescence.* 1994;29(116):865-873.
8. Jenkins AP, Treasure J, Thompson RP. Crohn's disease presenting as anorexia nervosa. *Br Med J (Clin Res Ed).* 1988;296(6623):699-700.
9. Mallett P, Murch S. Anorexia nervosa complicating inflammatory bowel disease. *Arch Dis Child.* 1990;65(3):298-300.
10. Metcalfe-Gibson C. Anorexia nervosa and Crohn's disease. *Br J Surg.* 1978;65(4):231-233.
11. Mackner LM, Crandall WV. Oral medication adherence in pediatric inflammatory bowel disease. *Inflamm Bowel Dis.* 2005;11(11):1006-1012.
12. Towler R, Silcock J, Raynor DK, Moayyedi P. Users reviews about compliance with rectally administered medicines. *Intern Journ Pharm.* 2003;11:abstract R13.
13. Simoni JM, Montgomery A, Martin E, New M, Demas PA, Rana S. Adherence to antiretroviral therapy for pediatric HIV infection: a qualitative systematic review with recommendations for research and clinical management. *Pediatrics.* 2007;119(6):e1371-1383.
14. Gearry RB, Barclay ML. Azathioprine and 6-mercaptopurine pharmacogenetics and metabolite monitoring in inflammatory bowel disease. *J Gastroenterol Hepatol.* 2005;20(8):1149-1157.
15. Ooi CY, Bohane TD, Lee D, Naidoo D, Day AS. Thiopurine metabolite monitoring in paediatric inflammatory bowel disease. *Aliment Pharmacol Ther.* 2007;25(8):941-947.
16. Engstrom I. Parental distress and social interaction in families with children with inflammatory bowel disease. *J Am Acad Child Adolesc Psychiatry.* 1991;30(6):904-912.
17. Kurina LM, Goldacre MJ, Yeates D, Gill LE. Depression and anxiety in people with inflammatory bowel disease. *J Epidemiol Community Health.* 2001;55(10):716-720.
18. Magni G, Bernasconi G, Mauro P, et al. Psychiatric diagnoses in ulcerative colitis: a controlled study. *Br J Psychiatry.* 1991;158:413-415.
19. Fuller-Thomson E, Sulman J. Depression and inflammatory bowel disease: findings from two nationally representative Canadian surveys. *Inflamm Bowel Dis.* 2006;12(8):697-707.

20. Akobeng AK, Suresh-Babu MV, Firth D, Miller V, Mir P, Thomas AG. Quality of life in children with Crohn's disease: a pilot study. *J Pediatr Gastroenterol Nutr.* 1999;28(4):S37-S39.

21. Nicholas DB, Otley A, Smith C, Avolio J, Munk M, Griffiths AM. Challenges and strategies of children and adolescents with inflammatory bowel disease: a qualitative examination. *Health Qual Life Outcomes.* 2007;5:28.

22. Graff LA, Walker JR, Lix L, et al. The relationship of inflammatory bowel disease type and activity to psychological functioning and quality of life. *Clin Gastroenterol Hepatol.* 2006;4(12):1491-1501.

23. Compton WM, Thomas YF, Stinson FS, Grant BF. Prevalence, correlates, disability, and comorbidity of DSM-IV drug abuse and dependence in the United States: results from the national epidemiologic survey on alcohol and related conditions. *Arch Gen Psychiatry.* 2007;64(5):566-576.

24. Karban A, Eliakim R. Effect of smoking on inflammatory bowel disease: is it disease or organ specific? *World J Gastroenterol.* 2007;13(15):2150-2152.

25. Moody G, Eaden JA, Mayberry JF. Social implications of childhood Crohn's disease. *J Pediatr Gastroenterol Nutr.* 1999;28(4):S43-S45.

26. Mackner LM, Crandall WV. Brief report: psychosocial adjustment in adolescents with inflammatory bowel disease. *J Pediatr Psychol.* 2006;31(3):281-285.

27. A consensus statement on health care transitions for young adults with special health care needs. *Pediatrics.* 2002;110(6 Pt 2):1304-1306.

28. Rosen DS, Blum RW, Britto M, Sawyer SM, Siegel DM. Transition to adult health care for adolescents and young adults with chronic conditions: position paper of the Society for Adolescent Medicine. *J Adolesc Health.* 2003;33(4):309-311.

29. Baldassano R, Ferry G, Griffiths A, Mack D, Markowitz J, Winter H. Transition of the patient with inflammatory bowel disease from pediatric to adult care: recommendations of the North American Society for Pediatric Gastroenterology, Hepatology and Nutrition. *J Pediatr Gastroenterol Nutr.* 2002;34(3):245-248.

CHAPTER 10

TRANSITION OF CARE

John M. Russo, MD and Wallace V. Crandall, MD

Adolescence represents an important, but often difficult, period of transition from childhood to adulthood. This transition includes increasing independence and decision making on the part of the adolescent, as well as an increasing regard for the opinions of peers, with less reliance on family members. At times, adolescents may manifest this growing independence in ways that are, or are perceived to be, "rebellious" if their wishes conflict with those of parents and others.

Adolescence is also a time when "fitting in" with peer groups is particularly important. Dealing with a chronic illness such as inflammatory bowel disease (IBD) during this difficult period can make children feel "different" from their peers. They may be embarrassed by the symptoms of their disease, or by the diagnosis itself, and may therefore behave as if no problem exists. As a result, patients may become less adherent to medical therapy. As such, maintaining adequate disease control and achieving good health may be particularly challenging during adolescence.

It is in this developmental context that transition of care occurs. This chapter will focus on the transition of medical responsibility from the parents and physicians to the adolescent in preparation for the subsequent transfer of care to an adult gastroenterologist.

Defining Transition of Care

A position paper from the Society for Adolescent Medicine defines transition as "the purposeful, planned movement of adolescents and young adults with chronic physical and medical conditions from child-centered to adult-oriented health care system."[1] Note that this differs from transfer of care. Transfer of care is an event (ie, the transfer of a patient to another provider for future medical care). In contrast, transition of care is a process of preparation and education that includes the subsequent transfer of care. We do our patients a disservice if transfer of care occurs without the appropriate transition of care.

Scherl EJ, Dubinsky MC.
The Changing World of Inflammatory Bowel Disease:
Impact of Generation, Gender, and Global Trends (pp 127-136)
© 2009 SLACK Incorporated.

Differences Between
the Pediatric and Adult Medical Setting

When discussing the transition from pediatric to adult medicine, it is important to understand the fundamental differences that exist between the two disciplines.[2] In 1995, Rosen[3] reviewed some perceptions of the differences between pediatricians and internists. Overall, pediatricians were described as warm and friendly, whereas internists were considered thoughtful and inquisitive. Additionally, internal medicine was described as more cerebral, with the pursuit of knowledge and a differential diagnosis the driving force. As such, patients of internists might feel neglected if the doctor is focused on solving individual problems and, in the process, losing focus on the patient as a whole. In contrast, the relationship between a pediatrician and a patient was described as more emotional and less methodical and therefore would temper the physician's enthusiasm to relentlessly pursue a diagnosis. The patient would be less likely to get lost in the process of the work-up.

Rosen further commented on the developmental focus of pediatricians. Pediatricians are trained in normal development and developmental milestones. They observe patients' growth and maturation and are trained to recognize when patients are delayed or stray from normal development. In contrast, the growth and development of adults should be complete, and therefore they are not prominent concerns of the internist. For those with a chronic illness whose development may be delayed, a pediatrician would be more prone to evaluate and address developmental concerns.

Another fundamental aspect of pediatric care, as described by Rosen, is that it is family oriented, with the active involvement of the parents being a critical and expected component. Parents are not only involved in their child's care, but they also typically have the responsibility of medical decision making on behalf of their children. Given this dynamic, pediatricians must gather information from both the adolescents and their parents, and parents' views and histories may be prioritized over those of the patient. Decisions may be made on behalf of the child by the parents and pediatrician, with the patient essentially acting as a bystander, having limited input into decisions affecting his or her care. Nonadherence may be viewed as typical of adolescence or blamed on immaturity, thus taking the responsibility off of the patient.

In contrast, internists speak directly with their patients in a private manner, expecting them to make joint decisions regarding their medical care. Adult patients are expected to be responsible for themselves and to make their own decisions in conjunction with their physician. They are expected to follow through with their mutually agreed-upon plan of care. Adult physicians may therefore be less tolerant of poor adherence. Families may be there to assist but are considered to be peripheral in their care.

Rosen and others have noted another key difference between internal medicine and pediatrics in the care of individuals with chronic illnesses—the use of multidisciplinary teams.[3,4] It is not uncommon for a pediatric subspecialty practice to have the involvement of multiple health care professionals, such as the managing physician, social worker, dietician, and psychologist, all available at a single visit. This facilitates communication among the multiple caretakers and allows the family ease of access to all aspects of their child's health care. This is rarely the case in adult medicine where multidisciplinary care will involve different members of the team at different times and often at different locations, making it more challenging for the patient and affording less direct communication among the caregivers.

While opinions may differ on Rosen's description of the differences between adult and pediatric practices, certainly real and substantial differences do exist. These differences may contribute to a failure in successful transfer of care. Anecdotal experience suggests that when patients leave the pediatric practice, they will often not keep the scheduled appointment with their new physician or will not schedule subsequent appointments. As a result, their next contact with a physician, often with the pediatric gastroenterologist, will not occur until a relapse has taken place.

Other Barriers to Successful Transition

In addition to the inherent differences in adult and pediatric practices, other factors may impede a successful transition. The pediatrician and the adolescent's parents may directly contribute to the difficulty of transitioning by failing to properly encourage self-management.[2,5] By not allowing the patient to become more independent and assume a greater role in his or her care, they may slow the necessary development and maturation that is required for the adolescent to function independently. For example, patients may not have learned or developed even basic skills such as communicating with their physician, scheduling appointments, refilling prescriptions, or taking medication without parental reminders.

Furthermore, pediatricians may be hesitant to transfer a patient that they have known for years and with whom they have built a strong relationship. They may feel that an adult physician will not understand their patient or be able to give them adequate care. They may even feel a sense of abandoning their patients and families as they transfer care to an internist. Similarly, families may feel a sense of abandonment when they are forced to move on from the pediatric practitioner. Feelings of abandonment on the part of either the physician or the patient/patient's family may delay efforts to encourage self-management and subsequent transfer of care.

The successful transition needs to address these issues to allow the patient to grow into an independent and well-educated adult who can successfully manage his or her disease with a meaningful and therapeutic relationship with his or her new adult practitioner.

Existing Research on Transition and Transfer of Care

There is a paucity of literature on the transition of care or even the transfer of care from a pediatric specialist to an adult specialist. This is true for chronic childhood illnesses generally, but particularly so for IBD. Despite a number of reviews and recommendations,[4,6,7] there have been very few studies examining different strategies or methods to facilitate the transition from a pediatric practice into an adult practice. This paucity of information on transition of care is being increasingly recognized, but efforts to better define the transition process and assure a more successful transition are needed.

Given the lack of data regarding the transition process in adolescents with IBD, we will review some of the research on transitioning in other adolescent disorders, specifically select studies in diabetes and rheumatic disease.

Kipps et al examined methods of transfer of 229 young people with Type I diabetes to adult services in the United Kingdom.[8] The authors compared 4 districts in the Oxford region, each using a different method to transfer care. They performed a retrospective review of patient records, as well as interviews of patients (164) with a recent transfer of care. The methods of transfer were 1) direct transfer from a pediatric to adult clinic, 2) transition through a young adult clinic either at a different hospital or 3) at the same hospital where they were introduced to the adult physician in the pediatric clinic prior to transfer, or 4) transition to an adolescent clinic held in the same hospital but run jointly by the pediatrician and the adult physician prior to transfer to the adult clinic. The mean age at transfer was 17.9 years (range 13.3 to 22.4 years). There was large interdistrict variation in clinic attendance post-transfer. There were lower rates of follow-up and higher rates of dissatisfaction from those transferred directly to the adult clinic. The authors concluded that mode of transfer, specifically using an intermediate young adult clinic, was more important than age at transfer and that personal contact with the staff from the adult clinic prior to transfer appears to be a key factor in the success of the transfer.

Using interviews and a qualitative phenomenological approach, Karlsson et al studied the transition toward autonomy in self-management in 32 Swedish adolescents with Type I diabetes.[9] They described a stage in which teenagers "hover" between separating from parents and retaining parental support, which leads to uncertainty about responsibilities and may complicate the process of transition. Acquiring experiential knowledge by gathering information, making one's own decisions, and practicing complex decision making was felt to be crucial to success. The encouragement, acceptance, and support of others were also thought to contribute to a successful transition to autonomy. Autonomy should include expanding the circle of support to include others and not be seen as a separation from family relationships. The authors emphasize the importance of supporting and offering security to teenagers who are "hovering."

Another study from Sweden by Lundin et al examined the transition of adolescents with diabetes through participant observations of patient visits and 10 semistructured interviews with care providers in 2 pediatric and 2 adult diabetes outpatient clinics.[10] They also found that the way the transition process is undertaken will affect its success. Professional meetings between the health care providers appeared to be of "vital importance" to allow for the proper communication between the pediatric and adult caretakers. They also observed that having a nurse and/or physician who could share time between both pediatric and adult care may be an option to facilitate the integration of care.

Van Walleghem et al[11] described the feasibility and acceptability of a Canadian administrative support and systems navigation service for young adults (16 to 30 years) with diabetes during the transition into the adult health care system. The project provided a nonmedical administrative coordinator, the "Maestro," to provide a centralized, coordinated, community-based navigation system for the care, education, and support of young adult patients with diabetes in the region. The coordinator maintained biannual telephone and e-mail contact with eligible participants in order to inquire about access to care and services and to help facilitate follow-up and referrals. Seventy-nine percent (373/473) of eligible individuals participated in the program. The authors concluded that the Maestro project did demonstrate the feasibility and acceptability of a coordinated "navigation" service for young adults with diabetes.

Recognizing the paucity of literature on the subject, McGill outlined factors that might help facilitate a smooth, effective transition from pediatric to adult diabetes care.[12] She described young adults as classic nonattenders who have not been well prepared for the transition and suggests that the early initiation of the transition process is essential. Key components of a transition plan would include discussions of self-advocacy, independent care behaviors, sexual health, psychosocial support, education and vocational planning, as well as lifestyle counseling. She also advocates the idea of adolescent transition clinics attended by both pediatric and adult teams, as well as the use of a transition coordinator.

The rheumatology literature is similar to that found for diabetes. There is no generally utilized method for the transition of children into adult settings and there is considerable variation in the styles practiced. Funding, staffing, and resources for transition programs are lacking.[13]

In the United Kingdom, a survey of health professionals and clinical staff involved in the implementation of a transition of care program found that there was a lack of information and teaching materials, lack of overall training in adolescent issues, and limited time in clinic to spend with adolescent patients. These represent potential areas for improvement in the development of transition programs.[14]

McDonagh et al described the development and initial evaluation of a multicenter, evidence-based, transition of care program for adolescents with juvenile arthritis.[15] The authors conducted focus groups of young patients with juvenile arthritis and their parents; a national survey of relevant professionals; a Delphi study of patients, parents, and health care professionals; a chart review; and a literature review. Results of these studies were combined to form the conceptual framework for a transition program.

The authors identified multiple principles that were felt to be key components of the format and content of a transition program. These principles included multidimensional, age-appropriate, adolescent-focused information that promotes self-advocacy in health care. Peer support and independent visits were to be included in preparing the adolescent to transfer to an adult service. The program was to be coordinated, individualized, and comprehensive, including plans to address disease education, psychosocial health, parental concerns, education, and vocation.

Key components to the program were a departmental transition policy to guide care, a local program coordinator (primarily a nurse) to help direct the adolescent, an individual transition plan to facilitate the transition process, and printed resources to support not only the patient, but also parents and health professionals. Meeting the needs of parents was also identified as important because parents need accurate information as they themselves are a key information resource for the adolescents.

Participants evaluated the acceptability and utilization of program components through questionnaires and focused group discussion, with the authors presenting their 6-month results. They found that the local program coordinator received higher acceptability scores compared to the paper-based resources ($p<0.001$), although both received scores indicating that they were felt to be helpful.

In Canada, a Young Adults with Rheumatic Disease (YARD) clinic was developed to provide age/developmentally appropriate rheumatology care to those over 18 years with childhood-onset disease to facilitate the transfer to the adult specialist.[13] The clinic is staffed by both pediatric and adult rheumatologists, along with a clinical nurse specialist and social worker. This clinic also has access to physical and occupational therapy, vocational and sexual counseling services, and "youth friendly" adult medicine specialists.

The transition process begins at age 14 or 15 when patients begin to spend some portion of their visit alone with the staff. They are introduced to the concept of the YARD clinic at 16, and transfer to the YARD clinic occurs at age 18. To ease the transition, parents can attend a portion of the first visit but are not invited to later visits. Parents are encouraged to let the patient handle all aspects of his or her care and all information parents obtain must be from the patient. This can be difficult for some families. Patients are usually transitioned over 3 to 5 years, once they have stable disease, an understanding of their disease and treatments, the ability to make and keep appointments, a mature relationship with the staff, and a primary care physician whom they use appropriately. Not all patients succeed, and if they have not done so by age 23, they are not likely to benefit from the program and are transitioned to adult care at that time.

Transitioning in Inflammatory Bowel Disease

Over the past few years, transition of care for adolescents with IBD has begun to receive more attention[2,16-18]; however, there is no primary literature on the subject. While some of the research regarding effective transition of care in other diseases must certainly apply to patients with IBD, there are also specific aspects of IBD that could affect the transition process. For example, symptoms and complications of IBD such as chronic diarrhea, fecal incontinence, poor growth, and altered body appearance may result in diminished psychosocial functioning.[19-22] In fact, a meta-analysis of different chronic childhood diseases found that IBD had the most profound effect on mental health of the diseases reviewed.[23] The recommendations regarding the transition of care of adolescents and young adults with IBD are based on the available literature from other disease states, as well as expert opinion, and are summarized next.

A medical position statement from the North American Society for Pediatric Gastroenterology, Hepatology and Nutrition (NASPGHAN)[2] states that the goal of a transition program is to achieve a "continuum of care that includes normalization of social and emotional development and acquisition of independent living skills. A successful program should result in improved compliance with therapy and effective planning for long-range needs."[2]

The authors suggested initiating the process of transition to an adult gastroenterologist during early or middle adolescence and provided several recommendations to facilitate the transition process. For example, adolescents should be seen without their parents to build a relationship promoting independence and self-reliance. The physician should discuss with the patient and family the benefits of transitioning to an internal medicine gastroenterology practice, help the patient identify an adult gastroenterologist knowledgeable in caring for adolescents and young adults with childhood-onset IBD, and encourage the development of a relationship with that physician. The authors also emphasized the importance of providing the patient with a brief medical summary and providing the internist/gastroenterologist all necessary medical records and summaries, thus helping the family to realize that all providers are indeed collaborating to provide optimal care.

Hait et al outlined a timeline and skills checklist for both patients and the medical team that allows them to work on transition through progressive developmental stages.[17] Beginning at age 11 and continuing through adulthood, the patient and medical team have developmentally appropriate tasks and teaching to complete. Each stage requires the patient to become more independent and responsible. At ages 11 to 13, the patient should be able to identify his or her condition, medications, and impact on school and daily life. The patient gradually becomes more independent and responsible and by age 20 to 23, he or she should be able to independently schedule and have an individual visit with an adult gastroenterologist.

Recommendations

The transition of adolescents with IBD must be carefully planned and individualized. The concept of transition should be introduced in early adolescence. Once the patient is capable of abstract thinking and visualizing the future, he or she may be introduced to the idea of transition.[17] Key aspects of the successful transition to an adult gastroenterologist are willingness, knowledge, maturity, and the ability of the patient, parents, and health care providers to work together toward this common goal.

NASPGHAN surveyed its members and found that the majority of practices do not have a structured transition process in place but would be interested in one if it were available (NASPGHAN survey 2006, personal communication).

In response to this need, NASPGHAN and the Children's Digestive Health and Nutrition Foundation (CDHNF) developed a series of checklists to help guide both the patient and the health care team through the transition process. These checklists can be downloaded for use from the NASPGHAN Web site (www.naspghan.org). They provide recommendations for patients in early adolescence (ages 12 to 14) continuing through late adolescence (age 17+). Areas of emphasis include knowledge, independence and assertiveness, and health and lifestyle (Figure 10-1).

While these checklists are valuable tools, they should be used as part of a more integrated transition program in order to maximize the chance of success. Components of a comprehensive transition program might include the following:

* Assessment of readiness to begin the various stages of transition. The patient must be able and willing to begin and continue through each of the transition steps.

* Recognition of barriers to successful transition (eg, perceived differences between pediatric and internal medicine-based practices, feelings of abandonment, failure to identify an adult gastroenterologist knowledgeable about pediatric onset IBD, and failure to facilitate appropriate self-management skills) and an individualized plan to address those concerns.

* The early and ongoing teaching of developmentally appropriate self-management and self-advocacy skills such as those outlined in the NASPGHAN/CDHNF checklists or other printed materials.

Healthcare Provider Transitioning Checklist

AGE	PATIENT	HEALTH CARE TEAM
12-14	**EARLY ADOLESCENCE** *New knowledge and responsibilities* □ I can describe my GI condition □ I can name my medications, the amount and times I take them □ I can describe the common side effects of my medications □ I know my doctors' and nurses' names and roles □ I can use and read a thermometer □ I can answer at least 1 question during my health care visit □ I can manage my regular medical tasks at school □ I can call my doctor's office to make or change an appointment □ I can describe how my GI condition affects me on a daily basis	□ Discuss the idea of visiting the office without parents or guardians in the future □ Encourage independence by performing part of the exam with the parents or guardians out of the examining room □ Begin to provide information about drugs, alcohol, sexuality and fitness □ Establish specific self-management goals during office visit
14-17	**MID ADOLESCENCE** *Building knowledge and practicing independence* □ I know the names and purposes of the tests that are done □ I know what can trigger a flare of my disease □ I know my medical history □ I know if I need to transition to an adult gastroenterologist □ I reorder my medications and call my doctor for refills □ I answer many questions during a health care visit □ I spend most of my time alone with the doctor during visit □ I understand the risk of medical nonadherence □ I understand the impact of drugs and alcohol on my condition □ I understand the impact of my GI condition on my sexuality	□ Always focus on the patient instead of the parents or guardians when providing any explanations and □ Allow the patient to select when the parent or guardian is in the room for the exam □ Inform the patient of what the parent or guardian must legally be informed about with regards to the patient condition □ Discuss the importance of preparing the patient for independent status with the parents or guardian and address any anxiety they may have □ Continue to set specific goals which should include: • Filling prescriptions and scheduling appointments • Keeping a list of medications and medical team contact information in wallet and backpack
17+	**LATE ADOLESCENCE** *Taking charge* □ I can describe what medications I should not take because they might interact with the medications I am taking for my health condition □ I am alone with the doctor or choose who is with me during a health care visit □ I can tell someone what new legal rights and responsibilities I gained when I turned 18 □ I manage all my medical tasks outside the home (school, work) □ I know how to get more information about IBD □ I can book my own appointments, refill prescriptions and contact medical team □ I can tell someone how long I can be covered under my parents' health insurance plan and what I need to do to maintain coverage for the next 2 years . □ I carry insurance information (card) with me in my wallet/purse/backpack.	**DISCUSS IN MORE DEPTH:** □ The impact of drugs, alcohol and non adherence on their disease □ The impact of their disease on sexuality, fertility □ Future plans for school/work and impact on health care including insurance coverage. □ How eventual transfer of care to an adult gastroenterologist will coordinate with future school or employment plans □ Remind patient and family that at age 18 the patient has the right to make his or her own health choices □ Develop specific plans for self-management outside the home (work/school) □ Provide the patient with a medical summary for work, school or transition □ Discuss plans for insurance coverage □ If transitioning to an adult subspecialist, provide a list of potential providers and encourage/facilitate an initial visit.

Digestive Health for Life

CDHNF — CHILDREN'S DIGESTIVE HEALTH & NUTRITION FOUNDATION

NASPGHAN — NORTH AMERICAN SOCIETY FOR PEDIATRIC GASTROENTEROLOGY, HEPATOLOGY AND NUTRITION

Figure 10-1. Checklist to help guide both the patient and the health care team through the transition process developed by NASPGHAN and CDHNF. (Used with permission of NASPGHAN.)

* A change from parental responsibility for medical care to family and peer support for the patient's medical decision making. Family and friends should take a supportive role instead of a management and decision-making role, providing emotional and psychological support and helping the patient access additional resources.

* Identification of a transition coordinator who will assume responsibility for oversight of the transition program and who will work directly with the patient and his or her family. This person not only helps to coordinate care issues but also provides teaching and direction to appropriate resources.

* If feasible, use of a multispecialty transition clinic that includes both pediatric and adult providers, nurses, dieticians, social workers, and psychologists and that is focused on the patient being actively involved in all aspects of his or her care.

* If a transition clinic is not feasible, an adult gastroenterologist(s) with expertise in pediatric-onset IBD should be identified and included in the transition plan.

* At transfer of care, communication in the form of a comprehensive medical summary, including all pertinent testing, should be given to the patient and his or her family as well as the adult gastroenterologist.

While the transition of a patient with IBD from a pediatric specialist to an adult specialist represents a challenge to all involved, awareness of this challenge is growing and the steps to meet it are beginning to take place. Organizations worldwide are working on identifying successful strategies for transitioning adolescents with chronic illnesses. The concepts of transition clinics and care coordinators seem to be attractive options in the early stages of evaluation. The next few years should prove to be exciting as we learn about and improve the transition process and ultimately improve the long-term care of our patients.

Acknowledgment

We would like to thank Dr. Susan Moyer for her expert review and valuable comments in the preparation of this chapter.

References

1. Blum RW, Garell D, Hodgman CH, et al. Transition from child-centered to adult health-care systems for adolescents with chronic conditions: a position paper of the Society for Adolescent Medicine. *J Adolesc Health*. 1993;14(7):570-576.
2. Baldassano R, Ferry G, Griffiths A, Mack D, Markowitz J, Winter H. Transition of the patient with inflammatory bowel disease from pediatric to adult care: recommendations of the North American Society for Pediatric Gastroenterology, Hepatology and Nutrition. *J Pediatr Gastroenterol Nutr*. 2002;34(3):245-248.
3. Rosen D. Between two worlds: bridging the cultures of child health and adult medicine. *J Adolesc Health*. 1995;17(1):10-16.
4. Transition of care provided for adolescents with special health care needs. American Academy of Pediatrics Committee on Children with Disabilities and Committee on Adolescence. *Pediatrics*. 1996;98(6 Pt 1):1203-1206.
5. David TJ. Transition from the paediatric clinic to the adult service. *J R Soc Med*. 2001;94(8):373-374.
6. A consensus statement on health care transitions for young adults with special health care needs. *Pediatrics*. 2002;110(6 Pt 2):1304-1306.
7. Reiss JG, Gibson RW, Walker LR. Health care transition: youth, family, and provider perspectives. *Pediatrics*. 2005;115(1):112-120.
8. Kipps S, Bahu T, Ong K, et al. Current methods of transfer of young people with Type 1 diabetes to adult services. *Diabet Med*. 2002;19(8):649-654.
9. Karlsson A, Arman M, Wikblad K. Teenagers with type 1 diabetes: a phenomenological study of the transition towards autonomy in self-management. *Int J Nurs Stud*. 2008;45(4):562-570.
10. Lundin CS, Danielson E, Ohrn I. Handling the transition of adolescents with diabetes: participant observations and interviews with care providers in paediatric and adult diabetes outpatient clinics. *International Journal of Integrated Care*. 2007;7:e05.
11. Van Walleghem N, MacDonald CA, Dean HJ. Building connections for young adults with type 1 diabetes mellitus in Manitoba: feasibility and acceptability of a transition initiative. *Chron Dis Can*. 2006;27(3):130-134.
12. McGill M. How do we organize smooth, effective transfer from paediatric to adult diabetes care? *Horm Res*. 2002;57(Suppl 1):66-68.
13. Tucker LB, Cabral DA. Transition of the adolescent patient with rheumatic disease: issues to consider. *Pediatr Clin North Am*. 2005;52(2):641-652, viii.
14. McDonagh JE, Southwood TR, Shaw KL. Unmet education and training needs of rheumatology health professionals in adolescent health and transitional care. *Rheumatology (Oxford)*. 2004;43(6):737-743.

15. McDonagh JE, Shaw KL, Southwood TR. Growing up and moving on in rheumatology: development and preliminary evaluation of a transitional care programme for a multicentre cohort of adolescents with juvenile idiopathic arthritis. *J Child Health Care.* 2006;10(1):22-42.
16. Mamula P, Markowitz JE, Baldassano RN. Inflammatory bowel disease in early childhood and adolescence: special considerations. *Gastroenterol Clin North Am.* 2003;32(3):967-995, viii.
17. Hait E, Arnold JH, Fishman LN. Educate, communicate, anticipate-practical recommendations for transitioning adolescents with IBD to adult health care. *Inflamm Bowel Dis.* 2006;12(1):70-73.
18. Adolescence into Adulthood in Inflammatory Bowel Disease (IBD) Meeting report. London, UK June 16, 2005.
19. Szigethy E, Levy-Warren A, Whitton S, et al. Depressive symptoms and inflammatory bowel disease in children and adolescents: a cross-sectional study. *J Pediatr Gastroenterol Nutr.* 2004;39(4):395-403.
20. Mackner LM, Crandall WV. Long-term psychosocial outcomes reported by children and adolescents with inflammatory bowel disease. *Am J Gastroenterol.* 2005;100(6):1386-1392.
21. Mackner LM, Crandall WV. Brief report: psychosocial adjustment in adolescents with inflammatory bowel disease. *J Pediatr Psychol.* 2006;31(3):281-285.
22. Mackner LM, Crandall WV, Szigethy EM. Psychosocial functioning in pediatric inflammatory bowel disease. *Inflamm Bowel Dis.* 2006;12(3):239-244.
23. Lavigne JV, Faier-Routman J. Psychological adjustment to pediatric physical disorders: a meta-analytic review. *J Pediatr Psychol.* 1992;17(2):133-157.

Financial disclosure: Dr. Crandall is a consultant for Centocor. He receives research support from Centocor and Abbott.

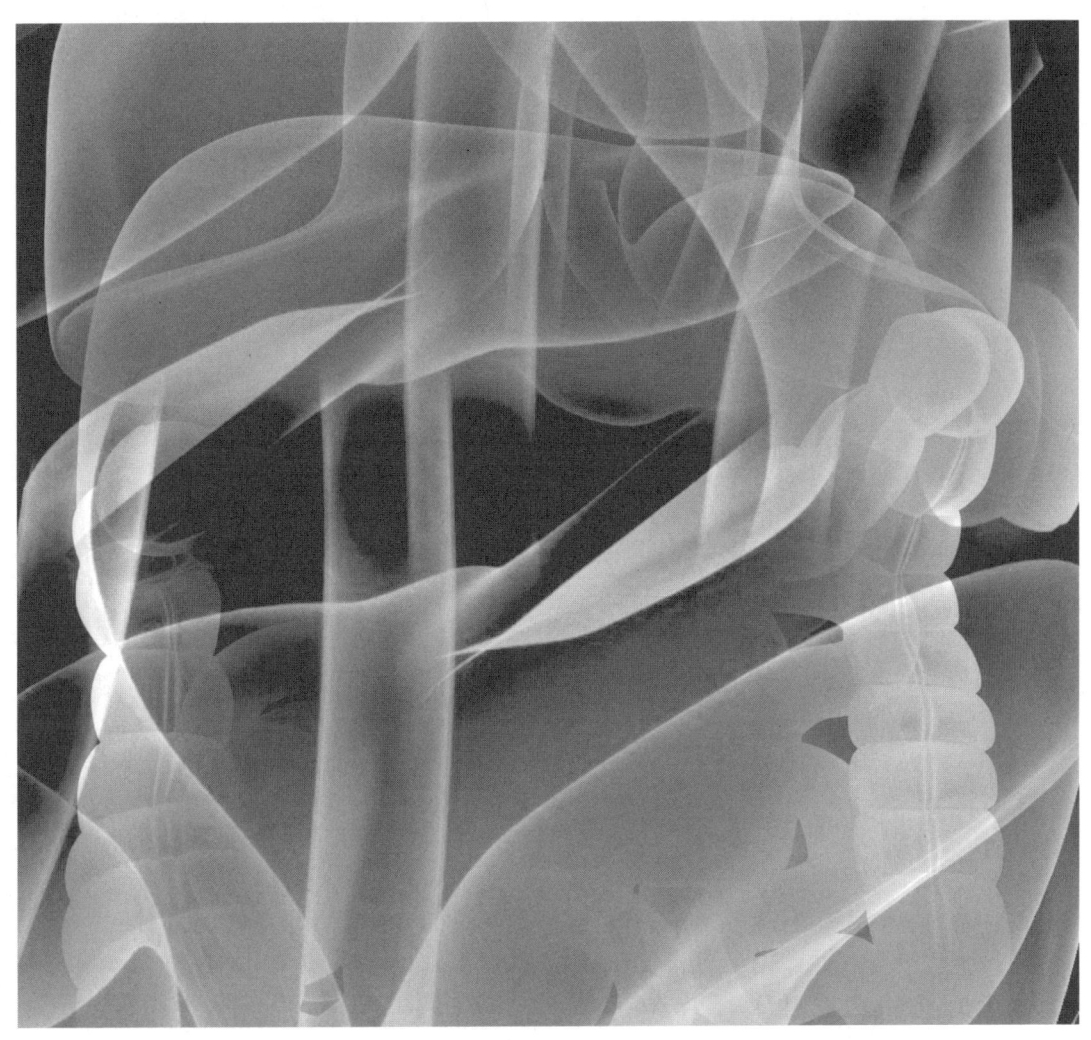

SECTION III

INFLAMMATORY BOWEL DISEASE AND THE YOUNG ADULT

INFLAMMATORY BOWEL DISEASE AND RELATIONSHIPS/SEXUAL HEALTH
AN OVERVIEW

Amy B. Trachter, PsyD, PhD

Inflammatory bowel disease (IBD) has an impact on quality of life in those living with this disease. Partner relationships and sexual health in IBD has received some attention in the literature devoted to psychological, relationship, and sexual functioning in recent years.[1-3] The purpose of this chapter is to provide an overview of the potential psychosocial impact of IBD on relationships and sexual health. Given that IBD typically has an onset in early adult years, effects on relationship and sexual health are not surprising. This chapter will provide an overview of the difficulties evaluating patient concerns, partner relationships, and sexual functioning; elucidate some of the difficulties identifying such problems; and provide prophylactic suggestions for physicians treating those who may experience such problems.

IBD, including both Crohn's disease (CD) and ulcerative colitis (UC), is a quite prevalent, distressing, and often misunderstood chronic illness that can impact patient sexuality and relationship health.[1-3] Yet, despite the increasing attention paid to most chronic diseases, these diseases have tended to be under-researched in both the behavioral medicine and sexuality literature. There are approximately 1 million reported individuals with IBD in the United States.[4-6] Among women in the general population, approximately 40% experience some type of sexual difficulty.[7] Due to the paucity of literature in this specialized area, the number of women with IBD in particular who have comorbid sexual difficulties can be estimated to be approximately 440,000. Due to the fact that typical age of onset is between 15 and 30 years of age, living with active IBD may impact the sexual health of the patient.[8,9] Sexual and relationship health of people living with IBD may be influenced by the disease itself and/or by the medical and surgical interventions used in treatment. Sexual health issues that may be impacted include growth and development, body image, intimacy, fertility, and pregnancy.

Scherl EJ, Dubinsky MC.
The Changing World of Inflammatory Bowel Disease:
Impact of Generation, Gender, and Global Trends (pp 139-146)
© 2009 SLACK Incorporated.

Psychological Impact
Pertaining to Relationships/Sexual Health

Individuals with IBD encounter some unique psychological issues in addition to the difficulties of living with a chronic disease. Although patients with IBD undergo an adjustment to chronic illness that individuals with other chronic illnesses encounter, those with IBD may feel an additional burden of shame. People with these diseases live with unpredictable symptoms that exact both a psychological and emotional toll.[1,10,11] Defecation is a natural physical function; however, when defecation occurs on a constant and/or unpredictable basis, these symptoms of IBD may facilitate feelings of shame, decreasing both body and sexual self-image.

Both direct (eg, fatigue, constant diarrhea, abdominal pain) and indirect (eg, side effects of medication, consequences of surgery, communication difficulties) effects of these diseases can disrupt body image, sexual functioning, and interpersonal relationships. Spending a significant amount of time during the day on a toilet may not promote a healthy body image or positive feelings regarding one's genitalia. The unpredictability of these diseases and the fear of unexpected symptoms may permeate self-esteem and psyche in an insidious manner.[12] Some medications may cause oral infections such as candidiasis, making the simple act of kissing aversive.[13] Additionally, symptoms themselves may be frightening due to their intensity.[14] For instance, the urgency of having to use a bathroom and "having an accident" in adulthood may significantly impact an individual's sense of psychological and sexual self-confidence.

The sexual self-image of women with IBD is influenced by the combination of societal attitudes generally[13,15] and by the insidious nature of experiencing socially unacceptable symptomatology. Women report greater symptom severity and have higher scores on patient concerns than do men.[16] Fears of being viewed as "sick" might also affect self-image and erode sexual confidence. Fears regarding conception, attractiveness, and potential partner relationship difficulties are common among women with IBD.[9,16] Women with spinal cord injuries, for example, reported that the greatest change after surgery was in their perceived attractiveness; they found themselves less attractive by 50% on average.[17] In most cases, the woman's overall appearance had not changed markedly, suggesting that one's sense of attractiveness is more dependent on internal feelings rather than outward appearance. A parallel may be drawn with IBD patients who rarely appear "sick," yet feel the ramifications of their disease permeate their daily living activities. For men, gaseous odors and flatulence, while undesirable, are almost expected by sociocultural norms. Women with similar symptoms, in contrast, may be viewed as unfeminine. Moreover, insecurity about fecal incontinence during sexual intercourse can strongly inhibit sexual motivation.[12,15,18] Physicians may provide validation and psychoeducational information by initiating discussion of the woman's relationship and sexual functioning and health.[13,15,19]

However, IBD tends not to be readily discussed either publicly or privately. Consequently, information on the impact of such illnesses on interpersonal relationships and sexuality is limited and often challenging to obtain for research purposes. Moreover, both sexuality and diarrhea are not commonly discussed independently of one another, much less together.

Although there is an abundance of research addressing the medical aspects of IBD, the psychosexual impact of these diseases is not commonly targeted for investigation.[1,12,16,20] Thus, obtaining quantifiable, comprehensive data may assist in the understanding of the individual's illness experience, as well as its impact on relationships and sexual health.[1,12,16,20] Despite the dubious role of psychological processes as a primary cause or contributor to the exacerbation of IBD, it is clear that these illnesses exact a psychological toll on the individual.[1-3,12,13,16,20-23] For instance, recent research suggests that those living with IBD who are depressed are more likely to have partner relationships and sexual functioning impacted.[8,9] Reviews of past research on frequency of psychiatric diagnosis in IBD patients demonstrate that such diagnoses range from 13% to 100%.[24] Additionally, disagreement in sample environments (eg, surveys in the community versus referrals in medical centers); lack of control groups; retrospective studies; small sample sizes; referral bias; and the use of different, inappropriate, and/or invalid assessment tools represent the methodological problems that exacerbate the difficulty in establishing conclusive, generalized results.[1,21,24,25] As a result of such difficulties, limited empirical studies pertaining to relationship and sexual difficulties exist. However, research investigating relationship and sexual difficulties is, while still uncommon, increasing.[9]

Implications of Psychological Impact and Difficulties Eliciting Information

Recent research indicates that including psychosocial evaluation during patient visits and considering psychological disturbances is helpful to patient care.[1-3,12,13,16,20,21,23] The assessment of relationship and sexual health among both men and women with IBD with sensitivity to gender-specific issues is integral in the implementation of a biopsychosocial approach to treatment[12,13,16,20] and essential to detecting sexual dysfunction. Sexual dysfunction cannot be treated unless it is identified. Unfortunately, women are less likely to volunteer such information to a primary care physician or gastroenterologist (especially if the physician is male); sexuality is almost as private as defecation. Hence, the burden lies on the physician to create the supportive environment and relationship that facilitates such discussions.

However, while relationship and sexual functioning is typically assessed as part of a psychological evaluation in the context of psychotherapy, it typically is not evaluated in a gastroenterologist's office. In addition, gynecologists may not typically inquire about the IBD activity among women. Due to the private nature of both sexuality and defecation and the obvious dichotomy of the 2 topics, patients are not likely volunteering information on either topic to the alternate physician and/or health professional.

Few studies have examined the impact of these diseases on interpersonal relationships or sexuality,[1] which may be due to an amalgam of reasons. First, physicians are quite busy and time constraints may hinder the physician's ability to evaluate such issues during the course of routine outpatient evaluation. Most physicians do not customarily address relationship or sexual concerns with their patients, even in the presence of known pathology. Second, most patients, especially those in a female patient-male doctor dynamic, do not volunteer problems with relationship and sexual functioning to their gastroenterologists. Consequently, difficulties identifying relationship and sexual health problems that are due, either directly or indirectly, to disease activity may be undetected. Third, due to the private nature of sexuality, both physicians and patients may feel uncomfortable discussing such issues. Fourth, those physicians who are comfortable discussing issues that pertain to partner relationships and sexuality may not feel appropriately trained to assess such issues and refer to a psychiatrist or psychologist, whom although trained to assess these issues, may not be not well versed in IBD. Consequently, difficulties with relationship and sexual functioning in women with IBD should ideally receive a multidisciplinary approach to treatment.

Relationship and sexual health needs to be evaluated in a manner that is not perceived as threatening or invasive, especially when there is a female patient-male doctor dynamic. After the disease activity has been medically evaluated, it should be considered in the context of relationships and sexual health. An algorithm for the assessment and treatment of sexual dysfunction in women with IBD is suggested in Figure 11-1. Additionally, the physician should be comfortable discussing such topics.

Additionally, many new patients initially see gastroenterologists with their partner. Assessing relationships and sexual health at the onset of diagnosis allows the physician to obtain information regarding current, historical, or potential difficulties through an integrated interview approach that is easily explained to the patient. The patient is less likely to view such invasive questioning

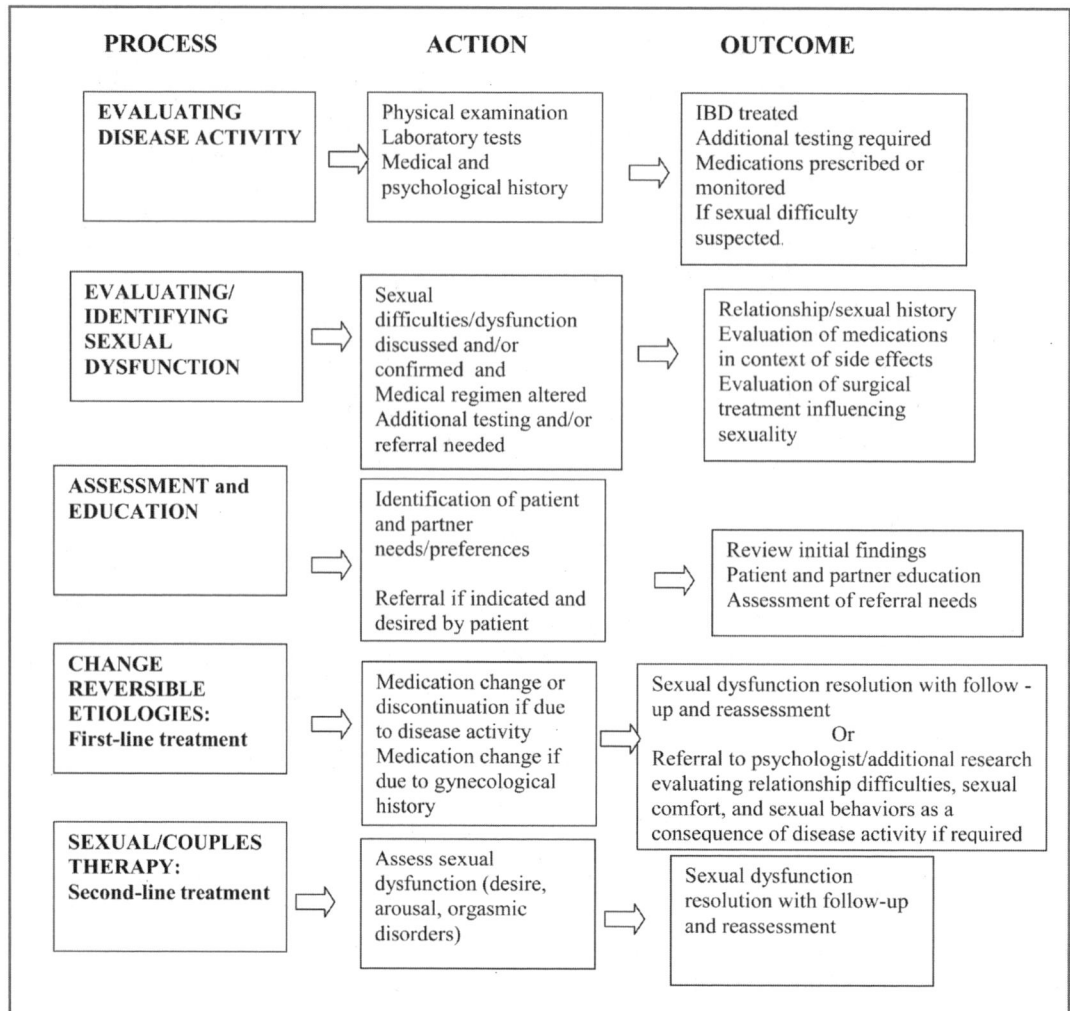

Figure 11-1. An algorithm for clinical decision making in the assessment and treatment of sexual dysfunction. Stages are identified in the model, with each stage reflecting specific "processes," "actions," and "outcomes." The importance of assessment and follow-up, as well as patient education and communication aspects, are depicted throughout the model. (Adapted from Trachter AB, Rogers AI, Leiblum SR. Inflammatory bowel disease in women: impact on relationship sexual health. *Inflamm Bowel Dis.* 2002;8(6):413-421.)

as unusual, and it facilitates questioning of relationship/sexual functioning by the physician at some future time. In addition to physician interviews, there are several assessment measures that are specifically utilized for evaluating relationships and sexual health and can be provided to the physician by a psychologist and/or psychiatrist.

There are ways for physicians to identify sexual/relationship issues in a subtle, appropriate manner (Table 11-1). For example, any identified depressed patient is more likely to have sexual/relationship difficulties as a result of depression as in any identified patient with any other form of psychopathology. People living with these diseases may find forming new relationships especially challenging and may be fearful of rejection.[15] Behaviors that are "hidden," such as chronic diarrhea and abdominal pain, are especially difficult to discuss given that it is unclear as to when to disclose such information. Some level of trust and closeness must be felt before disclosure can be contemplated,[15] regardless of whether disclosure is to a partner or a physician. Some women report that although disclosure is difficult, it increases intimacy and relieves anxiety.

Table 11-1

PROPHYLACTIC SUGGESTIONS FOR RELATIONSHIPS/SEXUAL HEALTH DIFFICULTIES

- Whenever possible, involve the partner of the patient. If the patient attends appointments alone, ask about a partner. Segue into relationship/sexual functioning.

- Give the partner the opportunity to ask questions after speaking with both the patient and partner about the disease, which assists in including the partner.

- When appropriate, educate both the patient and partner about pregnancy and fertility issues in as much detail as possible. Provide literature/brochures to further clarify and assist with remembering what you have said.

- Be aware of patients who have depression or other comorbid psychopathology as they are more likely to have difficulties with sexual/relationship functioning. Consider giving a brief depression screen to patients in your waiting room.

Sexual Functioning in Surgical Patients With Inflammatory Bowel Disease

For people who undergo surgical interventions for their disease, social and sexual functioning is also a concern.[12,26,27] Patients require reassurance as improved health postoperatively leads to improved quality of life and sexual/relationship functioning. Research shows that poor rapport between partners following surgery correlated with poor sexual relations prior to surgery,[28-35] indicating the importance of effective communication and support in interpersonal relationships. Gloeckner[36] reported that patients wished their partners had been included in sexual counseling postoperatively. Additionally, among IBD patients' concerns, uncertainty of disease activity, energy level, being a burden on others, and producing unpleasant odors were among the top 10 concerns[8,9]; "feelings about my body" and "attractiveness" were numbers 11 and 14, respectively.[8,9] Given these concerns, it is not surprising that relationship and sexual functioning may be affected. Nevertheless, operations do have a psychological and emotional impact on women. Research by Carlsson et al in 2003 revealed that the greatest concern for patients who underwent ileostomy was sexuality/intimacy.[37]

Summary

Interpersonal relationships, growth and development, body and sexual self-image, pregnancy, and surgery are topics that affect both men and women living with IBD, especially given the age group IBD afflicts. Patients need to explore and discuss their concerns with their physicians and significant others in order to facilitate adjustment to these diseases.[1-3,13] Effective communication not only between partners, but also between patient and physician, is essential to adequately address the psychosocial and emotional consequences of these patients in the context of their sexual identities and interpersonal relationships. The body is the most visible part of one's self, and—for women especially—occupies a central part of an individual's self-perception.[32,33] Alteration of one's body in any manner may affect an individual's self-perception, which may lead to difficulties with intimacy.

The loss of control over elimination is a blow to self-esteem and promulgates fears of rejection by family and friends and of being ostracized by society.[34] Feelings of isolation, social stigma, and depression may lead to loss of sexual desire and interest. Difficulties with personal acceptance, body and sexual self-image, sexual concerns, and potential operations may impact relationship and sexual functioning but can be ameliorated with appropriate counseling.[38] Moreover, sexual partners play key roles in helping the identified patient adjust to his or her illness through both psychological and sexual validation. When possible, partners should be included when addressing relationship and sexual issues that might be a consequence of disease activity. By addressing the problems and fears pertaining to relationship and sexual health at the onset of diagnosis, future difficulties may be circumvented and psychosocial adjustment might be facilitated.

References

1. Trachter AB, Rogers AI, Leiblum SR. Inflammatory bowel disease in women: impact on relationship and sexual health. *Inflamm Bowel Dis.* 2002;8(6):413-421.

2. Alstead EM. Inflammatory bowel disease in pregnancy. *Postgrad Med J.* 2002;78(915):23-26.

3. Timmer A, Bauer A, Dignass A, Rogler G. Sexual function in persons with inflammatory bowel disease: a survey with match controls. *Clin Gastroenterol Hepatol.* 2007;5(1):87-94.

4. Becker C. Will treat Crohn's disease, colitis. *Home News Tribune.* 1998. Available at http://www2.umdnj.edu/medpweb/caccofnj/new.html. Accessed April 20, 2009.

5. Adler D. Pregnancy, fertility, and contraception in inflammatory bowel disease. In: Korelitz BI, Sohn N, eds. *Management of Inflammatory Bowel Disease.* New York, NY: Mosby; 1992:34-44.

6. Sandler RS. Epidemiology of inflammatory bowel disease. In: Targan SR, Shanahan F, eds. *Inflammatory Bowel Disease—From Bench to Bedside.* Baltimore, MD: Williams and Wilkins; 1994:5-30.

7. Leiblum SR. Definition and classification of female sexual disorders. *Int J Impot Res.* 1998;10(Suppl 2):S104-S106.

8. Giese LA, Terrel L. Sexual health issues in inflammatory bowel disease. *Gastroenterol Nurs.* 1996;19(1):12-17.

9. Maunder RG, de Rooy EC, Toner BB, et al. Health-related concerns of people who receive psychological support for inflammatory bowel disease. *Can J Gastroenterol.* 1997;11(8):681-685.

10. Isaacs KL. Hormone therapy: beauty or beast? *Women's Issues in IBD From Menopause to Menarche.* 2001;9-13.

11. Steiner-Grossman P. Education, social support, and psychosocial issues. In: Targan SR, Shanahan F, eds. *Inflammatory Bowel Disease—From Bench to Bedside.* Baltimore, MD: Williams and Wilkins; 1994:451-456.

12. McCleod RS. Maintaining femininity through IBD surgery. *Women's Issues in IBD From Menopause to Menarche.* 2001;20-23.

13. Gerson LB, Triadafilopoulos G. Palliative care in inflammatory bowel disease. *Inflamm Bowel Dis.* 2000;6(3):228-243.

14. Brice JA. Psychological aspects of living with a chronic intestinal illness. In: James S, ed. *Surviving and Thriving With AIDS: Hints for the Newly Diagnosed.* New York, NY: People With AIDS Coalition; 1987:2-4.

15. Basson R. Sexual health of women with disabilities. *Can Med Assoc J.* 1998;159(4):359-362.

16. Hanauer SH. Setting a higher standard: caring for women with IBD. *Women's Issues in IBD From Menopause to Menarche.* 2001;4-8.

17. Kettle P, Zarefoss S. Female sexuality after spinal cord injury. *Sex Disabil.* 1991;9(4):287-295.

18. Counihan TC, Roberts PL, Schoetz DJ, Coller JA, Murray JJ, Veidenheimer MC. Fertility and sexual and gynecologic function after ileal-pouch-anal anastomosis. *Dis Colon Rectum.* 1994;37:1126-1129.

19. Leiblum SR. Female sexual dysfunction. In: Gebbard G, ed. *Treatment of Psychiatric Disorders.* Washington, DC: American Psychiatric Press; 1994:93-99.

20. Kane SV. Conception and pregnancy in women with IBD. *Women's Issues in IBD From Menopause to Menarche.* 2001;14-19.

21. Drossman DA. Inflammatory bowel disease. In: Spilker B, ed. *Quality of Life and Pharmacoeconomics in Clinical Trials.* Philadelphia, PA: Lippincott-Raven Publishers; 1996:925-935.

22. Ramchandani D, Schindler B, Katz J. Evolving concepts of psychopathology in inflammatory bowel disease: implications for treatment. *Med Clin North Am.* 1994;78(6):1321-1330.

23. Drossman DA. Psychosocial factors in ulcerative colitis and Crohn's disease. In: Kirsner JB, Shorter RG, eds. *Inflammatory Bowel Disease.* Baltimore, MD: Williamson & Wilkins; 1995:492-513.

24. Schwarz SP, Blanchard EB. Inflammatory bowel disease: a review of the psychological assessment and treatment literature. *Ann Behav Med.* 1990;12(3):95-105.

25. Helzer JE. Psychiatric aspects of inflammatory bowel disease. In: Kodner IJ, Fry RD, Roe JP, eds. *Colon, Rectal, and Anal Surgery: Current Techniques and Controversies.* New York, NY: Mosby; 1985.

26. McLeod R. The pelvic pouch procedure remains an excellent option for most patients with ulcerative colitis requiring surgery. In: Banks P, Present D, eds. *Inflammatory Bowel Diseases.* New York, NY: CCFA, Inc; 1997:236-238.

27. Sachar DB. Inflammatory bowel disease. Paper presented at the meeting of the American College of Gastroenterology Post Graduate Course; October 1997; Chicago, Illinois.

28. Bambrick M, Fazio VW, Hull TL, et al. Sexual function following restorative proctocolectomy in women. *Dis Colon Rectum.* 1996;39(6):610-614.

29. Damgaard B, Wettergren A, Kirkegaard P. Social and sexual function following ileal pouch-anal anastomosis. *Dis Colon Rectum.* 1995;38(3):286-289.

30. Metcalf AM, Dozios RR, Kelly KA. Sexual function in women after proctocolectomy. *Ann Surg.* 1986;204(6):624-627.

31. Scaglia M, Bronsino E, Canino V, et al. The impact of conventional proctocolectomy on sexual function. *Minerva Chir.* 1993;48(17):903-910.

32. Scaglia M, Delaini GG, Hulten L. Sexual dysfunctions after conventional proctocolectomy. *Chir Ital.* 1992;44(5-6):230-242.

33. Seidel SA, Peach SE, Newman M, et al. Ileoanal pouch procedures: clinical outcomes and quality of life assessment. *Am Surg.* 1999;65(1):40-46.

34. Tiainen J, Matikainen M, Hiltunen KM. Ileal J-pouch–anal anastomosis, sexual dysfunction, and fertility. *Scand J Gastroenterol.* 1999;34(2):185-188.

35. Huish M, Kumar D, Stones C. Stoma surgery and sexual problems in ostomates. *J Sex Mar Ther.* 1998;13(3):311-324.

36. Gloeckner M. Partner reaction following ostomy surgery. *J Sex Mar Ther.* 1983;9(3):182-190.

37. Carlsson E, Boseaus I, Nordgren S. What concerns subjects with inflammatory bowel disease and an ileostomy? *Scand J Gastroenterol.* 2003;38(9):978-984.

38. Walsh BA, Grunet BK, Telford GL, et al. Multidisciplinary management of altered body image in the patient with an ostomy. *J Wound Ostomy Continence Nurs.* 1995;22(5):227-236.

INFLAMMATORY BOWEL DISEASE AND FERTILITY

Kim L. Isaacs, MD, PhD

The incidence of inflammatory bowel disease (IBD) peaks during the childbearing years of most couples. As a result, questions regarding pregnancy and fertility rise as important concerns in men and women making decisions about starting a family. Concerns may include questions about the ability to conceive and carry out a healthy and safe pregnancy and about the impact of pregnancy on disease and disease impact on pregnancy. Once the decision is made to proceed with a pregnancy, many couples are faced with difficulties in conception. Even without the added complication of IBD, infertility is relatively common, affecting up to 15% of couples attempting to become pregnant.[1] This chapter will cover the issues of infertility in patients with IBD.

Multiple steps must occur for a couple to conceive. In the woman, there must be functioning ovaries with release of a mature egg from the ovary. The egg must then be picked up by the fallopian tube where it encounters sperm and is fertilized. The embryo must then travel through the fallopian tube, implant on the uterine lining, and develop. The sperm must reach and be able to penetrate the egg in order to fertilize it. Abnormal sperm motility, function, and amount may affect fertility. All of the above steps can be dysfunctional, leading to infertility. IBD presents a unique set of issues—active inflammation, surgical alteration, and medication therapy that may affect different parts of the conception process. Definitions of infertility are shown in Table 12-1.

Does Inflammatory Bowel Disease Affect Fertility?

CROHN'S DISEASE STUDIES

Studies have shown mixed results concerning whether Crohn's disease (CD) affects fertility. Studies range from showing no differences in fertility compared to a non-CD population to up to 53% infertility rates (Table 12-2).

Scherl EJ, Dubinsky MC.
The Changing World of Inflammatory Bowel Disease:
Impact of Generation, Gender, and Global Trends (pp 147-160)
© 2009 SLACK Incorporated.

Table 12-1

DEFINITIONS OF INFERTILITY

- Infertility: Inability to conceive within 1 year in the absence of contraception
- Primary infertility: Infertility in couples who have never conceived
- Secondary infertility: Infertility in couples who have had at least one successful conception
- Fecundability: The probability of becoming pregnant per month of unprotected intercourse

Table 12-2

FERTILITY AND CROHN'S DISEASE

Study	Disease	N	Infertility
Fielding and Cooke[2]	CD	77	32%
De Dombal et al[3]	CD	86	53%
Khosla et al[4]	CD	54	11%
Homan and Thorbjarnarson[5]	CD	78	47%
Mayberry and Weterman[6]	CD	224	42%
	Control	208	28%
Moody et al[7]	CD	284	19%
Baird et al[8]	CD	177	3%
	Control	216	4%
Hudson et al[9]	CD	123	14%
	Control	766	14%

CD = Crohn's disease
In studies that examined men and women, only the female infertility rates are reported.

Fielding and Cooke reported in 1970 on 77 married women with CD.[2] Of this group, 25 (32%) were infertile after 2 years of attempting to conceive. Infertility was more common in women with large bowel involvement (66.7%) than in those with small bowel involvement (25.8%). In the patients who were evaluated for infertility, the most common cause was bilateral occlusion of the fallopian tubes. In addition, vitamin B_{12} deficiency was prevalent in the population studied with resolution of infertility in 2 patients within 6 months of starting vitamin B_{12} supplementation.

De Dombal and colleagues studied 86 women with CD and found a high incidence of subfertility with overall 53.5% patients failing to conceive during the survey period.[3] There was a nonsignificant trend for patients with large bowel disease to exhibit higher infertility rates. Interestingly after surgical therapy for CD, fertility rates were not different than figures for the non-CD population. In examination of some of the reasons for subfertility, it was found that some patients had been advised not to get pregnant because of their CD and were infertile on that basis. It was also found that women tended to get pregnant while in remission.

No differences in the incidence of fertility were found by Khosla et al in a study of 54 women with CD.[4] Of the 54 women who were studied, 10 did not conceive during the 20-year study period. Of these 10 patients, only 6 had involuntary infertility for an overall infertility rate of 11%. Colonic disease appeared to be associated with infertility in this population.

A report by Homan and Thorbjarnarson contradicts these findings in that there was no significant difference in fertility rates between the patient groups with different sites of disease.[5] Overall, 78 women of childbearing age were studied, with 42 pregnancies occurring over the 20-year study period.

Many of the early studies looking at fertility in patients with CD have been limited by their retrospective or survey methodology and lack of normal population control group. Mayberry and Weterman carried out a case-control study using a European cohort of patients.[6] A total of 275 patients with age-matched controls were studied. There was a reduction in number of children born to cases after diagnosis compared to controls. Prior to a CD diagnosis, the obstetric history was similar. Patients used contraception to a lesser extent than did the controls, with 42% not conceiving compared to 28% of controls. Disease location did not affect the fertility rate. Of note, 40 patients with CD were counseled to avoid pregnancy compared with 8 controls. This advice did not affect contraceptive practice.

Moody and coworkers invited 1400 patients in Leicestershire, United Kingdom to participate in a questionnaire study designed to determine whether IBD patients had a similar fertility rate and a similar rate of congenital malformations to the background population in Leicestershire.[7] A total of 601 patients (52% male) with CD were enrolled into the study. Women with CD had an infertility rate of 19%. The total fertility rate for women with CD was 1.2 with a rate of 1.7 expected in the background population. In men, much of the infertility seen was associated with sulfasalazine therapy. Greater than 50% of women with CD experiencing a delay in conception were also taking sulfasalazine although the mechanism of this effect is not clear. Patients with CD had more births prior to diagnosis than after diagnosis.

These studies support subfertility in CD patients; however, due to the nature of the studies, it is difficult to identify patients who were actively trying to conceive, reasons for failure of conception, and the role of disease-related biological effects on fertility. Baird and coworkers reported on a case-control study in 1990 where the reproductive histories of 177 women with CD were compared to healthy control subjects nominated by the CD patients.[8] Fertility, as measured by the total number of pregnancies, was examined as well as a diagnosis of infertility, fecundability, and methods of birth control. Women whose first pregnancies occurred after disease onset had fewer total pregnancies than controls. Women who had first pregnancies prior to disease diagnosis had the same number of pregnancies as did the controls. Cases and controls were similar in proportions of those that had primary involuntary childlessness or secondary infertility (2% to 4%). Similar percentages of both groups had greater than 1 year of trying to conceive before conception was attained (15% to 20%). There was no significant reduction in fecundability in patients with IBD as compared to the controls. This well-controlled study suggests that there should be more optimism when counseling patients regarding fertility in patients with IBD.

A large survey study performed in northern Scotland also demonstrated no difference in the rate of involuntary infertility in patients with CD as compared to a control population.[9] Overall, there was a 14% (17/123) involuntary infertility rate in CD patients. The rate was also 14% in the control population. Interestingly, the voluntary infertility rate was much higher (30%) in the CD population than in controls (7%). Patients treated medically had lower infertility rates than those treated surgically (8% versus 20%); however, this finding in part was accounted for by higher numbers of voluntary infertility in patients treated medically (36%) compared to those treated surgically (23%). In the cases of patients with voluntary infertility, none were counseled against pregnancy because of their IBD. Unfortunately, factors leading to the decisions were not explored. There are multiple possibilities related to disease that may lead to a decision not to conceive, including changes in sexuality related to ill health, changes in body image, concerns about disease transmission, and worries about the effect of IBD medications on birth outcome. None of the studies to date have explored these issues.

ULCERATIVE COLITIS STUDIES

Whereas the fertility data are mixed in studies in CD, most studies suggest that fertility is maintained in patients with ulcerative colitis. The exception to this is in patients treated surgically for ulcerative colitis. This will be discussed separately. As with the CD studies, many of the early reviews do not report whether patients were actively trying to conceive, which would allow accurate fertility rates to be determined.

McDougall reported in 1956 that of 131 married women of childbearing age, a total of 100 patients had pregnancies.[10] Thirty-six of the pregnancies occurred before the onset of ulcerative colitis, 64 after developing the disease, 20 patients had no children, and 11 patients could not be traced. If all 20 patients who did not have children were infertile, the infertility rate would be 16%.

De Dombal et al reviewed data on 229 women with ulcerative colitis and found that 72 women had conceived, giving a fertility rate of 31%.[11] This study was limited in that the follow-up was short, there was not accurate marital information, desire for pregnancy was not known, and there was no information available regarding male infertility. This is the only ulcerative colitis study that suggested an overall fertility rate lower than what would be expected in the background population. With the major study limitations, the results are likely underestimating fertility in this population.[11]

In a review of the Mayo Clinic data, Webb and Sedlack reported a 10% infertility rate in the ulcerative colitis population.[12] A total of 61 married women were studied of whom 6 failed to get pregnant. Of note, only 26 patients conceived after the diagnosis of ulcerative colitis.

Willoughby and Truelove studied 147 married women of childbearing age with a history of ulcerative colitis attending the Oxford ulcerative colitis clinic over a 20-year period.[13] A total of 119 (81%) of the patients had conceived a child. Only 10 patients (6.8%) were involuntarily infertile. Pregnancy outcome and family size were comparable to the general British population.

In the study by Baird and colleagues involving 84 women with ulcerative colitis, there was no difference in fertility rate and fecundability ratios as compared to an age-matched nondisease population.[8] Two percent of patients were involuntarily childless (4% control), 3% secondarily infertile (4% control), and 17% had a pregnancy after greater than 1 year of attempting to conceive (15% control). The fecundability ratio was 1.1 in predisease pregnancies and 1.0 in postdiagnosis pregnancies compared to 1.0 in the control population.

In the large Leicestershire, United Kingdom questionnaire study, Moody et al reported that patients with ulcerative colitis had similar numbers of children to the background population in that area (Table 12-3).[7] There were, however, a large number of patients who had a significant delay in conceiving a child. Overall, 15% of patients experienced a delay of more than 12 months in achieving conception, 9% of men and 23% of women with UC. A large percentage of these patients were on sulfasalazine. Ultimately, many of those individuals with a delay in pregnancy were able to conceive, yielding an overall infertility rate of 15% in women with ulcerative colitis.

In the Scottish population described by Hudson and colleagues, an infertility rate of 15% in 138 patients with ulcerative colitis was reported.[9] Overall, the studies on patients with ulcerative colitis show remarkable similarity in fertility rates compared to background or control populations. Fertility rates in the earlier studies were affected by sulfasalazine therapy, which is known now to have an adverse effect on sperm in men. In all of the above ulcerative colitis studies, patients studied were receiving medical therapy for their disease process. Surgical therapy does affect the fertility of women with ulcerative colitis and is discussed in the next section.

Table 12-3

FERTILITY AND ULCERATIVE COLITIS

Study	Disease	N	Infertility
McDougall[10]	UC	120	16%
De Dombal et al[11]	UC	229	69%
Webb and Sedlack[12]	UC	61	10%
Willoughby and Truelove[13]	UC	147	6.80%
Baird et al[8]	UC	84	2%
	Control	216	4%
Hudson et al[9]	UC	138	15%
	Control	766	14%
Moody et al[7]	UC	352	15%

UC = ulcerative colitis

In studies that examined men and women, only the female infertility rates are reported.

Factors That May Affect Fertility

SEXUAL DYSFUNCTION

Sexual dysfunction may significantly impact reported fertility. The likelihood of conception is decreased in couples who have a low frequency of intercourse. This has not been well examined in studies on fertility in IBD. In patients with IBD, factors that may lead to sexual dysfunction include poor body image, ill health, and painful intercourse due to disease-related factors.

Sexual dysfunction is not commonly discussed at medical visits and may be under-recognized in the IBD population. Moody and colleagues performed a structured interview in 45 women with CD in stable relationships and compared them to an age-matched control population.[14] They found that 24% of patients had infrequent or no intercourse compared with 4% of controls. In those patients who were sexually active, intercourse frequency was similar. The reasons for decreased sexual activity included abdominal pain (24%), diarrhea (20%), and fear of fecal incontinence (14%). Dyspareunia was seen to a greater extent in patients (60%) than in controls. In this group, CD patients had a greater degree of difficulty in achieving conception with 22% experiencing a 2-year delay compared to 7% in the control group. Moody and Mayberry extended these studies by looking at similar issues in men with ulcerative colitis (54), women with ulcerative colitis (50), and men with CD (46).[15] In these populations, there was no difference in frequency of sexual intercourse. Dyspareunia was more common in patients (38%) than controls (18%). The concerns in this study population were similar to those voiced by the women with CD, including fear of incontinence (20%), abdominal pain (15%), and urgency (13%). The total number of pregnancies seen in these 3 groups were the same. In another survey of 165 sexually active women with CD by the same group, 30% were found to have dyspareunia.[16]

Body image perceptions also impact on sexual dysfunction in patients with IBD. This may result from perceived disfigurement from perineal disease or surgery. Steroids may lead to Cushingoid features and weight gain. Joachim and Milne found that 15% to 20% of IBD patients (n = 80) studied were unhappy with their sexuality and body image, whereas 42% felt that IBD had a negative impact overall on their life.[17] Perceptions of physical attractiveness after ostomy surgery have been studied with the finding that 60% of patients felt that they were less sexually attractive within the first year after surgery.[18] Patients felt disfigured or ugly; however, after the first year, this improved with most patients returning to prebaseline levels. Patients with longer illnesses preostomy tended to fare better with less impact on perceived sexuality. The United Ostomy Associations of America (www.uoaa.org) has a variety of resources available online that address the issues of sexuality and intimacy in patients with ostomies and that may be helpful to patients. The social impact of the unpredictable nature of this disease may lead to depression, which further affects sexual and personal relationships.[19]

SURGERY

For women to conceive, the fallopian tubes must be open and functional. Diseases involving the fallopian tubes are responsible for up to 35% of cases of infertility in women.[1] Obstruction of the fallopian tubes may result from a variety of causes, including sexually transmitted diseases and intra-abdominal inflammation, of which the latter is common in IBD. Peritubular adhesions affect the mobility of the tube, which may lead to impaired oocyte and sperm transport.[1] Partial obstruction of the fallopian tubes changes the immunochemical and hormonal balance of the tube, leading to altered sperm movement. Surgery for both ulcerative colitis and CD is associated with intra-abdominal adhesion formation and possible alteration in tubal anatomy. Of 662 patients who had undergone surgery for IBD studied at the Cleveland Clinic, 163 patients (25%) had difficulties with fertility with the cause being a tubal factor in 25%.[20] In this population, menstrual abnormalities were seen in 58% of patients and were thought to be due to the effects of the stress of chronic disease and poor nutrition on ovulation. Adhesion formation in IBD not only may play a role in the etiology of tubal infertility but also in the evaluation and surgical management of the tubal dysfunction.[21]

ILEAL POUCH ANAL ANASTOMOSIS FOR ULCERATIVE COLITIS

There is a growing body of literature that supports the impression that there are increased problems with fertility in patients who have undergone a total abdominal colectomy with ileal pouch anal anastomosis (IPAA) for ulcerative colitis. It is estimated that there is a 3-fold increase in infertility after IPAA.[22] This may not be limited to IPAA alone. Wikland and colleagues reported a 37% fertility rate (10/27) in patients attempting to conceive after a conventional proctocolectomy and end ileostomy for IBD (ulcerative colitis and CD).[23]

Since the mid to late 1980s, in an attempt to restore normal defecation and body image, restorative proctocolectomy with IPAA has become the surgical procedure of choice in patients with medically refractory ulcerative colitis. Oresland and colleagues performed a small study in 1994 that evaluated the effects of this procedure on gynecologic and sexual function in 21 women.[24] These women were evaluated by a gynecologic exam, hysterosalpingography, vaginography, and a detailed interview. Eleven women had either bilateral or unilateral tubal occlusion and 10 had tubes adhering to the bottom of the lesser pelvis. Of 14 patients trying to get pregnant in this group, only one was able to conceive. Of another 14 patients, not specifically studied in this group, 5 became pregnant after IPAA. This small study brought attention to the anatomic changes occurring after the extensive pelvic surgery in this population.

Two large Scandinavian studies from the University of Göteborg and Aarhus University Hospital evaluated further these observations in a larger population of patients. In the first study, preoperative and postoperative fertility were studied in 237 women and were compared to the number of births in the general population of that area.[25] A significant reduction in the observed number of births in the postoperative period was found. The birth rate was reduced to 49% of expected (p<0.001). Assisted reproduction with in vitro fertilization (IVF) occurred in 29% of the births, further lowering the birth rate of unassisted births to 35% of the expected. In this same study, the preoperative births were 87% of expected. The authors felt that the anatomic changes post-IPAA were the main reason for decreased fertility although in this study other factors such as advice against pregnancy or hesitancy to conceive due to worries about passing on ulcerative colitis to offspring were not evaluated.[25] This group proceeded to try to further clarify these issues with a structured telephone interview regarding reproductive behavior and waiting time to pregnancy in 290 patients and 662 women in a reference population.[26] Data were available on 98 patients for time to pregnancy (TTP) before diagnosis of ulcerative colitis, 84 before colectomy, and 149 after IPAA. The control patients provided information on 914 TTPs. Surgery reduced the fecundability rate of patients compared to the general population by 80%. There was no difference in fecundability in patients' prediagnosis of ulcerative colitis and postdiagnosis presurgery. The authors recommended that patients with IPAA who had difficulty conceiving should be referred for gynecologic evaluation and possible IVF early in the course of their difficulties.[26]

Other studies have shown an impact of IPAA surgery on fertility but not to the same extent as the Olsen study. Counihan et al reported a 16% (18/110) infertility rate in patients with IPAA for familial adenomatous polyposis and ulcerative colitis.[27] In this study, not all 110 patients were actively trying to conceive. There were 23 children born to 19 women after IPAA and 119 births to 57 women presurgery. The study did show a high incidence of persistent dyspareunia after surgery (27%).[27] In 1994, Gorgun and colleagues queried women of reproductive age in the Cleveland Clinic IPAA database regarding reproductive function before and after IPAA.[28] Of 300 patients identified, 206 patients had attempted to conceive. Before surgery, 38% (48/127) of patients were unsuccessful after 1 year of unprotected intercourse. The infertility rate increased to 56% (76/135) after surgery. The presurgery infertility rate is higher than that seen in the general population and may reflect a decrease in frequency of intercourse in this ill population. These authors also noted that intraoperative blood transfusion increased the infertility rate (21% rate with no transfusion versus 54% with transfusion). Blood transfusion may be a marker of a more complicated intraoperative course. There was no noticeable difference in fertility rate seen with use of oophoropexy or antiadhesion barriers at the time of surgery. In a Canadian study, the infertility rate in patients with IPAA was 38.1% (59/153) compared to a rate of 13.3% (8/60) in patients managed with medical therapy.[29] Increasing maternal age adversely affected fertility as well in this study. After surgery, 30.3% of patients used fertility treatments. In the large Scottish survey study by Hudson et al, 6/20 (30%) surgically treated ulcerative colitis patients had involuntary infertility compared to 15/118 (13%) medically treated patients.[9] More recently, a Finish study reported a 33% infertility rate post-IPAA compared to an 18% infertility rate in the control group. This rate in the IPAA group dropped to 24% if all births were considered, including those with infertility treatments and those that occurred after greater than 1 year of trying to conceive.[30] None of these studies approach the 80% infertility rate seen in the Olsen study, but all clearly demonstrate an adverse effect of restorative proctocolectomy with IPAA on fertility.

Infertility issues should be addressed when discussing IPAA with young women. In a patient with steroid-dependant ulcerative colitis, it may be possible to support a patient through a pregnancy and delay surgical therapy until a family is complete. This is not possible in the severely ill patient who is not responding to medical therapy. Currently in our society, many women are having children at a later age due to job and social constraints. Since maternal age is a factor in decreasing fertility, patients with an IPAA may want to consider not delaying attempts at conception.

Pelvic cysts after proctectomy have been described due to descent of the ovary from an intraperitoneal to an extraperitoneal location related to the mechanics of the surgery. Techniques have been developed to perform an oophoropexy to help prevent this.[31] Unfortunately, this has not been shown to improve fertility in the one study that was examined.[28] It may help prevent the descent of the ovary into the extraperitoneal location but the pexy may not put the ovary in an anatomically correct position for ova transfer to the fallopian tube. The data for this technique in patients with IPAA are limited due to small numbers and lack of prospective evaluation. Since tubal factors play a large role in infertility after IPAA, techniques to decrease adhesions in the pelvis may be useful. Gels and membranes placed at the time of surgery may decrease the incidence of postoperative adhesions. Glycerol hyaluronate/carboxymethylcellulose membranes placed under the midline incision have been studied in patients undergoing proctocolectomy with IPAA for ulcerative colitis and familial polyposis.[32] This membrane significantly decreased adhesions between the omentum and the small bowel compared to no therapy; however, 67% of patients with the membrane were found to have adhesions compared to 90% of patients with no treatment. For this to be useful in the pelvis, the membrane would need to be placed low in the tubal area. This may or may not be useful. Sodium hyaluronate/carboxymethylcellulose (Seprafilm, Genzyme Corporation, Cambridge, MA) has also been studied in this population and demonstrated 51% of treated patients free of adhesions compared to 6% of controls.[33] Dense adhesions are also reduced with 15% seen in treated patients compared to 58% of controls. Fertility issues have not been examined prospectively using these techniques but do deserve further study.

Laparoscopic IPAA (LAP-IPAA) has become more feasible with advances in laparoscopic techniques and instruments. There are now several large studies comparing laparoscopic and open techniques in terms of complications. Larson and colleagues report operative and postoperative outcomes on 100 consecutive LAP-IPAA patients compared to 200 open IPAA patients and found that the procedures were equivalent in terms of safety and feasibility.[34] Reoperation was required in 3% of LAP-IPAA and 6.5% of open IPAA (NS) patients during the first 90 days. There was an improvement in short-term recovery outcomes such as length of stay, time to a regular diet, and time to ileostomy output. The mean operative time was approximately 100 minutes longer in the LAP-IPAA group. As this technique gains more use, effects of postoperative infertility should be examined. It is possible that there may be a difference in adhesion rate is this group, although clearly adhesions remain a problem in laparoscopic surgery.

Male Infertility

In the general population, approximately 20% of infertile couples have a male factor as the primary etiology and 30% to 40% more as a contributing etiology.[1] The male factor may be azoospermia, oligospermia, or abnormal sperm function. Evaluation initially involved looking at a semen sample for volume, sperm concentration, sperm motility, and sperm morphology. There is a suggestion that IBD may impair male fertility; however, many of the earlier observations show a strong relationship between treatment with sulfasalazine and subsequent male infertility.[7,35] Burnell et al looked at 70 men with CD and age-matched controls and found a decrease in family size that was independent of steroid or sulfasalazine therapy.[36] Farthing and Dawson found oligospermia in 46% of men with CD not receiving sulfasalazine.[37] They suggested that factors such as disease activity, nutritional status, and other drugs should be considered as etiologic in male infertility in CD. In a case-control study of 106 men with CD and 62 with ulcerative colitis, a significantly lower number of pregnancies were found in CD patients compared to controls but not for men with ulcerative colitis.[38] There was no difference in fecundability in spouses of IBD patients and controls, suggesting that the overall reproductive capacity of men with IBD was not diminished. Specific drug therapies and disease activity were not examined in this study. From these studies and observations, it is clear that one must consider drug therapy, disease activity, and the effects of the disease when evaluating male fertility issues in IBD.

Common Inflammatory Bowel Disease Medications and Effect on Sperm

SULFASALAZINE

Sulfasalazine and its active metabolite 5-aminosalicylic acid are the mainstay of maintenance drug therapy in chronic ulcerative colitis. The effects of sulfasalazine on sperm density, motility, and morphology have been clearly documented to play a role in infertility in IBD patients on this drug. In 1979, Levi and colleagues reported 4 men with ulcerative colitis on sulfasalazine with oligospermia and infertility.[35] The drug was withdrawn and semen analysis improved, with pregnancies in 3 of the men's partners. The drug was reintroduced and in 2 patients there was a rapid change in the semen quality. Based on these observations, subsequent studies have evaluated the effect of sulfasalazine on semen. Toovey et al reported gross semen abnormalities in patients on sulfasalazine for greater than 2 months.[39] This included abnormal sperm density, abnormally low sperm motility, and increased percentage of abnormal forms. The changes seen have been shown to be reversible on sulfasalazine withdrawal. Since these initial descriptions, it has been shown that 5-aminosalicylic acid does not impair fertility. Rats fed the sulfapyridine moiety of sulfasalazine had impaired fertility, which was not evident when they were fed 5-aminosalicyclic acid.[40] Mesalamine substitution for sulfasalazine restores sperm motility, sperm count, and morphology.[41,42]

AZATHIOPRINE/6-MERCAPTOPURINE

The antimetabolites azathioprine and 6-mercaptopurine have become an important therapy to maintain remission in patients with refractory IBD. These drugs are used over long periods of time due to long-term efficacy and increased chance for relapse after withdrawal. The effects of azathioprine on male fertility have been evaluated. Dejaco et al evaluated the semen quality of 23 IBD patients treated with azathioprine.[43] In 10 patients, semen was evaluated before and after initiation of azathioprine. Sperm density, motility, morphology, total count, and volume were found to be unaffected by azathioprine therapy. There have been some concerns that azathioprine and 6-mercaptopurine may increase congenital abnormalities in offspring.[44] In a study in male rats, treatment with 6-mercaptopurine did not affect sperm morphology or sperm production.[45] There was an increase in resorption rates in the treatment groups (45% to 50% versus 21%) but not an increase in congenital malformations. It is possible that this class of drugs may cause occult damage to sperm in rats. This will need careful long-term observation and monitoring in men who conceive while on this class of drugs.

METHOTREXATE

Methotrexate is an antimetabolite and folic acid antagonist that is used as an alternative to azathioprine and 6-mercaptopurine in patients with IBD. It can cause chromosomal anomalies and point mutation that result in mutagenesis. In rats, methotrexate causes degeneration of spermatocytes, Sertoli cells, and Leydig cells. Sussman and Leonard reported a male treated with methotrexate for severe psoriasis who developed severe oligospermia associated with the drug. Withdrawal of methotrexate lead to normalization of sperm concentration.[46] The reversible oligospermia that methotrexate causes in humans is due to mitosis inhibition and flagellum damage.[47] There have been no reports of an increased risk of congenital defects in offspring of men treated with methotrexate. Men who are taking methotrexate should have a sperm analysis prior to attempts at conception. If there is oligospermia, the methotrexate should be discontinued at least 3 months prior to the attempt at conception.

INFLIXIMAB

Anti-TNF inhibitors are being used with increasing frequency in patients with active IBD. There is little information available on the effects of these agents on fertility. Mahadevan and colleagues evaluated the semen quality of men receiving infliximab for IBD.[48] Seven patients were on maintenance infliximab and 3 were receiving their first dose of infliximab. Semen samples were studied preinfusion (2 weeks) and postinfusion (1 week). The patients on maintenance infliximab had normal preinfusion and postinfusion semen volume, sperm concentration, and forward progression; however, sperm motility and percent normal oval forms were below the normal range. There was a significant volume increase in semen postinfusion and a significant decrease in normal oval forms. Infliximab-naïve patients showed a decrease in sperm motility postinfusion. Of note, prior to infusion, the number of normal oval forms was below normal and this number did not decrease further with infliximab infusion. These findings are not unexpected in that TNF-α dependent capsase family proteases may be important in sperm development. Whether these changes in sperm motility and morphology lead to abnormal fertility is not known. In the absence of other etiologies of infertility in a couple in which the male is receiving infliximab, changing therapy may be considered.

ZINC DEFICIENCY

Zinc deficiency is a common nutritional abnormality in patients with CD.[49] Zinc has an important role in all of the components of male reproduction and may impact on impaired fertility in men with IBD. Abbasi et al demonstrated that 24 to 40 weeks of dietary zinc restriction induces oligospermia with improvement after reintroduction of zinc into the diet.[50] Patients with CD may have zinc deficiency as a result of poor absorption or increased zinc loss. Zinc urinary losses postexercise are higher in CD patients than in nondisease controls.[51] Zinc deficiency should be considered in CD patients with abnormal sperm as another factor that may play a role in infertility.

Summary

Studies suggest that there may be a lower fertility rate in patients with CD; however, much of this may be due to voluntary infertility. Factors that may affect voluntary infertility in this population include abdominal pain, pelvic pain, fear of incontinence, decreased sexuality, and body image problems. These issues should be addressed with patients in the clinical setting.

Patients with ulcerative colitis do not appear to have lower fertility rates compared to the nondisease population. The one exception to this is the increased incidence of fertility problems after restorative proctocolectomy with IPAA. Women who require surgical therapy of their ulcerative colitis should be counseled about the increased infertility rates in this setting. Assisted reproductive technology techniques generally are successful in this population.

Men who are attempting to conceive need to be taken off sulfasalazine prior to attempts at conception. In men taking methotrexate, semen analysis should be performed to look for oligospermia. If present, then the methotrexate should be discontinued for 90 days prior to attempts at conception. Men who are on anti-TNF inhibitors also should have a semen analysis performed if they are experiencing fertility difficulties.

Disease activity should be controlled and nutritional deficiencies should be corrected prior to attempts at conception to optimize the chance of success.

References

1. Adamson G, V Baker V. Subfertility: causes, treatment and outcome. *Best Pract Res Clin Obstet Gynaecol.* 2003;17:168-185.
2. Fielding J, Cooke W. Pregnancy and Crohn's disease. *BMJ.* 1970;2:76-77.
3. De Dombal F, Burton I, Goligher J. Crohn's disease and pregnancy. *BMJ.* 1972;3:550-553.
4. Khosla R, Willoughby C, Jewell D. Crohn's disease and pregnancy. *Gut.* 1984;25:52-56.
5. Homan W, Thorbjarnarson B. Crohn disease and pregnancy. *Arch Surg.* 1976;111:545-547.
6. Mayberry J, Weterman I. European survey of fertility and pregnancy in women with Crohn's disease: a case control study by European collaborative group. *Gut.* 1986;27:821-825.
7. Moody G, Probert C, Jayanthi V, Mayberry J. The effects of chronic ill health and treatment with sulfasalazine on fertility amongst men and women with inflammatory bowel disease in Leicestershire. *Int J Colorectal Dis.* 1997;12:220-224.
8. Baird D, Narendranathan M, Sandler R. Increased risk of preterm birth for women with inflammatory bowel disease. *Gastroenterology.* 1990;88:987-994.
9. Hudson M, Flett G, Sinclair TS, et al. Fertility and pregnancy in inflammatory bowel disease. *Int J Gynaecol Obstet.* 1997;58:229-237.
10. McDougall I. Ulcerative colitis and pregnancy. *Lancet.* 1956;271:641-643.
11. De Dombal F, Watts J, Watkinson G, Goligher J. Ulcerative colitis and pregnancy. *Lancet.* 1965;2:599-602.
12. Webb M, Sedlack R. Ulcerative colitis in pregnancy. *Med Clin North Am.* 1974;58:823-827.
13. Willoughby C, Truelove S. Ulcerative colitis and pregnancy. *Gut.* 1980;21:469-474.
14. Moody G, Probert C, Srivastava E, et al. Sexual dysfunction amongst women with Crohn's disease: a hidden problem. *Digestion.* 1992;52:179-183.
15. Moody G, Mayberry J. Perceived sexual dysfunction amongst patients with inflammatory bowel disease. *Digestion.* 1993;54:256-260.
16. Lichtarowicz A, Mayberry J. Sexual dysfunction in women with Crohn's disease. *Br Med J.* 1987;295:1065-1066.
17. Joachim G, Milne B. Inflammatory bowel disease: effects on lifestyle. *J Adv Nurs.* 1987;12:483-487.
18. Gloeckner M. Perception of sexual attractiveness following ostomy surgery. *Res Nurs Health.* 1984;7:87-92.
19. Trachter A, Rogers A, Leiblum S. Inflammatory bowel disease in women: impact on relationship and sexual health. *Inflamm Bowel Dis.* 2002;8:413-421.
20. Weber A, Ziegler C, Belinson J, et al. Gynecologic history of women with inflammatory bowel disease. *Obstet Gynecol.* 1995;86:843-847.
21. Arkuran C, McComb P. Crohn's disease and tubal infertility: the effect of adhesion formation. *Clin Exp Obstet Gynecol.* 2000;27:12-13.
22. Waljee A, Waljee J, Morris A, Higgings PD. Threefold increased risk of infertility: a meta-analysis of infertility after ileal pouch anal anastomosis in ulcerative colitis. *Gut.* 2006;55:1575-1580.
23. Wikland M, Jansson I, Asztély M, et al. Gynaecological problems related to anatomical changes after conventional proctocolectomy and ileostomy. *Int J Colorectal Dis.* 1990;5:49-52.
24. Oresland T, Palmblad S, Ellström M, et al. Gynaecological and sexual function related to anatomical changes in the female pelvis after restorative proctocolectomy. *Int J Colorectal Dis.* 1994;9:77-81.
25. Olsen K, Joelsson M, Laurberg S, Oresland T. Fertility after ileal pouch-anal anastomosis in women with ulcerative colitis. *Br J Surg.* 1999;86:493-495.
26. Olsen K, Juul S, Berndtsson I, et al. Ulcerative colitis: female fecundity before diagnosis, during disease and after surgery compared with a population sample. *Gastroenterology.* 2002;122:15-19.
27. Counihan T, Roberts P, Schoetz DJ, et al. Fertility and sexual and gynecologic function after ileal pouch-anal anastomosis. *Dis Colon Rectum.* 1994;37:1126-1129.
28. Gorgun E, Remzi F, Goldberg J, et al. Fertility is reduced after restorative proctocolectomy with ileal pouch anal anastomosis: a study of 300 patients. *Surgery.* 2004;136:795-803.
29. Johnson P, Richard C, Ravid A, et al. Female infertility after ileal pouch-anal anastomosis for ulcerative colitis. *Dis Colon Rectum.* 2004;47:1119-1126.
30. Leipisto A, Sarna S, Tiitinen A, Jarvinen H. Female fertility and childbirth after ileal pouch-anal anastomosis for ulcerative colitis. *Br J Surg.* 2007;94:478-482.
31. Matthews J, Kodner I, Fry R, Fazio V. Entrapped ovary syndrome. *Dis Colon Rectum.* 1986;29:341-343.
32. Cohen Z, Senagore A, Dayton M, et al. Prevention of postoperative abdominal adhesions by a novel, glycerol/sodium hyaluronate/carboxymethylcellulose-based bioresorbable membrane: a prospective, randomized, evaluator-blinded multicenter study. *Dis Colon Rectum.* 2005;48:1130-1139.
33. Becker J, Dayton M, Fazio V, et al. Prevention of postoperative abdominal adhesions by a sodium hyaluronate-based bioresorbable membrane: a prospective, randomized, double-blind multicenter study. *J Am Coll Surg.* 1996;183:297-306.
34. Larson D, Cima R, Dozois E, et al. Safety, feasibility and short-term outcomes of laparoscopic ileal-pouch-anal anastomosis. *Ann Surg.* 2006;243:667-672.

35. Levi A, Fisher A, Hughes L, Hendry W. Male infertility due to sulfasalazine. *Lancet.* 1979;2:276-278.
36. Burnell D, Mayberry J, Calcraft B, et al. Male fertility in Crohn's disease. *Postgad Med J.* 1986;62:269-272.
37. Farthing M, Dawson A. Impaired semen quality in Crohn's disease—drugs, ill health or undernutrition. *Scand J Gastroenterol.* 1983;18:1983.
38. Narendranathan M, Sandler R, Suchindran C, Savitz D. Male infertility in inflammatory bowel disease. *J Clin Gastroenterol.* 1989;11:403-406.
39. Toovey S, Hudson E, Hendry W, Levi A. Sulfasalazine and male infertility: reversibility and possible mechanism. *Gut.* 1981;22:445-451.
40. O'Moráin C, Smethurst P, Doré C, Levi A. Reversible male infertility due to sulfasalazine: studies in man and rat. *Gut.* 1984;25:1078-1084.
41. Riley S, Lecarpentier J, Mani V, et al. Sulfasalazine induced seminal abnormalities in ulcerative colitis: results of mesalazine substitution. *Gut.* 1987;28:1008-1012.
42. Kjaergaard N, Christensen L, Lauritsen J, et al. Effects of mesalazine substitution on salicylazosulfapyridine-induced seminal abnormalities in men with ulcerative colitis. *Scand J Gastroenterol.* 1989;24:891-896.
43. Dejaco C, Mittermaier C, Reinisch W, et al. Azathioprine treatment and male fertility in inflammatory bowel disease. *Gastroenterology.* 2001;121:1048-1053.
44. Rajapakse R, Korelitz B, Zlatanic J, et al. Outcome of pregnancies when fathers are treated with 6-mercaptopurine for inflammatory bowel disease. *Am J Gastroenterol.* 2000;95:684-688.
45. Ligumsky M, Badaan S, Lewis H, Meirow D. Effects of 6-mercaptopurine treatment on sperm production and reproductive performance: a study in male mice. *Scand J Gastroenterol.* 2005;40:444-449.
46. Sussman A, Leonard J. Psoriasis, methotrexate and oligospermia. *Arch Dermatol.* 1980;116:215-217.
47. Grunewald S, Paasch U, Glander HJ. Systemic dermatological treatment with relevance for male fertility. *J Dtsch Dermatol Ges.* 2007;5:15-21.
48. Mahadevan U, Terdiman J, Aron J, et al. Infliximab and semen quality in men with inflammatory bowel disease. *Inflamm Bowel Dis.* 2005;11:395-399.
49. El-Tawil A. Zinc deficiency in men with Crohn's disease may contribute to poor sperm function and male infertility. *Andrologia.* 2003;35:337-341.
50. Abbasi A, Prasad A, Rabbani P, DuMouchelle E. Experimental zinc deficiency in man: effect on testicular function. *J Lab Clin Med.* 1980;96:544-550.
51. D'Inca R. Effect of moderate exercise on Crohn's disease patients in remission. *Ital J Gastroenterol Hepatol.* 1999;31:205-210.

Financial disclosure: Dr. Isaacs receives grant support from Abbott, Otsuka, UCB, and Ocera; DSMB from Centocor; and is a speaker for Centocor, Abbott, and UCB.

CHAPTER 13

PREGNANCY AND POSTPARTUM

Sonia Friedman, MD

The peak age of inflammatory bowel disease (IBD) onset coincides with the peak age of fertility, and many patients with IBD want advice regarding pregnancy. As little as a decade ago, we did not have good data on the effect of many essential IBD medications during pregnancy and until this year, there was scanty data on the effect of disease activity on pregnancy outcomes. New publications have explored the safety of azathioprine (AZA) and 6-mercaptopurine (6-MP) during pregnancy and have also attempted to separate out medication use as a confounder when measuring the impact of disease activity upon pregnancy outcomes. The issue of continuing biologic therapies such as infliximab and adalimumab during pregnancy is very much in the forefront of clinical research and hopefully, there will soon be published recommendations for pediatricians of babies whose moms used biologic therapy during pregnancy. Nursing while taking immunomodulators and biologics is another topic of heated debate, mostly because we have only scanty evidence-based medical literature on the subject. Other drugs we know even less about during pregnancy are budesonide and rifaximin as there are no data in pregnant women. Overall, however, pregnancy outcomes in Crohn's disease (CD) and ulcerative colitis (UC) patients are almost as good as in the general population, and women with IBD should be optimistic about having a successful pregnancy.

Effect of Disease Activity Upon Pregnancy

Perhaps the most important thing doctors should remember when counseling an IBD patient about a potential pregnancy is that the patient should be in remission at the time of conception. This remission should be durable, for at least 3 to 6 months on stable medications, prior to conception. Most IBD medications are safe during pregnancy and the biggest problem most patients have is stopping their long-term medications prior to conception. A frank discussion about pregnancy, reinforced at each office visit, helps both doctor and patient anticipate any potential problems.

Scherl EJ, Dubinsky MC.
The Changing World of Inflammatory Bowel Disease:
Impact of Generation, Gender, and Global Trends (pp 161-176)
© 2009 SLACK Incorporated.

It is fairly well-documented that babies born to women with CD and UC are at greater risk for adverse pregnancy outcomes, including premature birth and low birth weight when compared to controls in the general population.[1-10] Women with IBD, and probably CD in particular, are at greater risk for having a cesarean section. A meta-analysis of 12 prior studies encompassing 3907 patients with IBD (CD 1952 [64%] and UC 1113 [36%]) and 320,531 controls was published in 2007.[11] Overall, there was a 1.87-fold increase in the incidence of prematurity (<37 week gestation, 95% confidence interval [CI], 1.52 to 2.31, p<0.001) compared with controls. The incidence of low birth weight (<2500 grams) was over twice that of normal controls (95% CI, 1.38 to 3.19, p<0.001). Women with IBD were 1.5 times more likely to undergo cesarean section (95% CI, 1.47 to 3.82, p<0.001) and the risk of congenital anomalies was found to be 2.37-fold increased (95% CI, 1.47 to 3.82, p<0.001). The greater risk of low birth weight and cesarean section was significant only in patients with CD. The greater risk of congenital anomalies was found only in women with UC in a single study.[12] All types of congenital anomalies, including ones of minor significance, were included in this particular study, and the authors did not take disease activity or medications into consideration. When just the higher quality studies were analyzed, there was no greater risk of congenital anomalies. Neither disease activity nor medication use was used as a confounder in this meta-analysis.

There is even newer and more specific information about the impact of CD activity per se on pregnancy outcomes. A recent paper examined all births by women with CD in North Jutland County, Denmark from January 1977 to December 2005.[13] All individual medical records were reviewed. The authors found 71 pregnancies in women with disease activity and 86 pregnancies in women with inactive disease. There was no increased incidence of low birth weight, low birth weight at term, or congenital abnormalities among the 2 groups of women. However, there was an increased risk of preterm birth in women with moderate to high disease activity (RR, 3.4; 95% CI, 1.1 to 10.6). The authors controlled for the influence of drug therapy, particularly immunomodulator use, as a confounder.

Another recent, even more comprehensive paper looked at pregnancy outcomes in women with IBD in a large health maintenance organization in northern California.[14] This was a cohort study of 461 pregnant women with IBD matched to 493 pregnant women without IBD. All medical records were reviewed and data were gathered on many factors, including disease activity and IBD medications during pregnancy. Very few patients were on biologics or immunomodulators (4%) during pregnancy and conception, whereas 21% had some corticosteroid exposure and 51% had some aminosalicylate exposure. Pregnant women with IBD were less likely to have a live birth (60% versus 68%, p = 0.01) and more likely to have a cesarean section (13.8% versus 9.5%, p = 0.05) than women without IBD. The rate of therapeutic abortion and congenital anomalies were similar between the 2 groups. There was no difference in the rate of congenital anomalies between children born to mothers with UC or CD (p = 0.45). Women with IBD were also more likely to have an adverse conception outcome (spontaneous abortion, abortion for unknown reason) (23% versus 17%, p = 0.03), an adverse pregnancy outcome (preterm birth, small for gestation age, still birth) (25% versus 19%, p = 0.058), or a complication of pregnancy (25% versus 16%, p <0.01) compared with women without IBD. There was no statistically significant difference in newborn outcomes between the 2 groups (10% versus 7%, p = 0.18). Low birth weight was also more common among IBD patients than among non-IBD patients (7.4% versus 3.6%, p = 0.04).

Among all patients, predictors of an adverse conception outcome in a multivariate model included the presence of IBD, non-White ethnicity, a history of IBD surgery, and increasing maternal age (odds ratio [OR] per year of age, 1.10; 95% CI, 1.05 to 1.14). Predictors of an adverse pregnancy outcome were non-White ethnicity and the presence of IBD. Predictors of a pregnancy complication were a diagnosis of IBD, CD, and a history of IBD surgery. The only predictor of a newborn adverse outcome was a diagnosis of CD.

Disease activity, any IBD medication use, and moderate to severe disease activity were not associated with adverse outcomes. The majority of patients (about 80%) with both CD and UC had inactive or mild disease throughout pregnancy. Although limited by its homogeneous study population, this study should reassure us that women in remission should have healthy pregnancies. Since only 4% of patients were on immunomodulators or biologics, we need to look elsewhere for the safety of these specific medications during pregnancy.

Impact of Pregnancy Upon Disease Activity

Women with IBD are as likely to flare during pregnancy as they are to flare when not pregnant. Nielsen et al reported an exacerbation rate of 34% per year during pregnancy and 32% per year when not pregnant in women with UC.[15] Pregnant women with CD also had similar rates of exacerbation.[16] For a patient with UC in remission at the time of conception, there is about a one-third chance that she will flare during the 12 months of gestation and the puerperium. This is similar to a relapse rate of nonpregnant colitics followed for 1 year. In UC patients with active disease at the time of conception, roughly 50% will get worse while 25% will improve and 25% will remain unchanged. Thus, virtually 3 out of 4 patients will have active disease during the course of their pregnancy with a subsequent ill effect on the fetus. For patients with CD in remission at conception, about 25% will relapse in the following 12 months, no different than the nonpregnant CD patient. For patients with active disease at the time of conception, one-third will improve and one-third will worsen. Thus, two-thirds will have to contend with active disease during pregnancy.[17]

It is common for disease activity to vary from pregnancy to pregnancy in a particular individual despite the fact that disease may be inactive at conception. The only paper examining this question investigates the effect of human leukocyte antigen (HLA) mismatch on disease activity.[18] The authors studied 50 pregnancies in 38 women with CD or UC. Both mother and child were HLA tested. Thirty of the 50 pregnancies were disparate at both the DRB1 and the DQ loci. Twelve pregnancies were mismatched at the DRB1 locus and 4 at the DQ locus. Four were disparate at neither. When comparing the calculated average disease score for pregnancies disparate at one versus both loci, an OR of 22 (95% CI, 3.4 to 34, p = 0.007) was seen. By logistic regression analysis, HLA disparity at both DRB1 and DQ predicted a lower postpartum disease activity score. Thus, maternal immune response to paternal HLA antigens may play a role in pregnancy-induced remission of IBD.

There is some evidence that pregnancy may impact upon future disease course. A recent European study looked at data obtained at a 10-year follow-up study of 173 female UC patients and 93 female CD patients.[19] Researchers reported data from a chart review and a patient questionnaire. Five hundred eighty pregnancies, 403 occurring before the diagnosis of IBD and 177 after the diagnosis of IBD, were analyzed. The rate of spontaneous abortions increased after IBD was diagnosed (6.5% versus 13%, p = 0.005), whereas the rate of elective abortions was not significantly different. The significant increase in the number of spontaneous abortions was seen mainly in CD patients (OR, 5.5; 95% CI, 1.9 to 16.3, p<0.001). The use of cesarean section increased after IBD diagnosis (8.1% versus 28.7% of pregnancies). CD patients pregnant during the disease course did not differ from patients who were not pregnant during the disease course regarding the development of stenosis (37% versus 52% p = 0.13) and resection rates (mean number of resections 0.52 versus 0.66, p = 0.37). For the 40 patients followed before, during, and at least 3 years after their pregnancies, the rate of relapse decreased in the years following pregnancy in both UC (0.34 versus 0.18 flares/year, p = 0.008) and CD patients (0.76 versus 0.12 flares/year, p = 0.004). Thus, being pregnant may be associated with future reduced disease flares.

Management of Inflammatory Bowel Disease During Pregnancy

Patients with active disease should be considered high-risk pregnancies and should be followed by the appropriate obstetric service. Unlike many other diseases in pregnancy, delivery will rarely cure an IBD flare, although early delivery in some situations may protect the fetus and allow for more aggressive treatment of the mother. Disease activity should be monitored carefully prior to conception and throughout the pregnancy. Patients should be encouraged to be compliant with treatment if needed for flares or for maintenance as active disease is the greatest threat to a pregnancy. As patients with IBD can develop other gastrointestinal (GI) complications during pregnancy, an evaluation for infection, ulcer disease, nausea and vomiting associated with pregnancy, and biliary disease should be undertaken before starting treatment for a flare.

Disease assessment during pregnancy in IBD patients should rely heavily on clinical features, and patients should be questioned about abdominal pain, stool frequency, nocturnal stools, and blood and mucus in the stool. Laboratory parameters will often not be accurate since during gestation, hemoglobin and albumin levels will fall as a result of hemodilution and erythrocyte sedimentation rate (ESR) will rise. During pregnancy, the C-reactive protein level is a more accurate measure of IBD activity than the ESR. The pulse rate and temperature should be recorded and stool cultures and stool *C. difficile* toxin performed in the event of diarrhea. Maintaining adequate nutrition, hydration, and electrolyte balance is critical for the patient and the fetus. Antidiarrheal therapy can be used as an adjunct to IBD treatment to help avoid hospitalization in patients with refractory diarrhea.

Diagnostic Radiology During Pregnancy

Various imaging modalities are available for diagnostic use in the IBD patient during pregnancy. These include x-ray, ultrasonography, magnetic resonance imaging (MRI) in the second and third trimesters, and computed tomography (CT) after 25 weeks of gestation.[20] In humans, growth retardation, microcephaly, and mental retardation are the most common adverse effects from high-dose radiation. Based on data from atomic bomb survivors, it appears that the risk of central nervous system effects is greatest with exposure at 8 to 15 weeks of gestation, with no proven risk at less than 8 weeks of gestation or greater than 25 weeks of gestation. Thus, at 8 to 15 weeks of gestation, the fetus is at greatest risk for radiation-induced mental retardation and the risk appears to be at doses of at least 20 rad. Even multiple diagnostic x-ray procedures rarely result in ionizing radiation exposure to this degree. Fetal risks of anomalies, growth restriction, and abortions are not increased with radiation exposure of less than 5 rad, a level above the range of exposure of most diagnostic procedures. The risk of carcinogenesis as a result of in utero exposure to ionizing radiation is unclear but is probably very small. It is estimated that a 1 to 2 rad fetal exposure may increase the risk of leukemia by a factor of 1.2 to 2.0 over natural incidence and that an estimated 1 in 2000 children exposed to ionizing radiation in utero will develop childhood leukemia. This is increased from a background rate of 1 in 3000.[21-24] Table 13-1 details the estimated fetal exposure from some common radiologic procedures.

With MRI, magnets that alter the energy state of hydrogen protons are used instead of ionizing radiation. MRI is somewhat useful in establishing the diagnosis and/or evaluating the activity of CD in the second and third trimesters. Ultrasonography involves the use of sound waves and is not a form of ionizing radiation. It is less useful than MRI in evaluating IBD activity.[25]

Most intravenous contrast agents used with CT contain derivatives of iodine and have not been studied in humans; however, many have been studied in animals and do not appear to be teratogenic. Neonatal hypothyroidism has been associated with some iodinated contrast agents

Table 13-1

ESTIMATED FETAL EXPOSURE
FROM SOME COMMON RADIOLOGIC PROCEDURES

Procedure	Fetal Exposure
Chest x-ray (2 views)	0.02 to 0.07 mrad
Abdominal film (single view)	100 mrad
Intravenous pyelography	>1 rad
Hip film (single view)	200 mrad
Mammography	7 to 20 mrad
Barium enema or small bowel series	2 to 4 rad
CT scan of head or chest	<1 rad
CT scan of abdomen and lumbar spine	3.5 rad
CT pelvimetry	250 mrad
CT enterography	3.5 rad

taken during pregnancy and for this reason, these compounds are avoided unless essential for the correct diagnosis. Neonatal thyroid function should be checked during the first week if iodinated contrast media has been given during pregnancy. Paramagnetic contrast agents used during MRI have not been studied in pregnant women. Animal studies have demonstrated increased rates of spontaneous abortion, skeletal abnormalities, and visceral abnormalities when given at 2 to 7 times the recommended human dose. The agents should be used if the potential benefit justifies the potential risk. Only tiny amounts of iodinated or gadolinium-based contrast medium given to the lactating mother reach the milk and only a minute proportion is absorbed.[25]

Inflammatory Bowel Disease
Medications During Pregnancy

Perhaps the most controversial aspect of managing the pregnant IBD patient is convincing the patient (and referring obstetrician) not to stop IBD medications.

The greatest threat to a pregnancy is active disease, not the medications used to treat it. The safety of various IBD medications during pregnancy and nursing is outlined in Tables 13-2 and 13-3.

SULFASALAZINE AND 5-ASA MEDICATIONS

Sulfasalazine is a pregnancy category B drug (Table 13-4). It readily crosses the placenta, and fetal concentrations are nearly the same as maternal concentrations. It was formerly thought that sulfasalazine and bilirubin competed for the same binding site on albumin, potentially leading to unconjugated hyperbilirubinemia and an increased risk of kernicterus in the newborn. However, in vitro and human studies have not shown any decrease in the bilirubin-binding capacity of albumin in the presence of sulfasalazine and no increased risk of kernicterus.[26] In a cohort of 100 pregnancies exposed to sulfasalazine or 5-ASA drugs, there was no increased risk of birth defects, spontaneous abortions, or premature delivery. The average dose of sulfasalazine was 2 g/day.[27] In another cohort of 102 pregnancies, the use of sulfasalazine was not associated with an

Table 13-2

INFLAMMATORY BOWEL DISEASE MEDICATIONS DURING PREGNANCY

Category B	Category C	Category D	Category X
Mesalamine	Budesonide	Azathioprine†	Methotrexate
Balsalazide	Ciprofloxacin	6-mercaptopurine†	Thalidomide
Prednisone/prednisolone	Cyclosporine		
Sulfasalazine	Olsalazine		
Infliximab	Tacrolimus		
Metronidazole*	Diphenoxylate		
Adalimumab	Codeine		
Loperamide	Natalizumab		
Certolizumab			

*Safe during the second and third trimesters.
†Studies in women with IBD and renal transplants have shown that these medications are relatively safe during pregnancy (see text).

Table 13-3

INFLAMMATORY BOWEL DISEASE MEDICATIONS AND NURSING

Safe to Use When Needed	Limited Data Available But Likely Safe	Should be Avoided
Oral mesalamine	Azathioprine	Methotrexate
Balsalazide	6-mercaptopurine	Cyclosporine
Topical mesalamine	Anti-TNF	Metronidazole
Sulfasalazine		Ciprofloxacin
Prednisone/prednisolone		Tacrolimus

Table 13-4

PREGNANCY CATEGORIES

A	Controlled studies in pregnant women show no risk
B	Safe in animals, no studies in women or not safe in animals but safe in women
C	Adverse effects in animals, no studies in women
D	Evidence of human fetal risk but benefits may be acceptable
X	Contraindicated

increased risk of adverse pregnancy outcomes compared to women with IBD on no treatment.[28] A case-control study in the Hungarian population also found no significant teratogenic risk.[29] Sulfasalazine interacts with the cell-membrane transporter for natural folates. This interferes with folate absorption and may lead to folate deficiency. More aggressive folate supplementation with up to 2 mg of folic acid daily is therefore recommended for all pregnant female patients on sulfasalazine.[30,31]

Mesalamine and balsalazide are pregnancy category B drugs and olsalazine is a pregnancy category C drug. A retrospective study involving 123 pregnancies exposed to mesalamine showed that this drug is not associated with an increased risk of pregnancy-related complications, congenital anomalies, or stillbirths. The average dose of mesalamine in this study was 2.1 g/day.[32] In a prospective case-control study with 165 patients exposed to mesalamine, there was an increased risk of preterm delivery, less mean maternal weight gain, and a lower mean birth weight. Rates of spontaneous abortions, stillbirths, and congenital malformations were not significantly increased. The mean daily dose was 2 g/day.[33] Women who had active IBD or who were on numerous anti-IBD medications had higher rates of premature and low birth weight babies compared with women on mesalamine monotherapy. Like many of these studies of IBD drugs in pregnancy, the poorer birth outcomes were probably due to the disease activity not the 5-ASA medications.[34] Although there has been scanty clinical data on a 5-ASA dose of more than 2 to 3 g/day, years of postmarketing experience have shown doses of up to 4.8 g/day to be safe during pregnancy. Topical therapy with mesalamine enemas and suppositories is also pregnancy category B and can be a helpful adjunctive or primary therapy for those women with proctitis or proctosigmoiditis.[35] Only small amounts of 5-ASA are secreted into breast milk, but it has been associated with diarrhea in the nursing infant. Women can breastfeed on 5-ASA agents but the infants should be observed for a persistent change in stool frequency.[36,37]

CORTICOSTEROIDS

Prednisone and prednisolone, the biologically active form of prednisone, are pregnancy category B drugs during pregnancy and can be very helpful in treating moderate to severe IBD flares. There are a number of studies in which pregnant patients received either prednisone or prednisolone, and these corticosteroids apparently have little if any effects on the developing fetus.[38] A 20-year survey of pregnant women with active UC who were treated with corticosteroids alone, corticosteroids with sulfasalazine, or undetermined regimens resulted in no congenital anomalies in the corticosteroid group and one case of cerebral palsy in the combination group. The incidence of low birth weight infants was the same in the steroid and nonsteroid-treated groups.[39] A second study, which included 531 women with IBD, found no congenital anomalies in the corticosteroid-treated group.[40] Overall, there was not a statistically significant difference in complications between infants born to mothers receiving corticosteroids and infants born to mothers in the general population. Case-control studies of systemic corticosteroid use during the first trimester of pregnancy have noted an increased risk of oral clefts in the newborn.[41] This has not been replicated in other studies and the risk is thought to be very small. Neonatal adrenal insufficiency appears to be rare. A prospective study of 311 women did not demonstrate an increased risk of teratogenicity with use of corticosteroids during pregnancy.[42] Only trace amounts of prednisone are excreted into breast milk and the American Academy of Pediatrics has deemed it safe during breastfeeding. There are little data about the placental transfer of topical steroids, but postmarketing data have shown that hydrocortisone enemas, foam, and suppositories are safe during pregnancy and breastfeeding.[43]

While there are minimal risks to the fetus, the adverse maternal outcomes of prednisone include hypertension, edema, glucose intolerance, and pre-eclampsia. Women on prednisone should be monitored closely by their obstetricians.

Budesonide is helpful in treating CD of the terminal ileum and right colon. It is pregnancy category C because of 2 animal studies that have demonstrated an increased risk of spontaneous abortions, intrauterine growth retardation, and skeletal abnormalities with high doses of budesonide. Inhaled budesonide has been proven to be safe during pregnancy.[44-49] A recent human study in 8 pregnant CD patients showed no increased risk of adverse outcomes.[50]

AZATHIOPRINE/6-MERCAPTOPURINE

AZA/6-MP are Food and Drug Administration (FDA) pregnancy category D. However, decades of experience in IBD, transplant, and other immune diseases do not show a clear association with congenital anomalies.[51,52] The oral bioavailability of these agents is low in humans and the fetal liver in the first trimester lacks the enzyme inosinate pyrophosphorylase needed to convert AZA to 6-MP. Both of these factors may be protective to the fetus during organogenesis. There are only 2 retrospective IBD studies of the use of 6-MP in pregnancy that control for disease activity. One looked at the effect of 6-MP at conception and during pregnancy and found no statistical difference in conception failures (defined as a spontaneous abortion), abortion secondary to a birth defect, major congenital malformations, neoplasia, or increased infections among female or male patients taking 6-MP compared with controls (RR, 0.85 [0.47 to 1.55], p = 0.59).[53] There were 155 patients (79 female) and 325 pregnancies. This paper did not look at prematurity or low birth weight. All patients were in clinical remission at the time of conception with no patient moderately or severely ill during pregnancy.

Another paper by this same group looked at 6-MP and AZA in addition to other IBD medications taken during pregnancy.[27] These other medications used sometime during pregnancy included 5-ASA (100 of 207 conceptions), prednisone (49 conceptions), 6-MP or AZA (101), metronidazole (27), ciprofloxacin (18), and cyclosporine (2). Eighty-five of the conceptions were free of any medications. The authors reported that the "great majority of patients were in remission at the time of conception."[27] In multivariate analyses controlling for the age of the mother, there was no evidence that any type of drug therapy influenced pregnancy outcomes. Outcomes measured were spontaneous or therapeutic abortion, maternal or fetal illness resulting in abortion, premature birth, healthy full-term birth, multiple births, ectopic pregnancy, congenital abnormalities, birth weight, and type of delivery.

A more recent study found that among 20 women with IBD exposed to AZA/6-MP during pregnancy, the risk of preterm birth and congenital abnormalities was 4.2 (95% CI, 1.4 to 12.5) and 2.9 (95% CI, 0.9 to 8.9 NS), respectively.[54,55] However, the authors did not adequately control for disease activity.

Finally, the largest single study to date studied women who called a teratogen information service.[56] They compared 189 women exposed to AZA during pregnancy to 230 women who did not take any teratogenic medications during pregnancy. The rate of major malformations did not differ between groups with 6 neonates in each; the rate was 3.5% for AZA and it was 3.0% for the control group rate (P _ 0.775; OR, 1.17; CI, 0.37, 3.69). The mean birth weight and gestational age were lower in the AZA group 2995 g versus 3252 g (P _ 0.001, difference of mean: 257, 95% CI,: 106.3, 408.1) and 37.8 weeks versus 39.1 weeks (P _ 0.001, difference of mean: 1.3, 95% CI, 0.5, 2.0), respectively. The AZA group had more cases of prematurity (21.4% versus 5.2% [P _ 0.001; OR, 4.0; 95% CI, 2.0, 8.06]) and low birth weight (23% versus 6.0% [P _ 0.001; OR, 3.81; 95% CI, 2.0, 7.2]) as well, but this most likely reflects the patients' underlying disease state, which was not controlled. It is generally agreed that it is safer for women who need AZA/6-MP to stay on these drugs during pregnancy than to risk a flare and a potential pregnancy complication.[57,58] Breastfeeding has traditionally been discouraged, but recent data showing zero to minimal levels in breast milk and no detectable levels in the breastfeeding infant suggest that it may be safe.[59] However, more studies are needed before routinely recommending nursing on AZA/6-MP. The American Academy of Obstetricians and Gynecologists no longer advises women to stop thiopurines during breastfeeding.

INFLIXIMAB/ADALIMUMAB/CERTOLIZUMAB

The anti-tumor necrosis factor (TNF)-α agents infliximab and adalimumab are IgG1 antibodies and are pregnancy category B. IgG1 does not cross the placenta in the first trimester during organogenesis. However, these antibodies do cross highly efficiently in the third trimester. One paper reported on 133 infliximab exposures in women with CD or rheumatoid arthritis and there were data available on 96 pregnancies. Fetal adverse outcomes in women exposed to infliximab were no different than those outcomes in women who had not been exposed.[60] Another retrospective analysis of 10 women with CD treated intentionally with infliximab during pregnancy did not show any congenital anomalies, intrauterine growth retardation, or small-for-gestational age parameters.[61]

Infliximab has been detected in cord blood and levels are detectable in the infant up to 6 months after birth.[62] The effects of infliximab on the developing infant immune system and response to vaccines are not known, although limited data do not show harm. The recent recommendation is that the live rotavirus vaccine normally given in the second month of life should be avoided.[63] Common practice in the United States is to give the last dose of infliximab at the beginning of the third trimester and no later than 31 weeks and the next dose after delivery. If the mother flares during the third trimester, she may be given a dose of infliximab or prednisone if closer to the time of delivery. It is recommended that infliximab levels be checked in the infant around 7 months as well as consider testing for the infant's response to his or her vaccinations like tetanus toxoid and H. influenza b. The infant should be monitored until infliximab levels are undetectable, especially before the live vaccines varicella and MMR are given at 1 year of life. Limited data have shown that infliximab is not detectable in breast milk and mothers can probably safely nurse their infants.

Adalimumab and certolizumab pegol are listed as pregnancy category B drugs and are approved by the FDA for treatment of CD. Animal data have shown no evidence of harm to the fetus. There are several case reports of successful use of adalimumab during pregnancy in CD patients.[64,65] The Organization for Tetralogy Information Specialists reports 27 women enrolled in a prospective study of adalimumab in pregnancy and an additional 47 adalimumab-exposed pregnant women in a registry. The rates of spontaneous abortion, stillbirth, congenital malformation, and preterm delivery were not increased over the general population.[66] Adalimumab, like infliximab, will cross the placenta preferentially in the third trimester. To date, both adalimumab and certolizumab levels cannot be checked commercially and therefore it is difficult to know whether the infant has been exposed if the mother receives these medications during pregnancy. Investigations are underway to determine if pegylated medications do or do not cross the placenta.

NATALIZUMAB

Natalizumab has been recently approved for the induction and maintenance of remission of CD in patients failing anti-TNF therapies.[67] The drug is pregnancy category C and we need more data before recommending continuation of this drug during pregnancy.

CYCLOSPORINE AND TACROLIMUS

Cyclosporine is a pregnancy category C drug during pregnancy. A meta-analysis of 15 studies of pregnancy outcomes after cyclosporine therapy reported on a total of 410 patients with data on major malformations.[68-70] The calculated OR of 3.83 for malformations did not achieve statistical significance (95% CI, 0.75 to 19.6). In IBD, case reports have noted the successful use of intravenous cyclosporine during pregnancy.[71-73] In the setting of severe steroid refractory UC, cyclosporine is a better option than colectomy, which is associated with a 50% to 60% fetal mortality. Cyclosporine is excreted in the breast milk in high concentrations and is contraindicated during nursing.

Tacrolimus is also pregnancy category C. There is an increased incidence of perinatal hyperkalemia and prematurity. The reported malformation rate is 5.6% with no persistent anomalies seen.[74] There is a single case report of the successful use of tacrolimus in a pregnant patient with UC.[75]

ANTIBIOTICS

There are no studies of long-term antibiotic use during pregnancy. The safest antibiotics to use for CD in pregnancy for short periods of time (weeks, not months) are ampicillin and the cephalosporins.[43] These are pregnancy category B drugs, and human studies have not shown increased teratogenic risk. They are compatible with breastfeeding and may provide an alternative to ciprofloxacin or metronidazole. Metronidazole is a pregnancy category B drug, and multiple studies have suggested that it is not associated with birth defects. These include 2 meta-analyses, 2 retrospective cohort studies, and a prospective controlled study of 228 women exposed to metronidazole during pregnancy.[76-80] Metronidazole can be used in the second or third trimester. There is toxicity associated with long-term use of metronidazole and it is therefore not recommended for breastfeeding.

Ciprofloxacin causes cartilage lesions in immature animals and should be avoided because of the absence of data on its effects on growth and development in humans. Although a prospective study did not find any increased congenital anomalies, the effects on bone and cartilage may take years to develop and it is therefore not recommended during pregnancy.[81,82] It should also be held during breastfeeding due to lack of data.

Rifaximin is pregnancy category C. It has not been shown to effect fertility or pregnancy outcome in rats[83] but can cause teratogenic complications in rats and rabbits.[84] Safety in breastfeeding is unknown. There is limited evidence to suggest it works in IBD and thus is not recommended for use in pregnancy.

METHOTREXATE AND THALIDOMIDE

Methotrexate is pregnancy category X and a known teratogen. It is associated with multiple congenital abnormalities and should not be used during conception and pregnancy. Women should stop taking it at least 3 to 6 months prior to conception. Methotrexate is excreted in breast milk and may accumulate in neonatal tissues. It is contraindicated in breastfeeding.[85]

Thalidomide is also pregnancy category X and its teratogenicity has been extensively documented. It is contraindicated during pregnancy and in women of childbearing age who are not using 2 reliable methods of contraception for 1 month before starting therapy, during therapy, and for 1 month after therapy. There are no human data on breastfeeding but it is not advised.[85]

Surgery

Indications for surgery during pregnancy include uncontrollable bleeding, obstruction, perforation, fulminant disease refractory to medical management, or an intra-abdominal abscess that cannot be drained by other methods. Surgery during the second trimester carries a lower rate of miscarriage than the first trimester and is technically less complicated than the third trimester. Total colectomy for fulminant UC carries a 50% to 60% fetal mortality, and medical management with intravenous cyclosporine, infliximab, or early delivery is preferable.[86,87]

Flexible Sigmoidoscopy/Colonoscopy

The safety of flexible sigmoidoscopy has been demonstrated in multiple case reports and studies. It can be very helpful in assessing colitis activity, and the scope need only be inserted 10 or 15 cm. Flexible sigmoidoscopy has been performed without adverse outcome in all 3 trimesters of pregnancy. Most procedures are done without sedation and minimal bowel preparation. Tap water enemas are preferable due to a case report of bone demineralization in an infant due to Fleets (CB Fleets Co, Lynchburg, VA). MiraLAX (Schering-Plough Corp, Kenilworth, NJ) is pregnancy category C but safe to use during pregnancy both for constipation and to help with bowel preparation for sigmoidoscopy if needed. Although hemodynamic monitoring of the mother should always be a part of the procedure, most reported cases did not involve any fetal monitoring, although this may be considered, especially in cases of maternal hemodynamic instability. Colonoscopy is still an experimental procedure during pregnancy. There are not enough data to support its use and it should be reserved for life-threatening complications such as GI bleeding where the only alternative is laparoscopy.[88,89]

Mode of Delivery

In general, the mode of the delivery should be dictated by obstetric indication. Patients with active perianal disease report worsening of their disease after vaginal delivery and are generally recommended to undergo cesarean deliveries. Patients with fulminant UC should also undergo a cesarean section. Women in remission or with mild disease without perianal activity may deliver vaginally unless the circumstances of pregnancy dictate otherwise.[90,91] Women with ileoanal pouches report increased day and nighttime stool frequency during pregnancy but mostly revert back to "normal" after delivery. There is no contraindication to vaginal delivery for pouch patients, and a survey study showed successful outcomes with both vaginal deliveries and cesarean sections.[92-94] Women with ostomies have an increased risk of stomal prolapse and bowel obstruction during pregnancy but they revert back to "normal" after delivery.

Postpartum

The immediate postpartum period is a very stressful time for women, and there is an increased rate of IBD flares. A recent paper looked at medication use and breastfeeding in 122 women with IBD.[95] Forty-four percent of women breastfed their infants. Reasons for not breastfeeding included physician recommendation, fear of medication interactions, and personal choice. Seventy-four percent of women stopped taking their medications prior to breastfeeding and 43% of those who breastfed had a flare. Thus, the flare was due to medication cessation not the breastfeeding itself. This study emphasizes how imperative it is to encourage women to keep taking their medications during breastfeeding.

Summary

In general, women with IBD should have healthy pregnancies when they conceive in remission and remain on their IBD medications. Disease activity has a much greater impact on pregnancy outcome than the medications used to treat it. AZA/6-MP are now considered safe during pregnancy and should be continued in women who are dependent upon these medications. The biologics are generally safe during pregnancy but should be timed appropriately based on the placental transfer and the frequency of medication administration. Physicians should work with pediatricians and consider measuring infliximab levels in infants before administering the 1-year live vaccines. Radiologic imaging is generally safe during pregnancy, but CT scans should be done at 25 weeks or after if possible. Intravenous contrast dye should not be used during pregnancy unless absolutely necessary. Flexible sigmoidoscopy is safe during pregnancy, and necessary surgery should be performed if possible during the second trimester. Women with active perianal disease should have cesarean sections because vaginal delivery with episiotomy can cause a nonhealing wound. One of the most stressful times for women is immediately after delivery, and women who nurse—with the exception of those on AZA/6-MP—should not stop their medications. Overall, pregnancy outcomes are good as long as the physician is meticulous and experienced in his or her care and the patient reports symptoms and continues to adhere to recommended medications. Physicians should consider partnering with a high-risk obstetrician to manage the IBD patient during pregnancy.

References

1. Ludvigsson JF, Ludvigsson J. Inflammatory bowel disease in mother or father and neonatal outcome. *Acta Paediatr.* 2002;91(2):145-151.
2. Porter RJ, Stirrat GM. The effects of inflammatory bowel disease on pregnancy: a case-controlled retrospective analysis. *Br J Obstet Gynaecol.* 1986;93(11):1124-1131.
3. Elbaz G, Fich A, Levy A, et al. Inflammatory bowel disease and preterm delivery. *International Journal of Obstetrics and Gynecology.* 2005;90:193-197.
4. Fedorkow DM, Persaud D, Nimrod CA. Inflammatory bowel disease: a controlled study of late pregnancy outcome. *Am J Obstet Gynecol.* 1989;160(4):998-1001.
5. Larzilliere I, Beau P. Chronic inflammatory bowel disease and pregnancy: case control study. *Gastroenterol Clin Biol.* 1998;22(12):1056-1060.
6. Bush MC, Patel S, Lapinski RH, et al. Perinatal outcomes in inflammatory bowel disease. *J Matern Fetal Neonatal Med.* 2004;15(4):237-241.
7. Fonager K, Sorensen HT, Olsen J, et al. Pregnancy outcome for women with Crohn's disease: a follow-up study based on linkage between national registries. *Am J Gastroenterol.* 1998;93(12):2426-2430.
8. Moser MA, Okun NB, Mayes DC, et al. Crohn's disease, pregnancy, and birth weight. *Am J Gastroenterol.* 2000;95(4):1021-1026.
9. Kornfeld D, Cnattingius S, Ekbom A. Pregnancy outcomes in women with inflammatory bowel disease: a population-based cohort study. *Am J Obstet Gynecol.* 1997;177:942-946.
10. Norgard B, Fonager K, Sorensen HT, et al. Birth outcomes of women with ulcerative colitis: a nationwide Danish cohort study. *Am J Gastroenterol.* 2000;95:3165-3170.
11. Cornish J, Tan E, Teare J, et al. A meta-analysis on the influence of inflammatory bowel disease on pregnancy. *Gut.* 2007;56(6):830-837.
12. Dominitz JA, Young JCC, Boyko EJ, et al. Outcomes of infants born to mothers with inflammatory bowel disease: a population-based cohort study. *Am J Gastroenterol.* 2002;97:641-648.
13. Norgard B, Hundborg HH, Jacobsen BA, et al. Disease activity in pregnant women with Crohn's disease and birth outcomes: a regional Danish cohort study. *Am J Gastroenterol.* 2007;102:1947-1954.
14. Mahadevan U, Sandborn WJ, Li De-Kun, et al. Pregnancy outcomes in women with inflammatory bowel disease: a large community-based study from northern California. *Gastroenterology.* 2007;133:1106-1112.
15. Nielsen OH, Andreasson B, Bondesen S, et al. Pregnancy in ulcerative colitis. *Scand J Gastroenterol.* 1983;18(6):735-742.
16. Nielsen OH, Andreasson B, Bondesen S, et al. Pregnancy in Crohn's disease. *Scand J Gastroenterol.* 1984;19(6):724-732.
17. Miller JP. Inflammatory bowel disease and pregnancy: a review. *J R Soc Med.* 1986;79:221-225.
18. Kane S, Kisiel J, Shih L, et al. HLA disparity determines disease activity through pregnancy in women with inflammatory bowel disease. *Am J Gastroenterol.* 2004;99:1523-1526.
19. Riis L, Politi P, Wolters F, et al. Does pregnancy change the disease course? A study in a European cohort of patients with inflammatory bowel disease. *Am J Gastroenterol.* 2006;101:1539-1545.
20. ACOG Committee Opinion. Guidelines for diagnostic imaging during pregnancy. *Obstet Gynecol.* 2004;104(3):647-651.
21. Hall EJ. Scientific view of low-level radiation risks. *Radiographics.* 1991;13:347-368.
22. Cunningham FG, Gant NF, Leveno KJ, et al. General considerations and maternal evaluation. In: Wenstrom KD, ed. *Williams Obstetrics.* 21st ed. New York, NY: McGraw Hill; 2001:1143-1158.
23. Smits AK, Paladine HL, Judkins DZ. What are the risks to the fetus associated with diagnostic radiation exposure during pregnancy? *J Fam Pract.* 2006;55(5):441-443.
24. De Santis M, Di Gianantonio E, Straface G, et al. Ionizing radiations in pregnancy and teratogenesis: a review of the literature. *Reproductive Toxicology.* 2005;20:323-329.
25. Webb JA, Thomsen HS, Morcos SK, et al. The use of iodinated and gadolinium contrast media during pregnancy and lactation. *Eur Radiol.* 2005;15(6):1234-1240.

26. Jarnerot G, Andersen S, Esbjorner E, et al. Albumin reserve for binding of bilirubin in maternal and cord serum under treatment with sulphasalazine. *Scan J Gastroenterol.* 1981;16:1049-1055.

27. Moskovitz D, Bodian C, Chapman ML, et al. The effect on the fetus of medications used to treat pregnant inflammatory bowel disease patients. *Am J Gastroenterol.* 2004;99(4):656-661.

28. Mogdam M, Dobbins WO, Korelitz BI, et al. Pregnancy in inflammatory bowel disease: effect of sulfasalazine and corticosteroids on fetal outcome. *Gastroenterology.* 1981;80:72-76.

29. Norgard B, Czeizel AE, Rockenbauer M, et al. Population-based case-control study of the safety of sulphasalazine use during pregnancy. *Aliment Pharmacol Ther.* 2001;15:483-486.

30. Czeizel AE, Toth M, Rockenbauer M. Population-based case control study of folic acid supplementation during pregnancy. *Teratology.* 1996;53:645-651.

31. Jansen G, Van der Heijden J, Oerlemans R, et al. Sulphasalazine is a potent inhibitor of the reduced folate carrier: implications for combination therapies with methotrexate for rheumatoid arthritis. *Arthritis Rheum.* 2004;20:2130-2139.

32. Marteau P, Tennenbaum R, Elefant E, et al. Foetal outcome in women with IBD treated during pregnancy with oral mesalamine microgranules. *Aliment Pharmacol Ther.* 1998;12:1101-1108.

33. Diav-Cirton O, Park YH, Veerasuntharam G, et al. The safety of mesalamine in human pregnancy: a prospective controlled cohort study. *Gastroenterology.* 1998;114:23-28.

34. Norgard B, Fonager K, Pedersen L, et al. Birth outcome in women exposed to 5-aminosalicylic acid during pregnancy: a Danish cohort study. *Gut.* 2003;52:243-247.

35. Bell CM, Habal FM. Safety of topical 5-ASA in pregnancy. *Am J Gastroenterol.* 1997;92:2201-2202.

36. Briggs GG, Freeman, RK, Yaffe SJ. *Drugs in Pregnancy and Lactation.* 7th ed. Philadelphia, PA: Williams and Wilkins; 2005.

37. Caprilli R, Gassull MA, Escher JC, et al. European Crohn's and Colitis Organization. European evidence based consensus on the diagnosis and management of Crohn's disease: special situations. *Gut.* 2006;55(Suppl 1):136-158.

38. Rodriguez-Pinilla E, Martinez-Frias ML. Corticosteroids during pregnancy and oral clefts: a case-control study. *Teratology.* 1998;58:2-5

39. Willoughby CP, Truelove SC. Ulcerative colitis and pregnancy. *Gut.* 1980;21(6):469-474.

40. Reinisch JN, Simon NG, Karow WG, et al. Prenatal exposure to prednisone in humans and animals retards intrauterine growth. *Science.* 1978;202(4366):436-438.

41. Rolf BB. Corticosteroids and pregnancy. *Am J Obstet Gynecol.* 1966;95(3):339-344.

42. Yackel DB, Kempers RD, McConahey WM. Adrenocorticosteroid therapy in pregnancy. *Am J Obstet Gynecol.* 1966;96(7):985-989.

43. Mahadevan U, Kane S. American Gastroenterological Association Institute Technical review on the use of gastrointestinal medications in pregnancy. *Gastroenterology.* 2006;131:283-311.

44. Gur C, Diav-Citrin O, Shechtman S, et al. Pregnancy outcome after first trimester exposure to corticosteroids: a prospective controlled study. *Reprod Toxicol.* 2004;18:93-101.

45. Ekman L, Kihlstrom I, Ryrfeldt A. Toxicity study of the new glucocorticoid budesonide in rats. *Arzneimittelforschung.* 1987;37(1):37-42.

46. Kihlstrom I, Lundberg C. Toxicity study of the new glucocorticoid budesonide in rabbits. *Arzneimittelforschung.* 1987;37(1):43-46.

47. Gluck PA, Gluck JC. A review of pregnancy outcomes after exposure to orally inhaled budesonide. *Curr Med Res Opin.* 2005;21:1075-1084.

48. Rahimi R, Nikfar S, Abdollahi M. Meta-analysis finds use of inhaled corticosteroids during pregnancy safe: a systematic meta-analysis review. *Hum Exp Toxicol.* 2006;25:447-452.

49. Carmichael SL, Shaw GM. Maternal corticosteroid use and the risk of selected congenital anomalies. *Am J Med Genet.* 1999;86:242-244.

50. Beaulieu DB, Anathakrishnan AN, Issa M, et al. Budesonide induction and maintenance therapy for Crohn's disease during pregnancy. *Inflamm Bowel Dis.* 2009;15(1):25-28.

51. Penn I, Makowski E, Droegemueller W, et al. Parenthood in renal homograft recipients. *JAMA.* 1971;216(11):1755-1761.

52. Golby M. Fertility after renal transplantation. *Transplantation.* 1970;10(3):201-207.

53. Francella A, Dyan A, Bodian C, et al. The safety of 6-mercaptopurine for childbearing patients with inflammatory bowel disease: a retrospective cohort study. *Gastroenterology.* 2003;124:9-17.

54. Norgard B, Pedersen L, Christensen LA, et al. Therapeutic drug use in women with Crohn's disease and birth outcomes: a Danish Nationwide cohort study. *Am J Gastroenterol.* 2007;102:1406-1413.

55. Friedman S. Medical therapy and birth outcomes in women with Crohn's disease: what should we tell our patients? *Am J Gastroenterol.* 2007;102:1414-1416.

56. Goldstein LH, Dolinsky G, Greenberg R, et al. Pregnancy outcome of women exposed to azathioprine during pregnancy. *Birth Defects Res A Clin Mol Teratol.* 2007;79:696-701.

57. Alstead EM, Ritchie JK, Lennard-Jones JE, et al. Safety of azathioprine in pregnancy in inflammatory bowel disease. *Gastroenterology.* 1990;99:443-446.

58. Norgard B, Pedersen L, Fonager K, et al. Azathioprine, mercaptopurine and birth outcome: a population-based cohort study. *Aliment Pharmacol Ther.* 2003;17:827-834.

59. Sau A, Clarke S, Bass J, et al. Azathioprine and breastfeeding: is it safe? *BJOG.* 2007;114:498-501.

60. Katz JA, Antonini C, Keenen GF, et al. Outcome of pregnancy in women receiving infliximab for the treatment of Crohn's disease and rheumatoid arthritis. *Am J Gastroenterol.* 2004;99:2385-2392.

61. Mahadevan U, Kane S, Sandborn WJ, et al. Intentional infliximab use during pregnancy for induction or maintenance of remission in Crohn's disease. *Aliment Pharmacol Ther.* 2005;21:733-738.

62. Vasiliasuskas EA, Church JA, Silverman N, et al. Case report: evidence for transplacental transfer of maternally administered infliximab to the newborn. *Clin Gastroenterol Hepatol.* 2006;4:1255-1258.

63. Mahadevan U, Terdiman J, Church J, et al. Infliximab levels in infants born to mothers with inflammatory bowel disease. *Gastroenterology.* 2007;132A-144.

64. Mishkim DS, Van Deinse W, Becker JM, et al. Successful use of adalimumab (humira) for Crohn's disease in pregnancy. *Inflamm Bowel Dis.* 2006;21:827-828.

65. Vesga L, Terdiman JP, Mahadevan U. Adalimumab use in pregnancy. *Gut.* 2005;54:890.

66. Dubinsky M, Abraham B, Mahadevan U. Management of the pregnant IBD patient. *Inflamm Bowel Dis.* 2008;14(12):1736-1750.

67. Sandborn WJ, Colombel JF, Enns R, et al. Natalizumab induction and maintenance therapy for Crohn's disease. *N Engl J Med.* 2005;353:1912-1925.

68. Bar OZ B, Hackman R, Einarson T, et al. Pregnancy outcome after cyclosporine therapy during pregnancy: a meta-analysis. *Transplantation.* 2001;71:1051-1055.

69. Nagy S, Bush MC, Berkowitz R, et al. Pregnancy outcome in liver transplant recipients. *Obstet Gynecol.* 2003;102:121-128.

70. Jain A, Ventataeamanan R, Fung JJ, et al. Pregnancy after liver transplantation under tacrolimus. *Transplantation.* 1997;64:559-565.

71. Bertschinger P, Himmelmann A, Risti B, et al. Cyclosporine treatment of severe ulcerative colitis during pregnancy. *Am J Gastroenterol.* 1995;90:330.

72. Reindi W, Schmid RM, Huber W, et al. Cyclosporine A treatment of steroid-refractory ulcerative colitis during pregnancy: report of 2 cases. *Gut.* 2007;56:1019.

73. Angelberger A, Reinisch W, Dejaco C, et al. Prevention of abortion by cyclosporin treatment of fulminant ulcerative colitis during pregnancy. *Gut.* 2006;55:1364-1365.

74. Kainz A, Harabacz I, Cowlick IS, et al. Analysis of 100 pregnancy outcomes in women treated systemically with tacrolimus. *Transpl Int.* 2000;13(suppl 1):S299-S300.

75. Baumgart DC, Sturm A, Wiedenmann B, et al. Uneventful pregnancy and neonatal outcome with tacrolimus in refractory ulcerative colitis. *Gut.* 2005;54:1822-1823.

76. Burtin P, Taddio A, Ariburnu O, et al. Safety of metronidazole in pregnancy: a meta-analysis. *Am J Obstet Gynecol.* 1995;172:525-529.

77. Car-Paton T, Carvajal A, Martin de Diego I, et al. Is metronidazole teratogenic? A meta-analysis. *Br J Clin Pharmacol.* 1997;44:179-182.

78. Piper JM, Mitchel EF, Roy WA. Prenatal use of metronidazole and birth defects: no association. *Obstet Gynecol.* 1993;82:348-352.

79. Sorensen HT, Larsen H, Jensen ES, et al. Safety of metronidazole during pregnancy: a cohort study of risk of congenital abnormalities, preterm delivery, and low birth weight in 124 women. *J Antimicrob Chemother.* 1999;44:854-856.

80. Diav-Citron O, Shechtman S, Gotteiner T, et al. Pregnancy outcome after gestational exposure to metronidazole: a prospective controlled cohort study. *Teratology.* 2001;63:186-192.

81. Loebstein R, Addis A, Ho E, et al. Pregnancy outcome following gestational exposure to fluoroquinolones: a multicenter prospective controlled study. *Antimicrob Agents Chemother.* 1998;42:1336-1339.

82. Larsen H, Nielsen GL, Schonheyder HC, et al. Birth outcomes following maternal use of fluoroquinolones. *Int J Antimicrob Agents.* 2001;18:259-262.

83. Bertoli D, Borelli G. Fertility study of rifaximin (L/105) in rats. *Chemioterapia.* 1986;5:204-207.

84. Xifaxan (package insert). Morrisville, NC: Salix Pharmaceuticals, 2005.

85. Briggs GG, Freeman RY, Yaffe SJ. *Drugs in Pregnancy and Lactation: A Reference Guide to Fetal and Neonatal Risk.* 7th ed. Philadelphia, PA: Lippincott, Williams & Wilkins; 2005.

86. Malangoni MA. Gastrointestinal surgery and pregnancy. *Gastroenterol Clin North Am.* 2003;32(1):181-200.

87. Cohen-Kerem R, Railton C, Oren D, et al. Pregnancy outcome following non-obstetric surgical intervention. *Am J Surg.* 2005;190(3):467-473.

88. Siddiqui U, Proctor DD. Flexible sigmoidoscopy and colonoscopy during pregnancy. *Gastrointest Endosc Clin N Am.* 2006;16(1):59-69.

89. Qureshi WA, Rajan E, Adler DG, et al. ASGE guideline: guidelines for endoscopy in pregnant and lactating women. *Gastrointest Endosc.* 2005;61(3):357-362.

90. Ilnyckyji A, Blanchard JF, Rawsthorne P, et al. Perianal Crohn's disease and pregnancy: role of the mode of delivery. *Am J Gastroenterol.* 1999;94:3274-3278.

91. Brandt LJ, Estabrook SG, Reinus JF, et al. Results of a survey to evaluate whether vaginal delivery and episiotomy lead to perineal involvement in women with Crohn's disease. *Am J Gastroenterol.* 1995;90:1918.

92. Ravid A, Richard CS, Spencer LM, et al. Pregnancy, delivery, and pouch function after ileal pouch-anal anastomosis for ulcerative colitis. *Dis Colon Rectum.* 2002;45:1283-1288.

93. Juhasz ES, Fozard B, Dozois RR, et al. Ileal pouch-anal anastomosis function following childbirth: an extended evaluation. *Dis Colon Rectum.* 1995;38:159.

94. Nelson H, Dozois RR,, Kelly KA, et al. The effect of pregnancy and delivery on the ileal pouch-anal anastomosis functions. *Dis Colon Rectum.* 1989;32:384.

95. Kane S, Lemieux N. The role of breastfeeding in postpartum disease activity in women with inflammatory bowel disease. *Am J Gastroenterol.* 2005;100(1):102-105.

CHAPTER 14

MAINTAINING FEMININITY AFTER SURGERY

Maria T. Abreu, MD and Yuki Young, MD

Inflammatory bowel disease (IBD) is a chronic idiopathic inflammatory condition affecting more than 1 million Americans, at least half of whom are women. Clinicians face unique challenges when diagnosing and treating women with IBD as it relates to pregnancy, fertility, and psychosocial issues. This chapter is devoted to issues of sexuality and femininity after IBD surgery as fertility after IBD surgery is covered elsewhere in the book.

Women Have More Inflammatory Bowel Disease-Related Concerns as Compared to Men

Several retrospective studies have examined disease and sociodemographic factors associated with IBD-related concerns using a Rating Form of IBD Patients' Concerns, which was first developed by Drossman et al.[1] It is a survey designed to quantify the degree of concerns with specific issues related to IBD. In a study by Maunder et al[2] involving 343 subjects, women reported higher levels of IBD symptom severity and higher levels of concern about feelings related to their bodies, attractiveness, feeling alone, and having children compared with men. The model found that women and higher scores for depressive coping were independently associated with more intense IBD-related concerns. These results confirm that sex has a significant influence on a number of illness concerns, particularly concerns related to self-image and relationships.

Scherl EJ, Dubinsky MC.
The Changing World of Inflammatory Bowel Disease:
Impact of Generation, Gender, and Global Trends (pp 177-182)
© 2009 SLACK Incorporated.

Women With a Stoma

SEXUAL FUNCTION

Having a stoma in the abdominal wall and an external fecal pouch could significantly impact sexual function. A questionnaire[3] was sent to 113 female patients under long-term follow-up care, and 82 (73%) responded. The majority (93%) reported being happy with the stoma. Forty-seven percent reported no change in their sexual function, 7% reported an improvement, and 47% reported being affected negatively—14% severely, 11% moderately, and 22% mildly.

SEXUAL CONCERNS

Rolstad et al[4] sought to understand patient concerns regarding ileostomy. Fifty patients (25 women) with a permanent ileostomy who were routinely followed in the enterostomal therapy clinic at a university medical center were surveyed with a 14-item questionnaire. Sixty percent of the women felt sexually less desirable or attractive after surgery, but when asked whether they felt their partners agreed with this opinion, only 7% stated that their partners agreed. Thirty-two percent indicated that having a stoma made sexual intercourse more difficult physically, while 46% replied that it was made more difficult psychologically. Seventy-six percent viewed the appliance as a hindrance to sexual activity. Patients were asked to whom they talked when they needed advice about sexuality. Thirty-six percent cited the partner, 28% stated "no one," and only 6% cited a physician or a stoma therapist. When asked what methods they used to overcome sexual concerns, 60% did nothing. The remaining used pouch covers, good personal hygiene, and communication with the significant other. Therefore, clinicians should attempt to minimize appliance-related anxiety and make sure that patients are thoroughly educated in stoma care. An appliance that is nonintrusive, odor proof, and leak proof is essential. Studies have documented the importance of a significant other in providing ongoing support throughout rehabilitation. Clinicians should be prepared to facilitate sexual rehabilitation for the patient and the patient's significant other through education, counseling, or referral.

Women With Ileal-Pouch Anal Anastomosis

FUNCTIONAL OUTCOME AND QUALITY OF LIFE

The current preferred surgical option for the management of ulcerative colitis is an ileal pouch anal anastomosis (IPAA) because it removes the need for permanent stoma and an ileostomy bag. Several studies have reported in improvement in quality of life. The largest prospective study[5] collected follow-up information from 1156 consecutive patients, of whom 442 (42.5%) were women. Functional outcomes were comparable between men and women. Ninety-eight percent of patients would recommend the surgery to others. Long-term quality of life after ileal pouch surgery was excellent and the level of continence was satisfactory. This surgery was an excellent long-term option in patients requiring total proctocolectomy. There was no reduction in patient satisfaction with time.

SEXUAL FUNCTION

Farouk et al[6] assessed long-term functional outcomes among 692 women identified as having undergone IPAA for ulcerative colitis. Nocturnal stool frequency, fecal incontinence, protective pad use, and constipation medication requirements were higher in patients older than 45 at the time of IPAA. Before surgery, 16% reported complete abstinence from sexual activity and 20% had reduced sexual activity. After IPAA, 25% had improved levels of sexual activity and 19% reported restrictions in sexual activity. Pelvic pain and fear of soiling during intercourse were the primary concerns. Dyspareunia affected 8% of the women at 1 year and 11% at 12 years, whereas fecal leakage during intercourse affected 3%. Functional outcomes were comparable between men and women.

Damgaard et al[7] assessed sexual function after IPAA by interviewing 49 consecutive patients who underwent an IPAA at the University of Copenhagen. Twenty-three patients were women. About one-third of the women noted an increased frequency of intercourse after pouch surgery, while none reported a decreased frequency. However, in the period with diverting ileostomy, only 30% of the women had intercourse compared with 69% of the men. None of the women who were able to achieve orgasm preoperatively reported a postoperative disturbance of this ability, and 16% experienced an increased quality of orgasm. Postoperatively none reported dyspareunia, vaginal discharge, changes in their menstrual cycle, pain, soiling, or fecal leakage during intercourse. Only one woman reported some discomfort from the pouch during intercourse. None of the patients wanted to return to a life with an ileostomy. However, the study is limited by the small sample size and likely represents an underestimate as patients might have been uncomfortable in a personal interview.

Another questionnaire[8] survey involving 92 women who had undergone IPAA showed overall improvement in sexual relationships. The only significant differences in sexual function were vaginal dryness (27%), dyspareunia (27%), pain interfering with ability to feel sexual pleasure (31%), and fear of stool leakage limiting sexual activity (20%). Although 26% felt their relationship with their partner to be less satisfactory, only one woman felt her outcome limited her sexual activity to such an extent that she wished she had not undergone the surgery. There was no significant change in sexual desire, arousal, sensitivity, frequency of intercourse, or satisfaction with sexual relationship

GYNECOLOGIC FUNCTION

Counihan et al[9] attempted to address gynecologic issues by using a combination of data-base analysis and questionnaire. A questionnaire was sent to 206 female patients who underwent IPAA over a 10-year period. The questionnaire asked about menstrual, gynecologic, and obstetric history before and after IPAA. Additional information was obtained by retrospective review of the computerized registry of these patients. One hundred ten patients (53%) responded. The key findings showed that dyspareunia increased from 5% to 15%, fecal incontinence during intercourse increased from 3% to 7%, and menstrual problems increased from 23% to 31%. Cause of dyspareunia may be related to anatomic changes in the pelvis after proctectomy, for example deformity of the vaginal vault, dilation of the dorsal fornix, and displacement of the vagina toward the coccyx. These anatomic changes combined with sphincter impairment could affect sexual function such as dyspareunia and formation of pelvic cysts may be underestimated after IPAA.

References

1. Drossman DA, Leserman J, Li ZM, Mitchell CM, Zagami EA, Patrick DL. The rating form of IBD patient concerns: a new measure of health status. *Psychosom Med.* 1991;53(6):701-712.
2. Maunder R, Toner B, de Rooy E, Moskovitz D. Influence of sex and disease on illness-related concerns in inflammatory bowel disease. *Can J Gastroenterol.* 1999;13(9):728-732.
3. Awad RW, el-Gohary TM, Skilton JS, Elder JB. Life quality and psychological morbidity with an ileostomy. *Br J Surg.* 1993;80(2):252-253.
4. Rolstad BS, Wilson G, Rothenberger DA. Sexual concerns in the patient with an ileostomy. *Dis Colon Rectum.* 1983;26(3):170-171.
5. Fazio VW, O'Riordain MG, Lavery IC, et al. Long-term functional outcome and quality of life after stapled restorative proctocolectomy. *Ann Surg.* 1999;230(4):575-584; discussion 584-576.

6. Farouk R, Pemberton JH, Wolff BG, Dozois RR, Browning S, Larson D. Functional outcomes after ileal pouch-anal anastomosis for chronic ulcerative colitis. *Ann Surg.* 2000;231(6):919-926.
7. Damgaard B, Wettergren A, Kirkegaard P. Social and sexual function following ileal pouch-anal anastomosis. *Dis Colon Rectum.* 1995;38(3):286-289.
8. Bambrick M, Fazio VW, Hull TL, Pucel G. Sexual function following restorative proctocolectomy in women. *Dis Colon Rectum.* 1996;39:610-614.
9. Counihan TC, Roberts PL, Schoetz DJ Jr, Coller JA, Murray JJ, Veidenheimer MC. Fertility and sexual and gynecologic function after ileal pouch-anal anastomosis. *Dis Colon Rectum.* 1994;37(11):1126-1129.

Financial disclosure: Dr. Abreu is a consultant for Abbott, Procter & Gamble, and UCB; receives a research grant from Procter & Gamble; and is on the speaker's bureau at Abbott, Procter & Gamble, Prometheus, Salix, UCB, and Elan.

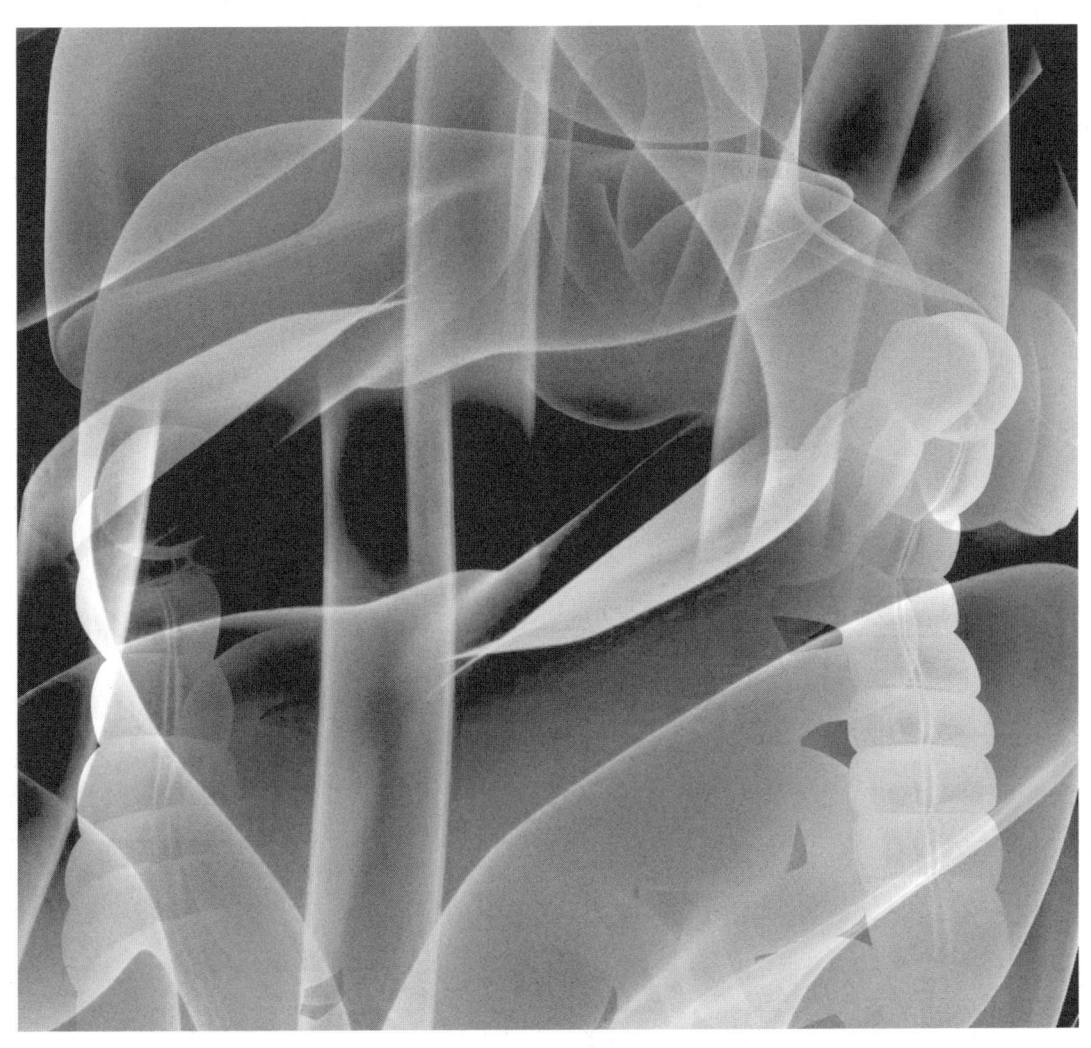

SECTION IV

INFLAMMATORY BOWEL DISEASE AND THE ELDERLY

THE EFFECT OF MENOPAUSE AND OTHER ISSUES IN THE OLDER PATIENT WITH INFLAMMATORY BOWEL DISEASE

Sunanda Kane, MD, MSPH, FACG, FACP, AGAF

Background

Inflammatory bowel disease (IBD) is a chronic disease with a typical age of onset in the early reproductive years. The effect of various stages in the reproductive cycle has been studied, but little is known about the effect of menopause on this chronic disease. In males, hormone changes manifested by erectile dysfunction (ED) and depression have been described but not well studied either. The effect of hormones and hormonal fluctuation on the gastrointestinal (GI) tract has been studied in animal models as well as humans. For example, there is symptomatic worsening of IBD symptoms during menses[1] and improvement in irritable bowel syndrome symptoms after disruption of menses through either medical (gonadotropin-releasing hormone analogs) or surgical means.[2,3]

The exact mechanism of how hormonal changes affect the GI tract and ultimate symptomatology in IBD has yet to be fully elucidated, but some plausible mechanisms have been proposed. One mechanism involves immunoresponses of cytokines; an imbalance between proinflammatory (IL-1, TNF-alpha) and immunoregulatory (IL-4, Interferon-gamma) cytokines and the presence of the appropriate antigen is thought to be involved in the pathogenesis of IBD. Estrogen has also been shown to disrupt this balance, while antiestrogen treatment in women helps restore this balance.[4] The hypoestrogen states in postmenopausal women could have a similar biologic effect in restoring the balance in cytokines, thus favoring an improvement in the disease course of IBD. Other mechanisms suggest changing levels of uterine prostaglandin concentration and levels of progesterone in various stages of reproductive cycle influence GI symptoms.[1]

However, estrogen has recently been found to have significant anti-inflammatory effects. Estrogen in the form of 17-B-estradiol suppresses the transcription of IL-2 from activated peripheral blood T cells and CD4+ T-cell lines through the suppression of transcription factors, including NF-kB. In multiple sclerosis, another autoimmune condition, exogenous estriol has been found

Scherl EJ, Dubinsky MC.
The Changing World of Inflammatory Bowel Disease:
Impact of Generation, Gender, and Global Trends (pp 185-192)
2009 SLACK Incorporated.

to inhibit activity.[5] Further, identification of pathway-selective estrogen receptor ligands that inhibit NF-kB transcriptional activity have been identified and tested on transgenic rat models of IBD.[6-8]

Menopause

EFFECT OF INFLAMMATORY BOWEL DISEASE ON MENOPAUSE

The only fully published data to date specific to the issue of menopause come from Lichtarowicz et al.[9] One hundred ninety-six women with Crohn's disease were surveyed via questionnaire regarding their menstrual and menopausal history. The age at menopause was compared to a sample of healthy controls from the same geographic area (South Wales). Thirty-four percent of the patient sample had a history of physiologic menopause and another 6% were status posthysterectomy. They found an association between a longer duration of disease and a later onset of menopause ($p<0.02$). For those women who had onset of disease in their 40s, menopause came 2 years earlier than healthy controls. The clinical significance of this finding correlates to an increased risk of osteoporosis and cardiovascular mortality.

EFFECT OF MENOPAUSE ON INFLAMMATORY BOWEL DISEASE

Until recently, there were no data regarding the effect of menopause on IBD. Kane et al presented an abstract examining disease activity pre- and postmenopause in women with either ulcerative colitis (UC) or Crohn's disease.[10] Twenty-three of 65 patients (35%) experienced active symptoms in the premenopausal time period, and 25 patients (38%) had disease indices consistent with a flare within the first 2 years after menopause ($p>0.05$). There was no apparent correlation between having a flare in the premenopausal state and postmenopause within any individual ($r = 0.32$, $p>0.05$). However, when stratified by hormone use, there appeared to be a significant protective effect for disease activity with hormone replacement therapy (HRT) use. HRT was associated with an 82% reduction in the likelihood of disease activity compared with women not taking any exogenous hormones ($p = 0.001$). When stratified by disease type, the odds ratios approached statistical significance, but the numbers of patients in each group were small. Of note, this study found that the age of menopause was similar to that of published healthy populations.

THE USE OF EXOGENOUS HORMONES ON DISEASE

The use of HRT has recently become more controversial with the findings that such agents increase the risk for certain cancers and do not carry as high a protective effect for cardiovascular events as once believed. The indications for use and duration are now individualized, with each woman's personal and family history taken into account.

Of the 25 women in the Kane study who experienced a flare of disease in the postmenopause, the 3 on HRT did not require escalation of therapy to an immunomodulator but rather an increase in mesalamine dosing. This was compared to only 23% (5/22) who could be treated without escalation of therapy to an immunomodulator. There also appeared to be a dose response to the protective effect against disease activity. The risk reduction was 55% with 1 year of use, which increased to 80% with use greater than 1 year. The odds ratio did not change when adjusted for use of concomitant immunomodulators or steroids, type of menopause (surgical versus natural), or type of preparation of hormonal therapy.

Dehydroepiandrosterone (DHEA) inhibits the activation of NF-kB and the secretion of IL-6 and IL-12[11] and has been shown to be effective in patients with lupus.[12] In a small phase II pilot trial in IBD, 6 of 7 patients with Crohn's disease and 8 of 13 patients with UC responded to treatment with 200 mg DHEA per day orally for 56 days.[13] The role of exogenous hormones to treat chronic inflammatory diseases is still in its infancy, and it is too early to say who is an appropriate candidate for such therapy.

OTHER CONSIDERATIONS

Menopause can be pharmacologic, surgical, or physiologic. Those women who undergo surgical menopause tend to be a younger age than those who experience menopause naturally. In this case, bone health must be considered and monitored. Menopause, either surgical or physiologic, is a significant risk factor for osteoporosis and in the setting of IBD, additional risk factors such as cigarette smoking, steroid use, and nutritional deficiencies increase this risk.

A 2-year prospective study of HRT for osteoporosis specifically in the setting of IBD demonstrated a significant change in bone mineral density in those patients treated with HRT.[14] There were no differences between those who had UC versus Crohn's disease or those who experienced a surgical versus physiologic menopause. In addition, no adverse events were noted nor did any patient have to stop therapy secondary to side effects.

Erectile Dysfunction

MEDICATIONS

A number of medications can cause ED. Among men in the general population who seek medical attention for impotence, it has been estimated that medications are responsible in up to 25% of cases.[15] Nevertheless, IBD medications per se do not appear to cause ED frequently. Among the medications commonly used to treat IBD, methotrexate is the one most often associated with impotence.[16-18] A single case of sulfasalazine causing impotence has been reported, but impotence resolved when the patient was switched to olsalazine.[19] ED has not been reported with the use of other commonly prescribed IBD agents, including azathioprine, 6-mercaptopurine (6-MP), infliximab, adalimumab, and prednisone. Although the medications used to treat IBD infrequently cause ED, it is important for the clinician to consider other medications when evaluating IBD patients with ED. For example, antidepressants and antianxiety medications are prescribed frequently for patients with IBD, and these medications often have sexual side effects.

SURGERY

Proctocolectomy is indicated to treat refractory colonic disease or dysplasia in IBD patients, often during their most sexually active stage of life. Ileal pouch anal anastomosis (IPAA) has been associated with sexual dysfunction in men. A large study of patients who had IPAA for the treatment of IBD found that 3% of men reported experiencing either retrograde ejaculation or no ejaculation at 10 years after the operation.[20] In this same study, the rates of other types of sexual dysfunction reported by men at 1 year (n = 762) and 12 years (n = 215) after surgery were 1% and 2%, respectively. Another study of 122 men who had IPAA (116 with IBD, 6 with familial adenomatous polyposis [FAP]) found that rates of retrograde ejaculation increased from 2/122 (<2%) preoperatively to 10/122 (8%) after IPAA, but that rates of ED were similar before and after surgery (complete ED in 4% preoperatively and 5% postoperatively; partial ED in 5% preoperatively and 7% postoperatively).[21] These investigators also evaluated male sexual function using a validated index that included 5 features: erectile function, orgasmic function, sexual desire, intercourse satisfaction, and overall satisfaction. The study found that, overall, there was a statistically significant improvement in 4 of those 5 features after IPAA, suggesting that any negative effect of the operation on sexual function was overshadowed by the beneficial effect of eliminating colitis. Two smaller studies of patients who had IPAA performed during childhood for the treatment of IBD or FAP found that none of the males experienced either impotence or retrograde ejaculation.[22,23] In a study with disparate findings, a group from the Netherlands studied 35 men who had IPAA for UC and found that the rate of sexual dysfunction—defined as impotence or retrograde ejaculation—was as high as 25%, but 90% of patients reported that overall they were satisfied with results of the operation.[24] A recent meta-analysis of 43 studies that evaluated patients after IPAA found the pooled incidence of sexual dysfunction to be 3.6%.[25] Lastly, there has been a randomized, placebo-controlled trial of sildenafil for ED following rectal excision performed either for cancer or IBD. In this study of 32 men with postoperative ED, a successful response to treatment as defined by erectile function questionnaire scores was noted in 79% of the sildenafil-treated group compared to only 17% of the group taking placebo.[26] In summary, the bulk of the available data suggest that we can reassure our male patients who have IPAA for the treatment of colitis that the rate of postoperative sexual dysfunction is low and, when it does occur, the sexual dysfunction can be treated successfully with sildenafil in most cases.

While IPAA often is prescribed for patients with UC, there are many IBD patients who have had, or who might be better served by, other colectomy/reconstruction procedures, including total colectomy with end-ileostomy, ileorectal anastomosis, ileoanal anastomosis without a pouch, and the Kock pouch. Unfortunately, the data on sexual function after these procedures are considerably more limited than those for IPAA. One study noted that patients who were converted from a traditional (or Brooke) ileostomy to a continent ileostomy (Kock pouch) reported improvement in the quality of their sexual life.[27] Other studies have found no significant differences between these 2 procedures in regards to sexual function.[28] One study found that patients with IPAA have fewer restrictions in sexual activities than those with Kock pouches or traditional ileostomies.[28] Considering that the pelvic dissection for colectomy with ileostomy is similar to that for colectomy with IPAA, it seems likely that any differences between the 2 procedures in sexual function would result from the surgery's effects on body image rather than from damage to the pelvic innervation.[29] Ileorectal anastomosis, in contrast, avoids extensive pelvic dissection and its potential for adverse sexual effects, but entails an increased risk for cancer development and for inflammatory disease in the retained rectum.[29]

Screening for Prostate Cancer

After proctocolectomy in men with IBD, digital rectal examination and rectal ultrasonography are no longer possible; consequently, screening for prostate cancer becomes more challenging. For such patients, prostate cancer screening is limited primarily to blood testing for serum prostate specific antigen (PSA) levels. If PSA levels are abnormal, then further, direct evaluation of the prostate is indicated. This is achieved by accessing the prostate through the perineum, both for ultrasonographic examination and for biopsy.[30-32]

Although there is no clear association between prostate cancer risk and IBD, a recent, large, population-based study from Sweden has suggested that, for men with UC, there may be a slightly increased relative risk of developing prostate cancer. The investigators identified 27,606 patients who were hospitalized for UC between 1964 and 2004 and found that 2058 had developed cancers. When standardized incidence ratios were calculated by comparing cancer rates in the UC patients with control subjects, the standardized incidence ratio for prostate cancer in UC patients was 1.14.[33] The authors speculate that this modest increase in prostate cancer frequency may be the result of increased rates of surveillance in UC patients rather than a true increase in prostate cancer incidence.

Summary

Menopause has not been well studied in the setting of IBD. Preliminary work suggests that menopause may be of earlier onset than healthy controls but it does not appear that it has any effect on disease course. Exogenous hormones may prove to have a therapeutic effect on disease activity based on their anti-inflammatory properties. In males, ED is not uncommon but not likely to be driven by hormone deficiency states. Prostate cancer screening remains an important part of health maintenance for older males.

References

1. Kane SV, Sable K, Hanauer SB. The menstrual cycle and its effect on inflammatory bowel disease and irritable bowel syndrome: a prevalence study. *Am J Gastroenterol.* 1998;93(10):1867-1872.
2. Mathias J, Ferguson K, Clench M. Debilitating "functional" bowel disease controlled by leuprolide acetate, gonadotropin-releasing hormone (GnRH) analog. *Dig Dis Sci.* 1989;34(5):761-766.
3. Prior A, Stanley K, Smith A, et al. Relation between hysterectomy and the irritable bowel: a prospective study. *Gut.* 1992;33(6):814-817.
4. Lahita RG. Sex hormones and systemic lupus erythematosus. *Rheum Dis Clin North Am.* 2000;26(4):951-968.
5. Zang YC, Halder JB, Hong J, Rivera VM, Zhang JZ. Regulatory effects of estriol on T cell migration and cytokine profile: inhibition of transcription factor NF-k B. *J Neuroimmunol.* 2002;124(1-2):106-114.
6. Chadwick CC, Chippari S, Matelan E, et al. Identification of pathway-selective estrogen receptor ligand that inhibit NF-k B transcriptional activity. *Proc Natl Acad Sci USA.* 2005;102(7):2543-2548.
7. Verdu EF, Deng Y, Bercik P, Collins SM. Modulatory effects of estrogen in two murine models of experimental colitis. *Am J Physiol Gastrointest Liver Physiol.* 2002;283:27-36.
8. Harnish DC, Albert LM, Leathurby Y, et al. Beneficial effects of estrogen treatment in the HLA-B27 transgenic rat model of inflammatory bowel disease. *Am J Physiol Gastrointest Liver Physiol.* 2004;286:18-25.
9. Lichtarowicz A, Norman C, Calcraft B, Morris JS, Rhodes J, Mayberry J. A study of the menopause, smoking and contraception in women with Crohn's disease. *Q J Med.* 1989;72(267):623-631.
10. Kane SV, Reddy D. Hormone replacement therapy after menopause is protective of disease activity in women with inflammatory bowel disease. *Am J Gastroenterol.* 2005;100(9)A:776 [Abstract].
11. Straub RH, Konecna L, Hrach S, et al. Serum dehydroepiandrosterone (DHEA) and DHEA sulfate are negatively correlated with serum interleukin-6, and DHEA inhibits IL-6 secretion from mononuclear cells in man in vitro: possible link between endocrinosenescence and immunosenescence. *J Clin Endocrinol Metab.* 1998;83(6):2012-2017.
12. van Vollenhoven RF, Park JL, Genovese MC, West JP, McGuire JL. A double-blind, placebo-controlled clinical trial of dehydroepiandrosterone in severe systemic lupus erythematosus. *Lupus.* 1999;8(3):181-187.
13. Andus T, Klebl F, Rogler G, et al. Patients with refractory Crohn's disease or ulcerative colitis respond to dehydroepiandrosterone: a pilot study. *Aliment Pharmacol Ther.* 2003;17:409-414.
14. Clements D, Compston JE, Evans WD, Rhodes J. Hormone replacement therapy prevents bone loss in patients with inflammatory bowel disease. *Gut.* 1993;34:1543-1546.
15. Beeley L. Drug-induced sexual dysfunction and infertility. *Adverse Drug React Acute Poisoning Rev.* 1984;3:23-42.
16. Thomas E, Koumouvi K, Blotman F. Impotence in a patient with rheumatoid arthritis treated with methotrexate. *J Rheumatol.* 2000;27:1821-1822.
17. Riba N, Moreno F, Costa J, et al. Appearance of impotence in relation to the use of methotrexate. *Med Clin (Barc).* 1996;106:558.
18. Blackburn WD Jr, Alarcón GS. Impotence in three rheumatoid arthritis patients treated with methotrexate. *Arthritis Rheum.* 1989;32:1341-1342.
19. Ireland A, Jewell DP. Sulfasalazine-induced impotence: a beneficial resolution with olsalazine? *J Clin Gastroenterol.* 1989;11:711.
20. Farouk R, Pemberton JH, Wolff BG, et al. Functional outcomes after ileal pouch-anal anastomosis for chronic ulcerative colitis. *Ann Surg.* 2000;231:919-926.
21. Gorgun E, Remzi FH, Montague DK, et al. Male sexual function improves after ileal pouch anal anastomosis. *Colorectal Dis.* 2005;7:545-550.
22. Hyams JS, Grand RJ, Colodny AH, et al. Course and prognosis after colectomy and ileostomy for inflammatory bowel disease in childhood and adolescence. *J Pediatr Surg.* 1982;17:400-405.
23. Parc YR, Moslein G, Dozois RR, et al. Familial adenomatous polyposis: results after ileal pouch-anal anastomosis in teenagers. *Dis Colon Rectum.* 2000;43:893-898.

24. Hueting WE, Gooszen HG, van Laarhoven CJ. Sexual function and continence after ileo pouch anal anastomosis: a comparison between a meta-analysis and a questionnaire survey. *Int J Colorectal Dis.* 2004;19:215-218.

25. Hueting WE, Buskens E, van der Tweel I, et al. Results and complications after ileal pouch anal anastomosis: a meta-analysis of 43 observational studies comprising 9,317 patients. *Dig Surg.* 2005;22:69-79.

26. Lindsey I, George B, Kettlewell M, et al. Randomized, double-blind, placebo-controlled trial of sildenafil (Viagra) for erectile dysfunction after rectal excision for cancer and inflammatory bowel disease. *Dis Colon Rectum.* 2002;45:727-732.

27. Nilsson LO, Kock NG, Kylberg F, et al. Sexual adjustment in ileostomy patients before and after conversion to continent ileostomy. *Dis Colon Rectum.* 1981;24:287-290.

28. Köhler LW, Pemberton JH, Zinsmeister AR, et al. Quality of life after proctocolectomy: a comparison of Brooke ileostomy, Kock pouch, and ileal pouch-anal anastomosis. *Gastroenterology.* 1991;101:679-684.

29. Hultén L. Proctocolectomy and ileostomy to pouch surgery for ulcerative colitis. *World J Surg.* 1998;22:335-341.

30. Fergany AF, Angermeier KW. A technique of transrectal ultrasound guided transperineal random prostate biopsy in patients with ulcerative colitis and an ileal pouch. *J Urol.* 2000;163:205-206.

31. Filderman PS, Jacobs SC. Prostatic ultrasound in the patient without a rectum. *Urology.* 1994;43:722-724.

32. Shinohara K, Gulati M, Koppie TM, et al. Transperineal prostate biopsy after abdominoperineal resection. *J Urol.* 2003;169:141-144.

33. Hemminki K, Li X, Sundquist J, et al. Cancer risks in ulcerative colitis patients. *Int J Cancer.* 2008;123(6):1417-1421.

Financial disclosure: Dr. Kane is a consultant for Abbott, Centocor, Elan, UCB, Shire, and Procter & Gamble and receives research support from Elan, UCB, Shire, and Procter & Gamble.

INFLAMMATORY BOWEL DISEASE AND AGING

SPECIAL CONSIDERATIONS AND MANAGEMENT

Darrell S. Pardi, MD

Although inflammatory bowel disease (IBD) occurs most commonly in young adults, a significant proportion presents initially in older subjects. In addition, IBD is a chronic disease without significant mortality, and the aging of younger patients will result in an increasing number of elderly patients with IBD. Although there is little specific information in the literature describing outcomes of treatment in elderly IBD patients, it appears that treatment responses in the elderly are similar to those of younger patients.[1,2] Specific issues related to the epidemiology, differential diagnosis, clinical course, and treatment of IBD in the elderly are discussed in this chapter, with a generalized approach to older patients with suspected IBD outlined in Figure 16-1.

Epidemiology

Ulcerative colitis and Crohn's disease are typically considered diseases of young patients, with a peak incidence in the second to fourth decades of life.[3,4] Some studies report a bimodal age distribution, with a second smaller peak in incidence in the sixth to eighth decades, although not all studies have shown this second peak.[3,4] Whether or not there is truly a second incidence peak, 8% to 16% of IBD is diagnosed in patients 60 years old or older.[3-5] Of these, 65% present in their 60s, 25% in their 70s, and 10% in their 80s.[6,7] In population-based cohorts, the incidence of Crohn's disease in patients over age 60 is 3 to 11 per 100,000 patient-years,[4,6,8] and the incidence of ulcerative colitis in patients over age 60 is 4 to 16 per 100,000 patient-years.[4,7,8] In the latter half of the last century, the incidence of Crohn's disease in elderly residents of Olmsted County, Minnesota rose initially but then stabilized[6] while the incidence of ulcerative colitis increased steadily.[7]

Scherl EJ, Dubinsky MC.
The Changing World of Inflammatory Bowel Disease:
Impact of Generation, Gender, and Global Trends (pp 193-202)
© 2009 SLACK Incorporated.

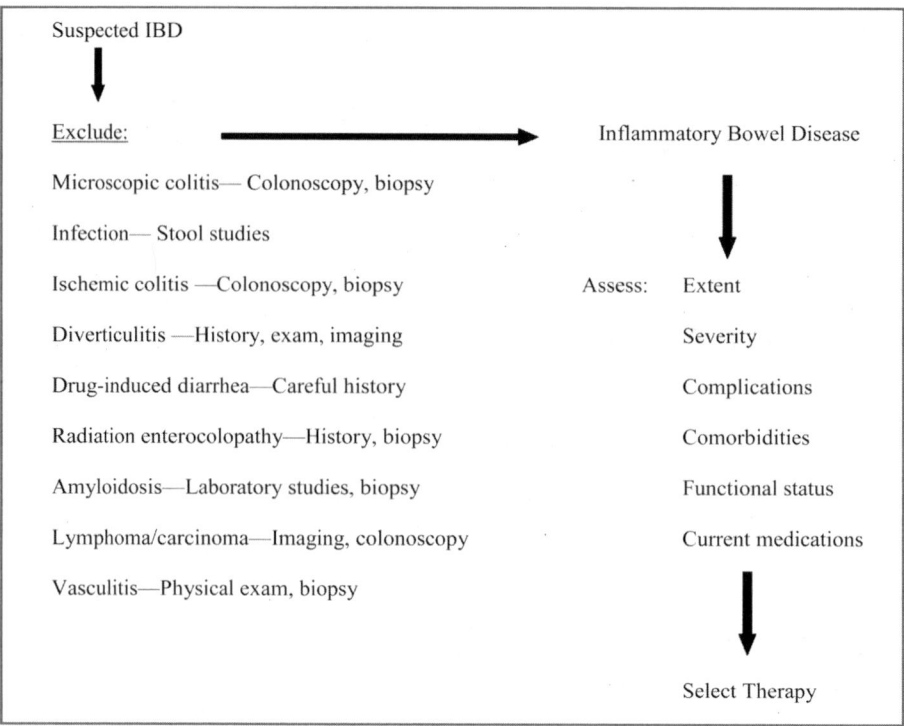

Suspected IBD

Exclude: Inflammatory Bowel Disease

Microscopic colitis— Colonoscopy, biopsy

Infection— Stool studies

Ischemic colitis —Colonoscopy, biopsy   Assess: Extent

Diverticulitis —History, exam, imaging   Severity

Drug-induced diarrhea—Careful history   Complications

Radiation enterocolopathy—History, biopsy   Comorbidities

Amyloidosis—Laboratory studies, biopsy   Functional status

Lymphoma/carcinoma—Imaging, colonoscopy   Current medications

Vasculitis—Physical exam, biopsy

                                                                       Select Therapy

Figure 16-1. Approach to IBD in the elderly. (Adapted from Pardi DS, Loftus EV Jr, Camilleri M. Treatment of inflammatory bowel disease in the elderly: an update. *Drugs Aging.* 2002;19:355-363.)

Differential Diagnosis

There are several causes of gastrointestinal symptoms that may mimic IBD and that occur more commonly in elderly patients, including microscopic colitis, infectious colitis, ischemic colitis, diverticular disease, medication-induced diarrhea and colitis, radiation colitis, and others (see Figure 16-1). Perhaps because of these alternative diagnoses, Crohn's disease is more often misdiagnosed in older patients compared to younger patients,[9] often with a significantly longer delay between the onset of symptoms and diagnosis,[1] suggesting that clinicians may have more difficulty diagnosing IBD in older patients. In addition to a careful history and review of the medication list, colonoscopy with biopsies and stool studies are usually helpful for distinguishing IBD from these other diagnoses.

Microscopic colitis is a common cause of diarrhea in the elderly, often accompanied by abdominal pain and weight loss.[10] Distinguishing this form of colitis from Crohn's disease and ulcerative colitis is important because treatment considerations are different.[10]

Infectious colitis is relatively common in elderly patients and should be considered high in the differential diagnosis, particularly for those patients with recent onset of bowel symptoms.[5,11] Stool culture (including specific testing for *Escherichia coli* 0157:H7) and fecal analysis for *Clostridium difficile* should be done in all elderly patients in whom the diagnosis of IBD is being considered. In one study, infection was found in 17% of patients with suspected IBD,[11] with infectious colitis more likely to present within 1 week of symptom onset and to be associated with fever.[12]

Ischemic colitis is also an important consideration in elderly patients presenting with bloody diarrhea, particularly in those with risk factors for vascular disease or conditions predisposing to colonic hypoperfusion, such as dehydration, hypotension, heart failure, and arrhythmias. However, many patients with ischemic colitis have no identifiable risk factors. Endoscopy and histology are often helpful in distinguishing ischemic colitis from IBD, although segmental Crohn's colitis may mimic ischemia. Rapid onset and spontaneous improvement are more suggestive of ischemia.

Diverticular disease is another common condition in the elderly,[13] including those with IBD.[14] Diverticulitis and diverticular bleeding can mimic symptoms of IBD, and diverticula-associated colitis is considered a form of IBD.[15] Given the high prevalence of diverticular disease in elderly patients, left-sided colonic Crohn's disease in this population is often misdiagnosed as diverticulitis.[6,9] Furthermore, patients operated on for presumed diverticulitis who are subsequently found to have Crohn's disease have an increased risk of postoperative complications.[16]

Finally, a careful history should seek other causes of bowel inflammation such as medications or a history of radiation therapy. Medications associated with colitis include nonsteroidal anti-inflammatory drugs, estrogens, digitalis, gold, sodium phosphate enemas, and methyldopa,[17] and many others can cause diarrhea without causing colitis.

Clinical Course

In general, IBD in elderly patients follows a similar clinical course to that in younger patients, although there are several notable differences.

The presenting signs and symptoms of IBD are generally the same, although elderly patients with Crohn's disease may be less likely to have abdominal pain and more likely to present with diarrhea and bleeding,[1,2,9,18,19] perhaps because elderly patients with Crohn's disease may be more likely to have isolated colonic disease,[1,5,6,14,20] although this difference was not observed in all reports.[9,16,18,19] The elderly patient with Crohn's disease is also less likely to have stricturing disease.[1,5] Compared to younger patients, older patients with Crohn's disease may[1] or may not[9] have a longer delay between the onset of symptoms and diagnosis, and they are more likely to have other medical problems, including cardiovascular disease. Elderly patients with Crohn's disease are less likely to need surgery,[5,20] and those who do may have a lower rate of postoperative recurrence than younger patients.[5,9] However, other studies comparing elderly and younger patients found similar indications for surgery and rates of surgery.[1,9,19] Predictably, the elderly have more postoperative complications, primarily cardiopulmonary,[21] and may have a higher overall mortality,[6,22] likely reflecting the higher prevalence of comorbidities. However, another report has shown lower mortality in the elderly patient with Crohn's disease, perhaps reflecting the higher prevalence of colonic disease in this study.[5]

Although in some studies ulcerative colitis may be more likely to be limited to the distal colon in elderly patients compared to younger patients,[2,5,7] other studies have shown no difference in disease location.[18] Ulcerative colitis in the elderly is more likely to present with a severe attack than in younger patients,[2,5,7] and therefore elderly patients presenting with ulcerative colitis have a higher mortality than younger patients.[4,5]

Older patients with Crohn's disease are less likely to have a family history of the disease, perhaps reflecting a greater environmental influence compared to younger patients.[9,19,20] This finding was not seen in patients with ulcerative colitis.[9] With regards to extraintestinal manifestations of IBD, there has not been a difference observed between elderly and younger patients.[9,18,19]

Treatment

In general, the treatment approach to IBD in the elderly is similar to that in younger patients, which is reviewed in detail in other chapters. Although some reports indicate that elderly patients are more likely to respond to medical therapy and to stay in remission than younger patients,[5,6] other studies comparing the course of Crohn's disease in elderly and younger patients found similar response rates to medical therapy.[1,9,19] Treatment options will be briefly reviewed here, with an emphasis on issues relevant to the older patient. Typically, elderly patients are more likely to have comorbidities and to be taking other medications, which must be considered when selecting an IBD therapy.

ULCERATIVE COLITIS

The extent and severity of inflammation help to determine the most appropriate therapy.[23] Ulcerative colitis can be divided into distal (distal to the splenic flexure) or extensive (extension proximal to the splenic flexure) disease. The severity can be defined as mild (<4 stools daily, no systemic signs, and a normal sedimentation rate), moderate (>4 stools daily with minimal signs of toxicity), severe (>6 bloody stools with signs of systemic toxicity), or fulminant (>10 bloody stools, with constant bleeding, pain, fever, and colonic dilatation on x-ray).[23]

For patients with mild to moderate distal disease, effective choices for therapy include oral aminosalicylates, topical mesalamine, or topical steroids,[23,24] although the elderly may be less responsive to topical therapy than younger patients.[23] This difference may be related to problems with adherence, as poor functional status, weak anal sphincter tone, physical incoordination, and baseline incontinence are important concerns in elderly patients. If topical therapy is prescribed, close follow-up is required to be sure the elderly patient is able to use it as directed.

Topical mesalamine may be more effective than oral therapy or topical steroids in patients with distal ulcerative colitis,[24] and the combination of oral and topical therapies is more effective than either therapy alone.[25] It should be noted that oral and topical aminosalicylates are effective for both induction and maintenance of remission, while topical steroids are effective for induction of remission only.[23] For patients with distal disease refractory to the above treatments, oral prednisone is effective for inducing remission, recognizing that the elderly are more susceptible to most steroid-associated side effects, including accelerated bone loss, fractures, hypertension, diabetes, and mental status changes.[26,27]

For patients with mild to moderate extensive disease, the usual therapy for induction and maintenance of remission is oral aminosalicylates, which are typically well tolerated, even in the elderly. Topical agents can be used in addition to oral therapy, particularly in patients with significant rectal symptoms, such as urgency or tenesmus, which are commonly associated with fecal incontinence in the elderly. For those patients who do not respond to oral aminosalicylates, an oral prednisone taper can be used to induce remission, with 6-mercaptopurine (6-MP) or azathioprine prescribed for maintenance of remission.[28] Important side effects of 6-MP and azathioprine include bone marrow suppression, infection, hepatitis, and pancreatitis, with no evidence that these side effects are more common in the elderly.

For patients with severe ulcerative colitis and those with moderate disease who do not respond to oral therapy, treatment with intravenous steroids is usually the next option. Severely ill elderly patients should also be considered for antibiotics, fluid resuscitation, nutritional support, blood transfusions, and early surgical consultation with close follow-up. Patients who do not respond to intravenous steroids in 5 to 7 days should be considered for intravenous cyclosporine, infliximab, or colectomy. Cyclosporine use may avoid colectomy in refractory ulcerative colitis,[29] but the possibility of side effects, which are probably more common in the elderly, needs to be considered.

Infliximab, a chimeric antibody against tumor necrosis factor alpha (TNF-α), is effective for induction and maintenance of remission in moderate to severe ulcerative colitis not responding to other medications[30] and is an alternative to surgery and cyclosporine. However, in one large open-label clinical experience with infliximab in Crohn's disease, the risk of serious side effects appeared to be higher in elderly patients.[31] Infliximab may also cause exacerbation of heart failure.[32] In addition, in a small study of severe colitis refractory to intravenous steroids, "rescue therapy" with infliximab was not statistically better than placebo for those patients with fulminant colitis.[33] Therefore, the role of infliximab and cyclosporine in the management of elderly patients with severe steroid-refractory ulcerative colitis needs to be further clarified, and the decision to use these drugs or to proceed to surgery should ideally be made in consultation with gastroenterologists and surgeons with familiarity with these medications and expertise in caring for these severely ill patients. Colectomy should be considered in patients who do not respond to medical therapy; those who have a complication of colitis such as severe bleeding, perforation, megacolon, carcinoma, or dysplasia[23]; and those with contraindications to infliximab or cyclosporine therapy.

CROHN'S DISEASE

Treatment of inflammatory Crohn's disease encompasses similar issues to those discussed previously for ulcerative colitis. Additional medications to consider include budesonide, methotrexate, adalimumab, and certolizumab. Although budesonide is a highly potent corticosteroid, the systemic toxicity is less than with conventional steroids due to high first-pass hepatic metabolism.[34] Thus, in elderly patients with mild to moderate ileal or ileocecal disease, budesonide is an appropriate induction agent. Methotrexate is an alternative immune modulator to azathioprine or 6-MP.[35] However, methotrexate may increase the risk of cardiovascular complications in the elderly, perhaps by increasing serum homocystine levels.[36] In addition, other methotrexate-associated complications may be more common in the elderly, perhaps as a result of declining renal function.[37] Therefore, this drug should be used with caution in elderly patients.

Adalimumab is a fully human anti-TNF antibody that is approved for the induction and maintenance of remission in Crohn's disease.[38,39] Certolizumab is a humanized, pegylated anti-TNF antibody that is also approved for the induction and maintenance of remission in Crohn's disease.[40,41] Although less is known about the safety profile of these drugs compared to infliximab, particularly in elderly patients, they are generally thought to have similar toxicity concerns as discussed previously for infliximab. In addition, since adalimumab and certolizumab are subcutaneous injections, the ability of an elderly patient to give an injection to him- or herself or to arrange to have it given must be considered.

For perianal Crohn's disease, the goal of treatment is to control local symptoms while preserving sphincter function and ideally, induce complete fistula closure.[40] Small fistulas with minimal drainage and few symptoms do not require treatment other than local hygiene. If there are significant symptoms, an abscess should be excluded before prescribing medical therapy. Metronidazole has been used extensively in patients with perianal disease, and ciprofloxacin is often used in conjunction or as an alternative.[42] Ciprofloxacin is generally well tolerated, metronidazole less so. The main side effects of metronidazole are gastrointestinal intolerance and peripheral neuropathy. The major drawback to antibiotic monotherapy is the high rate of recurrence when treatment is discontinued, such that prolonged therapy may be necessary. The concomitant use of an immunomodulatory medication such as azathioprine or 6-MP may allow maintenance of an antibiotic-induced remission of perianal Crohn's disease.[42] In addition, anti-TNF antibody therapy with infliximab[43] or adalimumab[44] has been reported to be effective for induction and maintenance therapy in fistulizing Crohn's disease.

DRUG-DRUG INTERACTIONS

Elderly patients with IBD are more likely to be on multiple medications than younger patients. Some of the commonly used medications in IBD have notable drug-drug interactions. The aminosalicylate compounds can reduce the effect of warfarin and digoxin. In addition, they increase the levels of the active metabolite of 6-MP and azathioprine.[45] The metabolism of 6-MP and azathioprine is significantly altered by allopurinol, which raises the level of active metabolites and increases the risk of serious leukopenia. Thus, the concomitant use of these medications should generally be avoided.[46] Significant anemia has been reported with the concomitant use of azathioprine and angiotensin-converting enzyme inhibitors, such that this combination should be avoided, or if necessary, close follow-up of hemoglobin levels is warranted.[47]

Corticosteroids have a number of established or probable drug-drug interactions that must be considered if these medications are used in the elderly. Cyclosporine also has a large number of established or probable drug-drug interactions. For example, it should not be used with other nephrotoxic drugs or with potassium-sparing diuretics. Finally, live attenuated vaccines should be avoided in patients receiving any immune-suppressing medications.

SURGERY

Ileal pouch anal anastomosis (IPAA) is the procedure of choice for patients with ulcerative colitis who need colectomy. In a study comparing IPAA outcomes in younger and older patients, postoperative complications, pouch failure rate, and quality of life after surgery were no different between age groups.[48] However, the risk of incontinence is higher in older patients, and some surgeons consider older age as a relative contraindication to IPAA.[49] A study of abdominal surgery in older Crohn's disease patients showed a higher risk of cardiopulmonary postoperative complications, but similar mortality and anastomotic leak rates compared to younger patients.[21]

METABOLIC BONE DISEASE

Osteopenia and osteoporosis are important considerations in many patients with IBD, even in the absence of corticosteroid therapy. Elderly patients with IBD are no exception, with a higher prevalence of osteoporosis in older patients.[50] All patients should receive education on lifestyle changes (weight-bearing exercise, tobacco cessation, avoiding excess alcohol).[50] Bone density should be measured in all patients with IBD at increased risk for osteoporosis (eg, steroid use, older age).[50] Calcium and vitamin D supplementation should be given at doses of 1200 to 1500 mg/day and 400 to 800 IU/day, respectively. Bisphosphonates should be considered in all patients with osteoporosis and perhaps prophylactically in patients who are expected to be treated with steroids for several months.[50]

Summary

A significant proportion of IBD is diagnosed in elderly patients, and with the aging of the population, an increasing number of elderly patients with IBD will be encountered in clinical practice. While the clinical course of IBD in the elderly is generally similar to that in younger subjects, there are specific differences in presentation and clinical course that need to be considered. An increased prevalence of comorbidities and increasingly common alternative diagnoses can make the diagnosis more challenging in the elderly. The treatment of IBD in the elderly should follow a similar strategy to that of the younger population, with attention to comorbidities, functional status, medication side effects, and drug-drug interactions. These considerations will become increasingly more relevant as the population ages. The Census Bureau projects that there will be 8 to 13 million Americans 85 years of age or older by the year 2040.[51] The diagnosis and treatment of IBD in the elderly will therefore become more common, and additional research on IBD in the old and very old is necessary. In addition, clinical trials involving new therapies for IBD will need to include patients in older age groups.

References

1. Harper PC, McAuliffe TL, Beeken WL. Crohn's disease in the elderly: a statistical comparison with younger patients matched for sex and duration of disease. *Arch Intern Med.* 1986;146:753-755.
2. Robertson DJ, Grimm IS. Inflammatory bowel disease in the elderly. *Gastroenterol Clin NA.* 2001;30:409-426.
3. Loftus EV Jr, Sandborn WJ. Epidemiology of inflammatory bowel disease. *Gastroenterol Clin NA.* 2002;31:1-20.

4. Bernstein CN, Blanchard JF, Rawsthorne P, Wajda A. Epidemiology of Crohn's disease and ulcerative colitis in a central Canadian province: a population-based study. *Am J Epidemiol*. 1999;149:916-924.

5. Softley A, Myren J, Clamp SE, et al. Inflammatory bowel disease in the elderly patient. *Scand J Gastroenterol*. 1988;23(suppl 144):27-30.

6. Loftus EV Jr, Silverstein MD, Sandborn WJ, et al. Crohn's disease in Olmsted County, Minnesota, 1940-1993: incidence, prevalence, and survival. *Gastroenterology*. 1998;114:1161-1168.

7. Loftus EV Jr, Silverstein MD, Sandborn WJ, et al. Ulcerative colitis in Olmsted County, Minnesota, 1940-1993: incidence, prevalence, and survival. *Gut*. 2000;46:336-343.

8. Piront P, Louis E, Latour P, Plomteux O, Belaiche J. Epidemiology of inflammatory bowel diseases in the elderly in the province of Liege: a three-year prospective study. *Gastroenterol Clin Biol*. 2001;25:157-161.

9. Wagtmans MJ, Verspaget HW, Lamers CB, et al. Crohn's disease in the elderly: a comparison with young adults. *J Clin Gastroenterol*. 1998;27:129-133.

10. Pardi DS. Microscopic colitis: an update. *Inflamm Bowel Dis*. 2004;10:860-870.

11. Tedesco FJ, Hardin RD, Harper RN, et al. Infectious colitis endoscopically simulating inflammatory bowel disease: a prospective evaluation. *Gastrointest Endosc*. 1983;29:195-197.

12. Schumacher G, Kollberg B, Sandstedt B. A prospective study of first attacks of inflammatory bowel disease and infectious colitis: clinical findings and early diagnosis. *Scand J Gastroenterol*. 1994;29:265-274.

13. Manousos ON, Truelove SC, Lumsden K. Prevalence of colonic diverticulosis in the general population of the Oxford area. *Br Med J*. 1967;3:762.

14. Heresbach D, Alexandre JL, Bretagne JF, et al. Crohn's disease in the over-60 age group: a population based study. *Eur J Gastroenterol Hepatol*. 2004;16:657-664.

15. Koutroubakis IE, Antoniou P, Tzardi M, Kouroumalis EA. The spectrum of segmental colitis associated with diverticulosis. *Int J Colorectal Dis*. 2005;20:28.

16. Tchirkow G, Lavery IC, Fazio VW. Crohn's disease in the elderly. *Dis Colon Rectum*. 1983;26:177-181.

17. Pardi DS, Loftus EV Jr, Camilleri M. Treatment of inflammatory bowel disease in the elderly: an update. *Drugs Aging*. 2002;19:355-363.

18. Greth J, Török HP, Koenig A, Folwaczny C. Comparison of inflammatory bowel disease at younger and older age. *Eur J Med Res*. 2004;9:552.

19. Triantafillidis JK, Emmanouilidis A, Nicolakis D, Ifantis T, Cheracakis P, Merikas EG. Crohn's disease in the elderly: clinical features and long-term outcome of 19 Greek patients. *Digest Liver Dis*. 2000;32:498-503.

20. Polito JM, Childs B, Mellits ED, et al. Crohn's disease: influence of age at diagnosis on site and clinical type of disease. *Gastroenterology*. 1996;111:580-586.

21. Norris B, Solomon MJ, Eyers AA, et al. Abdominal surgery in the older Crohn's population. *Aust N Z J Surg*. 1999;69:199-204.

22. Wolters FL, Russel MG, Sjibrandij J, et al. Crohn's disease: increased mortality 10 years after diagnosis in a European-wide population based cohort. *Gut*. 2006;55:510-518.

23. Kornbluth A, Sachar DB. Ulcerative colitis practice guidelines in adults (update): American College of Gastroenterology, Practice Parameters Committee. *Am J Gastroenterol*. 2004;99:1371-1385.

24. Cohen RD, Woseth DM, Thisted RA, Hanauer SB. A meta-analysis and overview of the literature on treatment options for left-sided ulcerative colitis and ulcerative proctitis. *Am J Gastroenterol*. 2000;95:1263.

25. Safdi M, DeMicco M, Sninsky C, et al. A double-blind comparison of oral versus rectal mesalamine versus combination therapy in the treatment of distal ulcerative colitis. *Am J Gastroenterol*. 1997;92:1867.

26. Thomas TPL. The complications of systemic corticosteroid treatment in the elderly. *Gerontology*. 1984;30:60-65.

27. Akerkar GA, Peppercorn MA, Hamel MB, et al. Corticosteroid-associated complications in elderly Crohn's disease patients. *Am J Gastroenterol*. 1997;92:461-464.

28. George J, Present DH, Pou R, Bodian C, Rubin PH. The long-term outcome of ulcerative colitis treated with 6-mercaptopurine. *Am J Gastroenterol*. 1996;91:1711-1714.

29. Cohen RD, Stein R, Hanauer SB. Intravenous cyclosporin in ulcerative colitis: a five-year experience. *Am J Gastroenterol*. 1999;94:1587-1592.

30. Rutgeerts P, Sandborn WJ, Feagan BJ. Infliximab for induction and maintenance therapy for ulcerative colitis. *N Engl J Med*. 2005;353:2462-2476.

31. Colombel JF, Loftus EV Jr, Tremaine WJ, et al. The safety profile of infliximab in patients with Crohn's disease: the Mayo clinic experience in 500 patients. *Gastroenterology*. 2004;126:19-31.

32. Curtis JR, Kramer JM, Martin C, et al. Heart failure among younger rheumatoid arthritis and Crohn's patients exposed to TNF-alpha antagonists. *Rheumatology (Oxford)*. 2007;46:1688-1693.

33. Järnerot G, Hertervig E, Friis-Liby I, et al. Infliximab as rescue therapy in severe to moderately severe ulcerative colitis: a randomized, placebo-controlled study. *Gastroenterology*. 2005;128:1805-1811.

34. Spencer CM, McTavish D. Budesonide: a review of its pharmacological properties and therapeutic efficacy in inflammatory bowel disease. *Drugs*. 1995;50:854-872.

35. Feagan BG. Methotrexate treatment for Crohn's disease. *Inflamm Bowel Dis*. 1998;4:120-121.

36. Landewe RB, van den Borne BE, Breedveld FC, et al. Methotrexate effects in patients with rheumatoid arthritis with cardiovascular comorbidity. *Lancet*. 2000;355:1616-1617.

37. Tett SE, Triggs EJ. Use of methotrexate in older patients: a risk-benefit assessment. *Drugs Aging.* 1996;9:458-471.

38. Sandborn WJ, Rutgeerts P, Enns R, et al. Adalimumab induction therapy for Crohn disease previously treated with infliximab: a randomized trial. *Ann Intern Med.* 2007;146:829-838.

39. Sandborn WJ, Hanauer SB, Rutgeerts P, et al. Adalimumab for maintenance treatment of Crohn's disease: results of the CLASSIC II trial. *Gut.* 2007;56:1232-1239.

40. Sandborn WJ, Feagan BJ, Stoinov S, et al. Certolizumab pegol for the treatment of Crohn's disease. N Engl J Med. 2007;357:296-298.

41. Schreiber S, Kaliq-Kareemi M, Lawrence IC, et al. Maintenance therapy with certolizumab pegol for Crohn's disease. *N Engl J Med.* 2007;357:239-250.

42. Lichtenstein GR. Treatment of fistulizing Crohn's disease. *Gastroenterology.* 2000;119:1132-1147.

43. Present DH, Rutgeerts P, Targan S, et al. Infliximab for the treatment of fistulas in patients with Crohn's disease. *N Engl J Med.* 1999;340:1398-1405.

44. Hinojosa J, Gomollón F, García S, et al. Efficacy and safety of short-term adalimumab treatment in patients with active Crohn's disease who lost response or showed intolerance to infliximab: a prospective, open-label, multicentre trial. *Aliment Pharmacol Ther.* 2007;25:409-418.

45. Lowry PW, Franklin CL, Weaver AL, et al. Leukopenia resulting from a drug interaction between azathioprine or 6-mercaptopurine and mesalamine, sulphasalazine, or balsalazide. *Gut.* 2001;49:656-664.

46. Brooks RJ, Dorr RT, Durie BG. Interaction of allopurinol with 6-mercaptopurine and azathioprine. *Biomed Pharmacother.* 1982;36:217-222.

47. Gossman J, Kachel HG, Schoeppe W, Scheuermann EH. Anemia in renal transplant recipients caused by concomitant therapy with azathioprine and angiotensin-converting enzyme inhibitors. *Transplantation.* 1993;56:585-589.

48. Chapman JR, Larson DW, Wolff BG, et al. Ileal pouch-anal anastomosis: does age at the time of surgery affect outcome? *Arch Surg.* 2005;140:534.

49. Delaney CP, Fazio VW, Remzi FH, et al. Prospective, age-related analysis of surgical results, functional outcome, and quality of life after ileal pouch-anal anastomosis. *Ann Surg.* 2003;238:221-228.

50. American Gastroenterological Association Medical Position Statement: Guidelines on Osteoporosis in Gastrointestinal Diseases. *Gastroenterology.* 2003;124:791.

51. Bureau of the Census. Current Population Reports. Special Studies. Sixty-five Plus in America. Washington, D.C.: Government Printing Office; 1993.

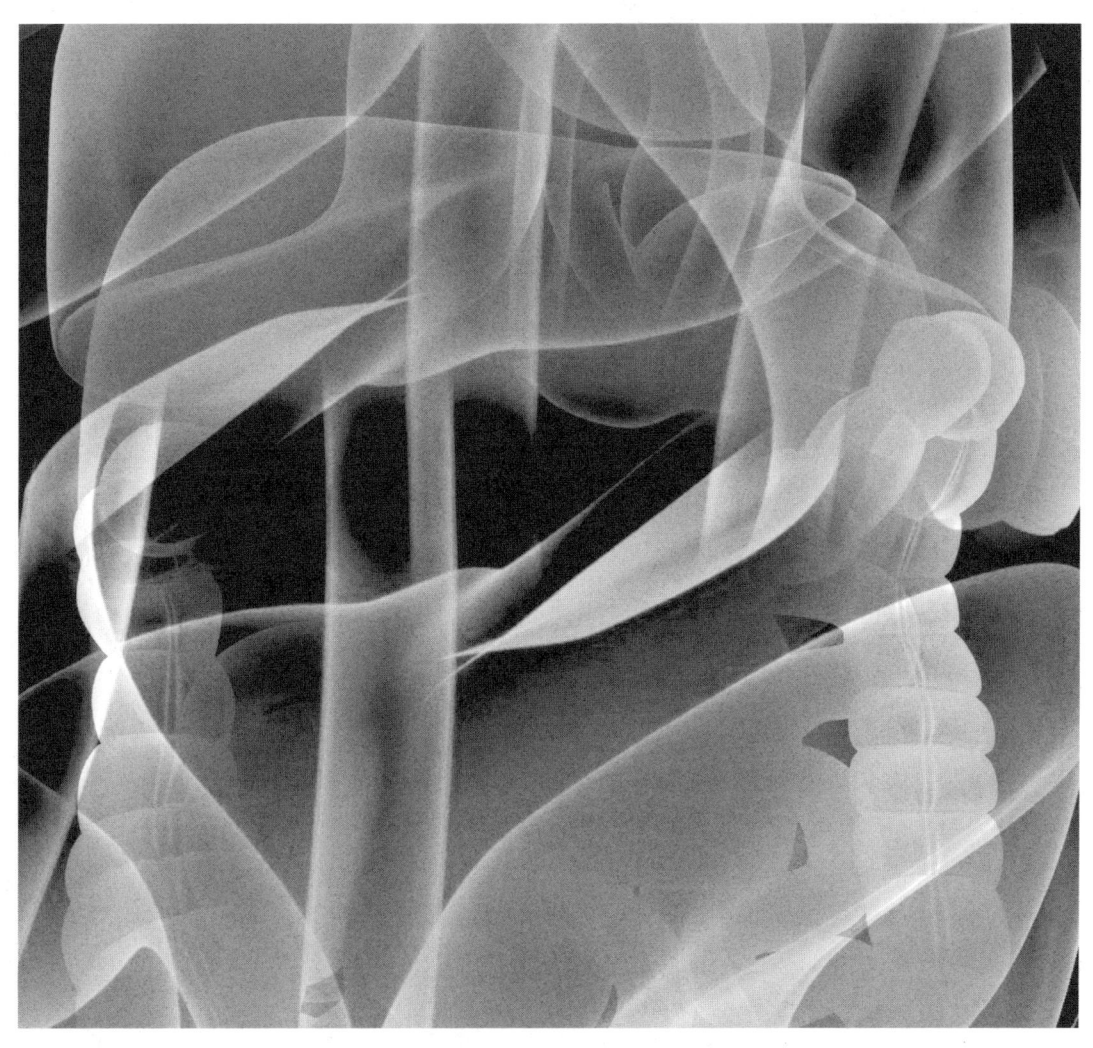

SECTION V

Special Considerations in the Management of the Inflammatory Bowel Disease Life Cycle

CHAPTER 17

CHRONIC CARE OF INFLAMMATORY BOWEL DISEASE

David T. Rubin, MD, FACG, AGAF

Inflammatory bowel disease (IBD) is recognized as a chronic condition classified broadly into 2 sister conditions—Crohn's disease and ulcerative colitis—and is characterized by various levels of disease activity, extent, and severity. A majority of patients suffer from characteristic relapsing and remitting disease activity (and therefore symptoms), but some have a single period of active inflammation followed by prolonged stable remission, while a smaller group apparently suffers from prolonged active inflammation and progression to bowel destruction and disability.[1-4] Current treatment goals of IBD include successful induction of remission, which is defined as a patient who is free of inflammatory symptoms, and long-term maintenance of steroid-free disease control (Table 17-1). Recognizing that IBD is, for most patients, a lifelong disease, management goals must incorporate long-term plans for health management, avoidance of complications, and improved quality of life (Table 17-2). This chapter will highlight those goals and suggest a practical approach to several different groups of patients for the clinician.

What Are the Outcomes of Inflammatory Bowel Disease Patients?

In order to develop an approach to the long-term care of patients with IBD, it is essential to review the available information about the progression and complications of IBD, which include such outcomes as surgery, hospitalizations, exposure to steroids, disability, and death. A majority of patients with Crohn's disease will require at least one surgery during their disease course, and a substantial number who have had surgery will suffer from disease recurrence and a need for repeat surgery.[5,6] It is estimated that approximately one-quarter to as much as one-third of patients with ulcerative colitis will require proctocolectomy, most due to medically refractory disease and a minority due to neoplasia.[7] In addition, it has been well-described that IBD is an expensive condition to treat, not only because it is a lifelong condition but also because it begins at a young age

Scherl EJ, Dubinsky MC.
*The Changing World of Inflammatory Bowel Disease:
Impact of Generation, Gender, and Global Trends (pp 205-214)*
© 2009 SLACK Incorporated.

Table 17-1

SHORT-TERM GOALS FOR THE
MANAGEMENT OF INFLAMMATORY BOWEL DISEASE

- Early and accurate diagnosis of the disease and its extent
- Rapid and safe induction of remission
- Steroid-free durable maintenance of remission
- Restoration of growth and development; correction of malnutrition
- Avoidance of drug-related and disease-related complications

---

Table 17-2

LONG-TERM GOALS FOR THE
MANAGEMENT OF INFLAMMATORY BOWEL DISEASE

- Establishment of an effective and preserved patient-health care team relationship, with emphasis on communication, trust, and respect for autonomy
- Sustained steroid-free remission with safe therapies
- Enrollment in a cancer prevention program
- Avoidance of work or school absence and disability
- Periodic "healthy visits" for routine review and monitoring
- Vaccination against preventable at-risk infections (not clearly defined yet)
- Avoidance of bone loss

---

in most patients. The majority of the direct costs of care in IBD are due to hospitalizations and surgeries, with a growing percentage of the direct expenditures coming from newer therapies.[8] However, effective disease control with antitumor necrosis factor therapies has demonstrated that these therapies can successfully reduce hospitalizations and surgeries and therefore become a cost-effective approach to management.[9,10] The indirect costs associated with IBD include those associated with lost time from work or school, unemployment, and disability. In one study, which relied primarily on Scandinavian data, approximately 5% to 10% of patients with IBD suffered from work disability.[8,11,12] In addition, the chronic nature of IBD as well as its often socially isolating nature results in an increased rate of depression and anxiety among patients.[13,14] It makes sense to appreciate that effective disease control would necessarily improve all of these outcomes, and in fact, some studies have begun to demonstrate improvements in quality of life and depression associated with therapies.[15-17]

Disease- and drug-related complications from IBD are well-known and have been increasingly clarified in recent years. In addition to surgery of the bowel, complications of IBD include infections, failure to grow or develop in an age-appropriate fashion, malnutrition including anemia, vitamin and trace element deficiencies, nephrolithiasis, and a variety of less common but important extraintestinal manifestations of bowel inflammation such as arthralgias, eye inflammation, and dermatologic manifestations. Despite clinicians' and patients' concerns about the potential short-term and longer-term complications of immune-modifying therapies, the patients who are steroid dependent have substantially worse outcomes than patients treated with thiopurines and biologic therapies.

Adenocarcinoma of the bowel and osteoporosis of the bones are well-described complications of IBD as well with unique disease-related and treatment-related contributions. Osteoporosis (and osteopenia) in IBD is multifactorial. The risk factors for this important problem include active inflammation of the bowel, malabsorption or poor intake of calcium and vitamin D, low body mass index, female gender, smoking tobacco, and corticosteroid exposure.[18,19] Adenocarcinoma of the colon and small bowel is a rare but well-described complication of chronic bowel inflammation. Established risk factors for adenocarcinoma of the colon and rectum include longer duration of disease, greater extent of colorectal involvement, primary sclerosing cholangitis (PSC), and a family history of colorectal cancer (CRC).[20] More recently, it has been shown that the degree of inflammation of the bowel is an independent risk factor for this complication, implying that effective anti-inflammatory therapy may alter this risk factor.[21-23] The impact of treating to "mucosal healing" or escalating therapy based on baseline inflammation remains theoretical but an important concern for future management strategies.

Additional long-term complications of IBD include recent reports of increased age-matched mortality in IBD and possibly increased risks of non-Hodgkin's lymphoma, with most recent data suggesting that this complication is more likely due to some therapies than from the disease itself, yet treatment benefit appears to outweigh this risk.[24-27]

Successful Induction and Maintenance of Remission Is the First Step to Successful Long-Term Care of the Inflammatory Bowel Disease Patient

Perhaps one of the most pressing and immediate problems facing the clinician managing a patient with IBD is addressing the active disease. The specific treatment strategies are outlined in more detail in other chapters of this book but must be briefly addressed here since it follows that successful induction of remission and stable maintenance of disease control are believed to result in much fewer downstream complications in the chronic care of patients with Crohn's disease and ulcerative colitis. How can a clinician best succeed in this regard? First, settle for nothing less than remission, defined as absence of symptoms or laboratory abnormalities due to active inflammation. Patients and their health care providers should not accept the misperception that a diagnosis of IBD is a life sentence of active disease requiring, for example, that social outings involve "bathroom mapping" or that IBD means ultimate disability or death due to complications. Confirmation of successful remission may involve re-evaluation of disease activity when it is not clear whether the patient is suffering from an irritable bowel or might better be served by a limited bowel resection rather than more anti-inflammatory therapies. Remember that surgery should be embraced as a very effective therapeutic option when patients have fibrotic disease or complications of inadequately controlled inflammation. The patient with persistent symptoms may require therapy escalation, addition of symptom-controlling (but not inflammation-masking) therapies, or a second opinion from a trusted colleague or expert. Second, steroid-responsive but steroid-dependent disease is not remission. Patients who are steroid dependent are at the highest risk for complications, including serious infections, death, bone disease, and other steroid-related complications.[28,29] Patients who are steroid dependent or who have relapsed through maintenance therapy more than once in a year should have their treatment plans reviewed and therapies escalated.

> **Table 17-3**
>
> ## SUGGESTED APPROACH TO CHRONIC CARE OF THE INFLAMMATORY BOWEL DISEASE PATIENT
>
> - Define the purpose of maintenance therapy and the rationale for long-term medication use
> - Schedule "healthy" follow-up visits to review disease control, monitor therapy, and schedule preventive exams
> - Address bone density in at-risk patients
> - Enroll at-risk patients in colorectal cancer prevention programs
> - Anticipate the future with the patient

Approach to the Chronic Care of the Inflammatory Bowel Disease Patient

A suggested approach to the chronic care of a patient with IBD is described below and summarized in Table 17-3.

DEFINE THE PURPOSE OF MAINTENANCE THERAPY AND THE RATIONALE FOR LONG-TERM MEDICATION USE

Once IBD patients achieve a successful remission of their condition, it is common for them to believe that they may not require long-term medical therapy to manage their condition. If a physician or health care provider does not discuss this issue, patients will undoubtedly stop their medication under the belief that either they are "cured" of the condition or, more often, because they do not understand the need or do not want to take chronic medical therapy. The concept of maintenance of remission is not to actively suppress symptoms but rather to reduce the likelihood of relapse. Explaining to patients that the purpose of chronic therapy is to prevent recurrence is an important component of the communication about chronic management. Unfortunately, nonadherence to medications is common and has been well-described for 5-ASA therapy in ulcerative colitis. This therapy is associated with a much greater likelihood of relapse when this occurs.[30] Reasons for nonadherence include believing the therapy is no longer needed or is not working, simple forgetfulness, fear of complications, and also the cost of medications.[31] It is essential to remind patients that IBD is a chronic condition and that as such, it requires chronic therapy. In routine clinic visits, anticipating the challenge of staying on medications is an important portion of the history taking. In a patient who is relapsing or who has not achieved stable steroid-free remission, assessment of adherence is essential. For patients on azathioprine or 6-mercaptopurine, monitoring levels of 6-thioguanine nucleotides and 6-methylmercaptopurine metabolites may be useful for the assessment of both optimization of dosing as well as adherence to therapy. It has been demonstrated repeatedly that episodic use of infliximab therapy is not effective and leads to a greater likelihood of infusion reactions and loss of response to the therapy compared to patients who are committed to scheduled maintenance infusions. It is believed that this phenomenon is true with the newer biologic therapies as well (ie, adalimumab, certolizumab pegol, and natalizumab). Given that adalimumab and certolizumab pegol are injectable therapies that are currently or may in the future be self-administered by patients, the impact of nonadherence to these therapies and disease relapse and loss of response remains an important consideration.

Finally, although an attractive concept, there is not good evidence that any duration of stable disease control warrants withdrawal of therapy or dose reduction.

SCHEDULE "HEALTHY" FOLLOW-UP VISITS TO REVIEW DISEASE CONTROL, MONITOR THERAPY, AND SCHEDULE PREVENTIVE EXAMS

The purpose of such visits is to avoid episodic or "crisis"-based care. Routine visits can also enable the clinician to review changes in the patient's social situation, update the patient on advances in the field of IBD or discuss new therapies or strategies that may be available, reinforce the importance of adherence to therapy, and to obtain routine laboratory investigations for the safety and monitoring of therapies. These tests are disease specific and therapy specific. For example, patients on chronic 5-ASA therapy should have periodic renal function assessments (this is every 6 months in my practice), patients on azathioprine and 6-mercaptopurine should have a complete blood count quarterly while on stable dosing and liver function tests twice yearly, and patients on the anti-TNF therapies should have annual testing for *Mycobacterium tuberculosis* infection. In our practice, we also routinely provide influenza vaccination to our patients on immunosuppression, although recent evidence suggests that many of these patients may not mount an effective immune response.[32,33] During these visits, patients are scheduled for their bone density testing and screening or surveillance colonoscopies. Recent evidence suggests that IBD patients on immunosuppressive therapy have an increased risk of abnormal Pap smears.[34] Although this has not yet been confirmed in additional studies, it is reasonable that female patients should be reminded to have annual follow-ups with their gynecologists.

Some clinicians find it useful to monitor disease activity in routine visits with C-reactive protein or erythrocyte sedimentation rate, but the use of these tests in the asymptomatic IBD patient is unclear.

ADDRESS BONE DENSITY IN AT-RISK PATIENTS

Part of the long-term management of IBD should include appropriate assessment of bone density and therapy to address low bone density. Current guidelines recommend that at-risk IBD patients who should be screened and monitored include postmenopausal women, patients with ongoing corticosteroid use, cumulative prior corticosteroid exposure of greater than 3 months, history of low trauma fractures, and those who are over 60 years old. Patients with low body mass index and those who smoke should also be considered at risk. Treatment should involve aggressive steroid avoidance therapies, smoking cessation programs, calcium and vitamin D supplementation, and in some patients, use of bisphosphonate therapy.[18,19] Follow-up bone density assessment is recommended and referral to an endocrinologist may be required for more severe or refractory situations.

ENROLL AT-RISK PATIENTS IN COLORECTAL CANCER PREVENTION PROGRAMS

Current guidelines identify patients who have had inflammation of the colorectum of greater extent than proctitis as at increased risk for dysplasia and CRC. Recent assessments suggest that the cumulative risk of CRC may be less than previously thought, and in a meta-analysis presented at Digestive Disease Week 2008, the overall risk of cancer was about 1% at 10 years, 4% at 20 years, and 14% with greater than 20 years of disease.[35] Current guidelines recommend a screening colonoscopy after 8 years of disease, and interval surveillance exams every 1 to 2 years subsequently.[36,37] Patients with concurrent PSC are at specific increased risk and should begin surveillance at the time of diagnosis of the PSC. During the examination, current guidelines still advise random biopsies throughout the colon (at least 33 biopsies) but also emphasize the importance of targeted biopsies of masses, polyps, and abnormal mucosa. Recent studies demonstrate that chromoendoscopy with or without magnification is more effective in the identification of dysplasia, but a uniform approach to it for practice and the impact of chromoendoscopy on outcomes and cost of care has not been determined.[38] There remains some evidence of chemoprevention with aminosalicylate therapy, and a meta-analysis of the case control and cohort studies in 2005 concluded that there was a 49% risk reduction of cancer and dysplasia for patients who were on chronic therapy.[39] However, there have been a number of studies subsequently that have demonstrated positive and negative results, so this issue remains incompletely answered. Nonetheless, a discussion of the possible chemopreventive effects of 5-ASA therapy is a reasonable strategy when discussing long-term management and the importance of adherence.[40]

ANTICIPATE THE FUTURE WITH THE PATIENT

The chronic care of a patient with IBD should include discussions about the patient's interests and goals so that together the clinician and the patient can customize the treatment plan and adjust it to the changing situations. For example, the patient who plans to travel around the world after graduating from college should have plans for therapy and emergencies. The patient planning to start a family should be advised of the effects sulfasalazine (sperm dysmotility) and methotrexate (abortive agent) have and these therapies should be avoided, while other effective disease-controlling therapies should be continued. An ongoing discussion of treatment options and an open discussion of the patient's thoughts, alternative therapies, and beliefs about the disease and its triggers will result in a strong doctor-patient relationship and successful partnership over many years.

Specific Scenarios for Special Patient Populations

APPROACH TO THE PEDIATRIC PATIENT WITH INFLAMMATORY BOWEL DISEASE

Management of the child with IBD requires attention to additional issues. First, growth failure or delayed puberty occurs in up to 40% of children with IBD, so fastidious attention to growth curves and weight gain as well as successful achievement of midparental height and puberty is essential.[41] Baseline height and weight and calculation of midparental height should occur, and this goal should be reviewed at each follow-up appointment. Radiography of the long bones and assessment of the status of the growth plates will provide information of the bone age of the child and the potential for "catch up" growth prior to fusion of the plates. The most effective way to achieve this is with therapy that achieves stable remission and maintenance of steroid-free disease control. Surgery is sometimes required to achieve this goal. Growth hormone therapy, once considered a viable option for many children with IBD, is avoided in favor of effective therapy for the underlying IBD and is now rarely used.

Another key issue for children with IBD is timing of vaccinations. Children on immunosuppressive therapies should not receive live virus vaccines. These vaccines include rotavirus, MMR, varicella, and the live version of polio. (For travelers, yellow fever is also a live vaccine.) Therefore, such vaccines should be administered before immunosuppression is administered and communication to the parents and pediatrician should occur. In the teenager, a discussion about the human papilloma virus (HPV) vaccine should be initiated along with a frank discussion about safe sexual relations. In the child with IBD already on immune suppression, there is increasing understanding of the possibility that conversion to active immunity may not occur, so follow-up titer assessment may be prudent.

Adolescents may be at increased risk for nonadherence with medical therapies. Education about the risks of nonadherence should occur and some of this discussion should occur between the gastroenterologist and the patient, with the parents respectfully absent from the examination room. The adolescent's autonomy and independence should be respected and encouraged. This time in a child's life can be very challenging, and living with a chronic disease makes it even more difficult, so patience and empathy are required. It may be prudent to schedule more frequent "healthy" visits in order to provide ongoing reinforcement of key principles of management and the need for maintenance therapy. Age-appropriate support groups may also be very helpful in this situation.[39]

APPROACH TO THE FEMALE PATIENT WITH INFLAMMATORY BOWEL DISEASE

There are a number of specific issues related to the chronic care of women with IBD. Women with significant weight loss or ineffectively treated IBD may have menstrual irregularity or even amenorrhea. Routine assessment of the patient's menstrual cycle should be performed and when irregular or there has been a change from a previously established healthy baseline, assessment of disease activity and adjustment of medical therapies are essential. Although commonly discussed, it is not yet clear whether menstrual cycles worsen disease activity, although it is well described that menses can affect the bowel symptoms of IBD patients. Review of oral contraceptive use and adjustments when necessary may help with this. A frank discussion regarding sexual activity and a woman's sexuality in the context of having IBD or previous surgery for IBD should occur in a sensitive and supportive manner. This is frequently an area that is insufficiently addressed or even ignored by the physician and not instigated by the patient. Referral to sex therapists may be helpful.

As mentioned above, there is evolving information to suggest that women with IBD and on immunosuppression are at increased risk for abnormal Pap smears.[34] Although not confirmed, the female patient who is prescribed immunosuppressives should be made aware that she needs annual Pap smears and is included in the American College of Obstetricians and Gynecologists' increased risk category for cervical dysplasia. At the time immunosuppression is considered, discussion about HPV vaccination should occur, with emphasis that this vaccine does not protect against all serotypes of HPV and does not prevent sexually transmitted diseases.

Women with IBD who are planning to have children (even in the distant future) should be provided information about the safety of their medications or surgical procedures in the context of this issue. Relying on the patient to ask about this issue later or to research it herself on the Internet will likely lead to misinterpretation or nonadherence to therapy without a full understanding of the current state of knowledge regarding stable remission and fertility rates, as well as the safety of the majority of IBD therapies.[43] This important issue is covered in more detail in additional chapters of this text.

Finally, women with IBD have the additional risk of loss of bone density associated with menarche. Careful attention to bone health and supplements with calcium and vitamin D should occur.[16]

APPROACH TO THE GERIATRIC PATIENT WITH INFLAMMATORY BOWEL DISEASE

There is increased appreciation that the older patient with IBD may have different needs than the adolescent or young adult. Although it remains unclear whether the immune system functions differently over time in these patients and whether treatment can be reduced or discontinued, there are some general considerations for the patient over 65 with IBD.

Older patients with IBD are more likely to have comorbid illnesses and be on additional medical therapies. Therefore, a careful review of all medications and potential drug-drug interactions should occur at each visit. Older patients are at increased risk for Varicella zoster reactivation (shingles) and may inquire about receiving a booster vaccination. This is a live virus vaccine, so it is contraindicated in the IBD patient on immunosuppressive therapy. Fastidious attention to bone health and colon cancer screening (even in the patient who does not have known colonic disease) is essential.

Given comorbid illnesses and limited reserve for complete recovery from severe illness, surgical options may be considered earlier in elderly patients. Therefore, careful consideration of risks and benefits of immunosuppression versus surgical treatment must occur. Older patients may be best served with permanent ostomies, given the likelihood of decreased sphincter tone or future cognitive impairments that may inhibit continence.

Summary

In today's rapidly changing field of IBD, the care for the patient involves a working knowledge of the range of effective induction therapies and an active strategy for long-term maintenance of disease control. Fortunately, the care of IBD patients has come a long way since the early days of episodic care and crisis management. However, effective care of any patient diagnosed with IBD now requires a healthy clinician-patient relationship and active plans to avoid long-term complications from the disease or from therapies. It is anticipated that these strategies may alter the natural history of IBD and result in profoundly better long-term outcomes. Clinicians must carefully consider the specific patient and his or her unique needs in their approach to management and treatment options. A customized plan for each patient will provide individualized care that achieves the optimal outcomes.

References

1. Cosnes J, Cattan S, Blain A, et al. Long-term evolution of disease behavior of Crohn's disease. *Inflamm Bowel Dis.* 2002;8(4):244-250.
2. Farmer RG, Easley KA, Rankin GB. Clinical patterns, natural history, and progression of ulcerative colitis: a long-term follow-up of 1116 patients. *Dig Dis Sci.* 1993;38(6):1137-1146.
3. Langholz E, Munkholm P, Nielsen OH, et al. Incidence and prevalence of ulcerative colitis in Copenhagen county from 1962 to 1987. *Scand J Gastroenterol.* 1991;26(12):1247-1256.
4. Langholz E, Munkholm P, Davidsen M, Binder V. Course of ulcerative colitis: analysis of changes in disease activity over years. *Gastroenterology.* 1994;107(1):3-11.
5. Mekhjian HS, Switz DM, Watts HD, Deren JJ, Katon RM, Beman FM. National Cooperative Crohn's Disease Study: factors determining recurrence of Crohn's disease after surgery. *Gastroenterology.* 1979;77(4 Pt 2):907-913.
6. McLeod RS, Wolff BG, Steinhart AH, et al. Risk and significance of endoscopic/radiological evidence of recurrent Crohn's disease. *Gastroenterology.* 1997;113(6):1823-1827.
7. Faubion WA Jr, Loftus EV Jr, Harmsen WS, Zinsmeister AR, Sandborn WJ. The natural history of corticosteroid therapy for inflammatory bowel disease: a population-based study. *Gastroenterology.* 2001;121:255-260.
8. Zisman TL, Cohen RD. Pharmacoeconomics and quality of life of current and emerging biologic therapies for inflammatory bowel disease. *Curr Treat Options Gastroenterol.* 2007;10(3):185-194.
9. Lichtenstein GR, Yan S, Bala M, Sands BE. Infliximab maintenance treatment reduces hospitalizations, surgeries, and procedures in fistulizing Crohn's disease. *Gastroenterology.* 2005;128(4):862-869.
10. Feagan BG, Panaccione R, Sandborn WJ, et al. Effects of adalimubab therapy on incidence of hospitalization and surgery in Crohn's disease: results from the CHARM study. *Gastroenterology.* 2008;135(5):1493-1499.
11. Feagan BG, Bala M, Yan S, Olson A, Hanauer S. Unemployment and disability in patients with moderately to severely active Crohn's disease. *J Clin Gastroenterol.* 2005;39(5):390-395.
12. Cohen RD, Thomas T. Economics of the use of biologics in the treatment of inflammatory bowel disease. *Gastroenterol Clin North Am.* 2006;35(4):867-882.
13. Gregor JC, McDonald JWD, Klar N, et al. An evaluation of utility measurement in Crohn's disease. *Inflamm Bowel Dis.* 1997;3:265-276.
14. Lix LM, Graff LA, Walker JR, et al. Longitudinal study of quality of life and psychological functioning for active, fluctuating, and inactive disease patterns in inflammatory bowel disease. *Inflamm Bowel Dis.* 2008;14(11):1575-1584.
15. Lichtenstein GR, Feagan BG, Yan S, Bala M, Bao W. The effects of infliximab maintenance therapy on health-related quality of life. *Am J Gastroenterol.* 2003;98(10):2232-2238.
16. Loftus EV, Feagan BG, Colombel JF, et al. Effects of adalimumab maintenance therapy on health-related quality of life patients with Crohn's disease: patient-reported outcomes of the CHARM trial. *Am J Gastroenterol.* 2008;103(12):3132-3141.

17. Rutgeerts P, Schreiber S, Feagan B, Keininger DL, O'Neil L, Fedorak RN. Certolizumab pegol, a monthly subcutaneously administered Fc-free anti-TNFα, improves health-related quality of life in patients with moderate to severe Crohn's disease. *Int J Colorectal Dis.* 2008;23(3):289-296.

18. American Gastroenterological Association. American Gastroenterological Association medical position statement: guidelines on osteoporosis in gastrointestinal diseases. *Gastroenterology.* 2003;124(3):791-794.

19. Bernstein CN, Katz S. Guidelines for osteoporosis and inflammatory bowel disease: a guide to diagnosis and management for the gastroenterologist (monograph). The American College of Gastroenterology. 2003.

20. Rubin DT, Kavitt RT. Surveillance for cancer and dysplasia in inflammatory bowel disease. *Gastroenterol Clin North Am.* 2006;35(3):581-604.

21. Rutter M, Saunders B, Wilkinson K, et al. Severity of inflammation is a risk factor for colorectal neoplasia in ulcerative colitis. *Gastroenterology.* 2004;126(2):451-459.

22. Gupta RB, Harpaz N, Itzkowitz S, et al. Histologic inflammation is a risk factor for progression to colorectal neoplasia in ulcerative colitis: a cohort study. *Gastroenterology.* 2007;133(4):1099-1105; quiz 1340-1091.

23. Rubin DT, Huo DZ, Rothe JA, et al. Increased inflammatory activity is an independent risk factor for dysplasia and colorectal cancer in ulcerative colitis: a case-control analysis with blinded prospective pathology review. *Gastroenterology.* 2006;130:A2.

24. Loftus EV, Sandborn WJ. Lymphoma risk in inflammatory bowel disease: influences of referral bias and therapy. *Gastroenterology.* 2001;121(5):1239-1242.

25. Lewis JD, Bilker WB, Brensinger C, Deren JJ, Vaughn DJ, Strom BL. Inflammatory bowel disease is not associated with an increased risk of lymphoma. *Gastroenterology.* 2001;121(5):1080-1087.

26. Lewis JD, Gelfand JM, Troxel AB, et al. Immunosuppressant medications and mortality in inflammatory bowel disease. *Am J Gastroenterol.* 2008;103(6):1428-1435.

27. Lewis JD, Schwartz JS, Lichtenstein GR. Azathioprine for maintenance of remission in Crohn's disease: benefits outweigh the risk of lymphoma. *Gastroenterology.* 2000;118(6):1018-1024.

28. Lichtenstein GR, Feagan BG, Cohen RD, et al. Serious infections and mortality in association with therapies for Crohn's disease: TREAT registry. *Clin Gastroenterol Hepatol.* 2006;4(5):621-630.

29. Summers RW, Switz DM, Sessions JT Jr, et al. National Cooperative Crohn's Disease Study: results of drug treatment. *Gastroenterology.* 1979;77(4 Pt 2):847-869.

30. Kane S, Huo D, Aikens J, Hanauer S. Medication nonadherence and the outcomes of patients with quiescent ulcerative colitis. *Am J Med.* 2003;114(1):39-43.

31. Loftus EV Jr. A practical perspective on ulcerative colitis: patients' needs from aminosalicylate therapies. *Inflamm Bowel Dis.* 2006;12(12):1107-1113.

32. Mamula P, Markowitz JE, Piccoli DA, Klimov A, Cohen L, Baldassano RN. Immune response to influenza vaccine in pediatric patients with inflammatory bowel disease. *Clin Gastroenterol Hepatol.* 2007;5(7):851-856.

33. Melmed GY, Frenck R, Barolet-Garcia C, et al. TNF blockers and immunomodulators impair antibody responses to pneumococcal polysaccharide vaccine (Ppv) in patients with inflammatory bowel disease. *Gastroenterology.* 2008;134:A68.

34. Kane S, Khatibi B, Reddy D. Higher incidence of abnormal Pap smears in women with inflammatory bowel disease. *Am J Gastroenterol.* 2008;103(3):631-636.

35. Lutgens MW, van der Hejden GJ, Vleggaar FP, et al. A comprehensive meta-analysis of the risk of colorectal cancer in ulcerative colitis and Crohn's disease. *Gastroenterology.* 2008;134:A33-A34.

36. Kornbluth A, Sachar DB. Ulcerative colitis practice guidelines in adults (update): American College of Gastroenterology, Practice Parameters Committee. *Am J Gastroenterol.* 2004;99(7):1371-1385.

37. Itzkowitz SH, Harpaz N. Diagnosis and management of dysplasia in patients with inflammatory bowel diseases. *Gastroenterology.* 2004;126(6):1634-1648.

38. Zisman TL, Rubin DT. Colorectal cancer and dysplasia in inflammatory bowel disease. *World J Gastroenterol.* 2008;14(17):2662-2669.

39. Velayos FS, Terdiman JP, Walsh JM. Effect of 5-aminosalicylate use on colorectal cancer and dysplasia risk: a systematic review and meta-analysis of observational studies. *Am J Gastroenterol.* 2005;100(6):1345-1353.

40. Rubin DT, Cruz-Correa MR, Gasche C, et al. Colorectal cancer prevention in inflammatory bowel disease and the role of 5-aminosalicylic acid: a clinical review and update. *Inflamm Bowel Dis.* 2008;14(2):265-274.

41. Mamula P, Markowitz JE, Baldassano RN. Inflammatory bowel disease in early childhood and adolescence: special considerations. *Gastroenterol Clin North Am.* 2003;32:967-975.

42. Kim SC, Ferry GD. Inflammatory bowel diseases in pediatric and adolescent patients: clinical, therapeutic, and psychosocial considerations. *Gastroenterology.* 2004;126:1550-1560.

43. Mahadevan U, Terdiman JP, Aron J, Jacobsohn S, Turek P. Infliximab and semen quality in men with inflammatory bowel disease. *Inflamm Bowel Dis.* 2005;11:395-399.

18

SURGICAL TREATMENT OF CROHN'S DISEASE THROUGH THE LIFE CYCLE

Sharon L. Stein, MD and Fabrizio Michelassi, MD

urgical therapy for inflammatory bowel disease is largely unchanged from practice 20 years ago. New advances in pharmacologic treatment of inflammatory bowel disease have been successful at reversing or abating symptoms of ulcerative colitis (UC) and Crohn's disease (CD), but for some patients there will still be progression of disease despite medical therapy. Patients may develop neoplasia, perforation, toxic megacolon, or unremitting bleeding. When these complications occur or when medical therapy fails, surgical interventions may be required.

Surgical indications and treatments are different for CD and UC. CD presents a challenge to the surgeon because the disease is not eradicated by surgery. Seventy percent of patients with CD will require surgical therapy at some point in their lives and 70% of these patients will have recurrence of their disease.[1,2] Over 60% of patients with recurrent disease will eventually require a second surgical intervention.[3] The recurrent nature of CD presents a problem for surgeons, as patients may require extensive and repeat resections of large and small bowel, leading to metabolic derangement or nutritional deficiencies. Surgical options for CD vary depending on the extent, location, and symptoms of disease. Surgery is tailored to the patient's specific disease process.

In UC, surgical options are more straightforward. Between 10% to 30% of patients require surgical intervention; in most cases a total proctocolectomy (TPC) is the procedure of choice.[4,5] Resection of the entire colon and rectum cures the intestinal manifestations of UC. Preoperative decision making is focused on the correct diagnosis of UC and whether offering a restorative proctocolectomy versus ileostomy is appropriate for an individual patient. Complications following ileal pouch anal anastomosis (IPAA) or J-pouch surgery can present difficult surgical dilemmas.

The prevalence, incidence, and distribution of inflammatory bowel diseases are well covered in preceding chapters of this book. This chapter will concentrate on surgical indications and surgical options, including laparoscopic and bowel sparing techniques for patients with inflammatory bowel disease, while concentrating on surgical considerations based on the patient's stage within the life cycle.

Scherl EJ, Dubinsky MC.
*The Changing World of Inflammatory Bowel Disease:
Impact of Generation, Gender, and Global Trends (pp 215-230)*
© 2009 SLACK Incorporated.

Surgical Indications

Common surgical indications for CD include obstruction and abscess. Toxic megacolon and hemorrhage are more common indications in UC. Both groups may require surgical intervention if disease escalates despite best medical treatment. Cancer is a clear indication for surgery in both populations.

The most common indication for surgery in inflammatory bowel disease is the failure of medical management. Chronic symptoms may progress despite maximal medical therapy; patients may refuse further escalation of medications or have intolerable side effects from medications. Patients with CD commonly present with chronic symptoms, including intestinal bloating, abdominal pain, and frequent bowel movements. Bleeding, profuse diarrhea, and incontinence are more common in UC. In an acute episode of UC requiring hospitalization, failure to improve after 5 to 7 days of maximal medical therapy is an indication for surgical intervention. Pregnant patients may be unable to escalate medications without risks to the pregnancy in either the acute or chronic period. Children may develop growth retardation, which may occur in up to 25% of patients secondary to malnutrition and pharmacotherapy.[6] Cochrane review of data regarding effectiveness of interventions for prepubertal patients with IBD recommended the use of enteral nutrition and judicious use of surgical intervention for prepubertal and pubertal patients with persistent growth retardation.[6]

Obstruction occurs frequently in patients with CD (Figure 18-1). Obstruction is typically subacute, with gradually progressing symptoms. Stricturing CD will typically require surgical intervention, but inflammatory disease may be treated nonoperatively with medications or endoscopic dilation. Failure to resolve is an indication for surgery but typically in a semielective setting. It is also important to remember that patients with inflammatory bowel disease may also develop adhesions or internal hernias after prior surgery. Bowel obstructions in this case may be treated nonoperatively in patients who are hemodynamic stable without signs of ischemia, sepsis, or hypotension. Nasogastric tubes and bowel rest are used, and computed tomography scans may show a transition point. Failure to resolve obstruction in 48 to 72 hours is usually indicative of a complete obstruction. In these cases, less than 20% of patients will go on to spontaneously resolve their obstruction and surgery may be indicated.

Fistulae are another indication for surgery in patients with CD. Although fistulae are found in up to 25% of patients intraoperatively, they are infrequently the cause of operative intervention.[7] When asymptomatic, fistulae may not require surgical intervention. Symptomatic fistula typically requires excision of the primary source of disease and repair or resection of the secondarily involved organ. Fistulae may occur between adjacent loops of bowel, between the bowel and other abdominal organs, and between the intestines and the skin. Enteroenteric fistula may cause bypass of significant lengths of intestine, leading to malabsorption and diarrhea, as in an ileosigmoid fistula. Fistulae between intestines and the bladder may present with pneumaturia, fecaluria, or urinary tract infections. Entero or colovaginal fistulae occur most frequently in patients who have had prior hysterectomies and may cause embarrassing vaginal discharge. Surgical options include reconstruction and the use of healthy tissue flaps as a buttress to prevent recurrence. Enterocutaneous fistula are typically seen in patients with multiple prior surgeries. These fistulae may cause significant skin irritation and wound care, drainage of associated abscess, and bowel rest to manage the fistula may be sufficient.

Abscesses are common complications from CD and may be intraloop, intramesenteric, intraperitoneal, or retroperitoneal. When accessible by interventional radiology and the patient is stable, initial percutaneous drainage has become the overwhelming treatment of choice. A subsequent sonogram or tube injection may be performed to determine if there is enteric communication with the abscess cavity, which occurs in most cases and typically requires definitive surgical treatment.[8] The use of appropriate antibiotic treatment and surgical drainage can alleviate symptoms and allows for physiologic improvement of the patient prior to definitive management. Patients

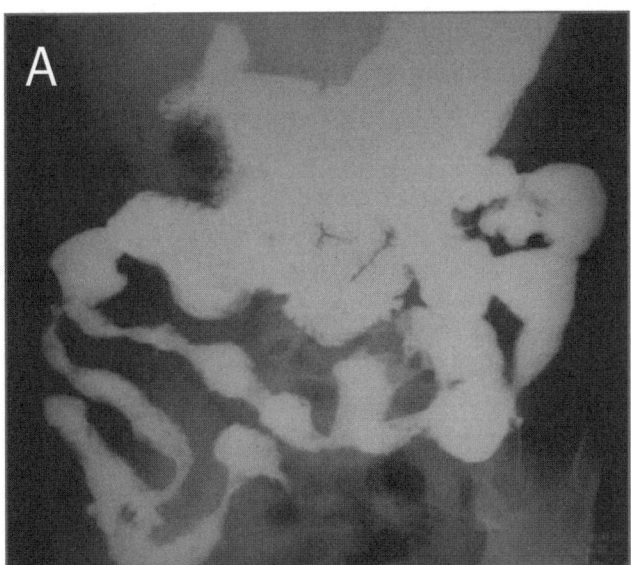

Figure 18-1. (A) This small bowel follow-through demonstrates numerous areas of narrowing and dilation throughout the small intestine consistent with severe pan-intestinal Crohn's stricturing. (B) An image from the operating room shows severely strictured segment of intestine. Other characteristic findings include thickened and foreshortened mesentery. (Reprinted with permission from Fabrizio Michelassi, MD.)

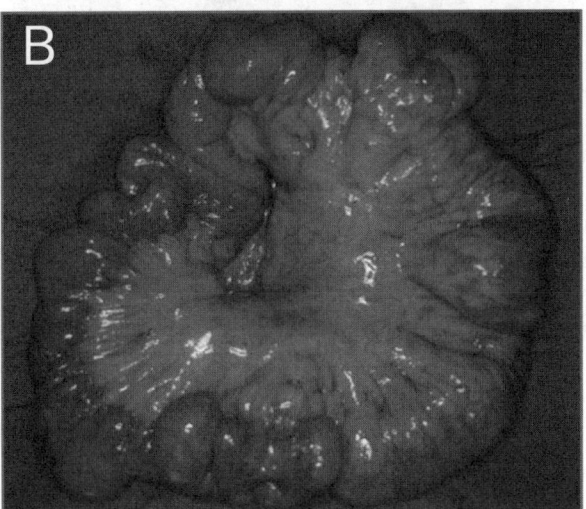

are less likely to develop recurrent disease after surgical treatment if they underwent preoperative percutaneous drainage.[9] Approximately 30% of patients require surgical treatment within 1 year of presentation with abscess (Figure 18-2).

While perforating CD causing abscesses, fistulae, and sinus tracts is common, free perforation is a rare and serious complication necessitating immediate surgical intervention. It occurs more commonly in patients with UC, and prevention of perforation is a key indication for urgent surgery in patients with severe acute colitis. Patients may present with severe abdominal pain and peritoneal signs, including tenderness and guarding. Fever, leukocytosis, and sepsis are late findings and signs of systemic infection and inflammation. An abdominal film demonstrating free air is diagnostic and enough to warrant an immediate exploratory laparotomy. Computed tomography (CT) scan has a higher sensitivity for diagnosis of perforation and may assist with localization of pathology but is not necessary in most cases. It is important to remember that patients with inflammatory bowel diseases are frequently on immunosuppressive medications, such as steroids, which may blunt physiological findings of peritonitis and complicate diagnosis. Morbidity may be significant in these patients.[7]

Figure 18-2. (A) A preoperative photo demonstrates a large right lower quadrant mass, consistent with an abscess. (B) CT scan of the patient demonstrates a rim-enhanced mass. The mass does not fill with contrast, differentiating this mass from a dilated loop of bowel. (Reprinted with permission from Fabrizio Michelassi, MD.)

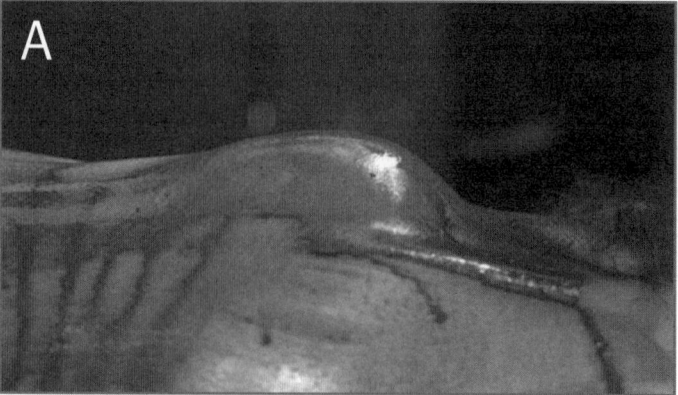

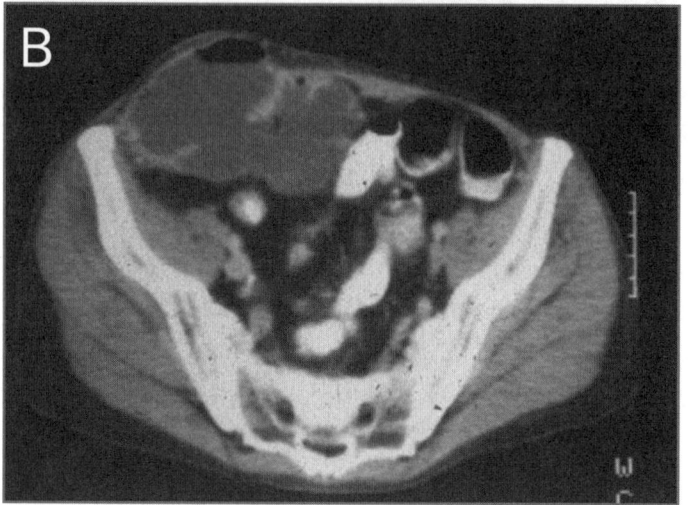

Risk of colon and small intestine cancers are increased in patients with inflammatory bowel disease and correlate with extent and duration of disease.[10] Relative risk of malignant transformation of the colon varies in the literature but is estimated to be 8% with 20 years of disease and 18% after 30 years of disease.[11] This translates to risk approximately 4 to 20 times the risk for the nonaffected population.[12] A low threshold for resection in the presence of colonic dysplasia, dysplasia-associated lesion or mass especially in patients on immunosuppression should be maintained. Any patient with surgical resectable colon or small intestine malignancy in the setting of CD should have a segmental resection with en bloc removal of the both the arterial and lymph node drainage. Patients with UC are recommended to undergo TPC secondary to the risk of synchronous or metachronous cancers.

Severe hemorrhage requiring surgical intervention is rare in CD but more common in UC. Hemorrhage of the small bowel in CD tends to be intermittent and chronic, requiring blood transfusion. Resection may be required ultimately for definitive management but rarely in the acute setting. Surgically significant bleeding occurs more frequently in the colon but is still a rare cause for surgical intervention in patients with CD.[13] Patients with UC may have chronic bleeding and anemia but can also develop acute episodes of bleeding, requiring surgical intervention.

Preoperative Evaluation

Prior to elective surgical intervention, it is essential to have an accurate assessment of the distribution and severity of patient disease. There are many diagnostic and evaluation tools available to appropriately assess patients with inflammatory bowel disease. Colonoscopy and endoscopy help to differentiate CD from UC and determine the extent of disease. They provide pathologic diagnosis and may identify the existence of malignancy. Radiographic imaging, including CT, small bowel follow-through, and magnetic resonance imaging (MRI), provides preoperative assessment of anatomic features and extent of disease and helps prepare both the patient and surgeon for operative findings. Imaging may diagnose perforation and typhlitis, which are indications for emergent intervention. Identification of abscess may be the determining factor in abandoning medical treatment in favor of surgery or indicating need for a temporizing drainage procedure. Extent of disease may determine surgical approach, need for fecal diversion, and whether surgical intervention is necessary. In addition, imaging and endoscopy may help differentiate difficult cases of indeterminate colitis, which has a clear bearing on surgical approach.

Although choice of imaging procedure is covered elsewhere in the book, it is warranted to say a few words regarding the use of repeated radiographic images. For most patients, the dosing of a single image or test is inconsequential. However, patients with CD will typically require repeat imaging throughout their lifetimes. Children, adolescents, and young adults of reproductive age or pregnant are of significant concern, as radiation can affect growth and reproductive capabilities. In addition, the cumulative dosing of radiation can be considerable and caution should be used for these patients who expect to have ongoing medical problems with probable repeated need for imaging. Shielding of the groin or uterus can help protect testicles ,ovaries, and embryos. Ultrasound and MRI are radiographic options that limit or eliminate radiation while still providing important anatomic information. Ultrasound can demonstrate abscess and inflammation, although the sensitivity of the ultrasound is highly dependent on the skills of the radiologist who performs and interprets the test. MRI provides abdominal imaging and is the test of choice for pregnant patients should abdominal imaging be required.

Another preoperative consideration includes the patient's metabolic and nutritional status. An accurate assessment of recent weight loss, anemia, nutritional deficiencies, and electrolyte imbalances is crucial to a successful operation. Patients with moderate to severe malnutrition may have improved outcomes after receiving preoperative nutrition, including parental nutrition.[14] Anemia and hypoalbuminemia have both been shown to be significant risk factors for postoperative complications in patients with inflammatory bowel disease. Preoperative resuscitation and repletion of electrolytes, even in the emergent setting, may be important prior to proceeding with general anesthesia and surgery.

Important consideration must be paid to any pharmacologic agents used preoperatively for patients as many may affect wound healing, infectious complication, and postoperative course. Steroids have been shown to negatively affect postoperative wound healing and can cause adrenal crisis in the setting of operative stress. There is growing concern among surgeons about the complications occurring in patients on biologics such as anti-TNF agents, including infectious complications and anastomotic leaks.[15,16] Recommendations are not yet available, but when possible waiting 4 to 5 half lives of the biologic to allow it to clear from the patient's system is preferable.

Elderly patients who undergo surgery are at higher risk for perioperative complications, a trend that persists in patients with inflammatory bowel disease even after multivariate analysis.[17] Recent data from the National Inpatient Sample show elderly patients were only half as likely to undergo surgery as their younger counterparts and trends were greater inpatients with UC and nonfistulizing and nonstricturing CD.[18]

General premises of surgery during pregnancy are that interventions necessary for the safety of the mother must be performed. However, surgeons attempt to avoid surgical intervention particularly during the embryonic sensitive stage in the first trimester of pregnancy, as well as the organogenesis that occurs in the third trimester of pregnancy. Minimizing length of surgical intervention is also considered. CD patients may have a drain placed by interventional radiology to delay surgery, while in the setting of UC a "blow-hole" colostomy can be created to alleviate toxic megacolon. The risks of surgery include the sedation of the patient, which can have significant effects on the fetus, and if viable, the fetus should be monitored by the obstetrics team perioperatively.

Operative Options in Crohn's Disease

Surgical management of CD should be individualized to fit the needs of the patient. Depending on the operative indications, prior surgical history, and disease state, a carefully tailored plan should be created for the patient, with special consideration of the current and future ramifications of surgical intervention. In general, patients who undergo surgery for CD initially should undergo thorough exploratory laparotomy or laparoscopy with full 4-quadrant abdominal exploration. This includes a full assessment of the intestine, measurement of viable quantity of small intestine, and identification of diseased segments. The small intestine should be "run" or inspected visually and using tactile senses from the ligament of Treitz to the terminal ileum. Up to 15% of patients with CD have multiple segments of diseased small bowel or skip lesions.[19] Areas of thickened mesentery and enlarged lymph nodes may indicate diseased segments and warrant careful evaluation. If an area of stenosis is suspected but not visualized, a partially inflated Foley catheter balloon may be passed through the segments of the small bowel to determine the presence of functional stenosis.

After determination of functionally limiting disease, an operative strategy is initiated to minimize resection of bowel and maximize functional results. The resection of microscopic disease does not decrease recurrence rates for patients with CD.[20] Thereby, segments with actively strictured, fistulizing, or obstructive disease are resected but other areas with "creeping fat" or thickened mesentery are generally left in situ if they are not causing active symptoms. As patients frequently require multiple resections during their lifetime, taking a slightly more liberal margin may culminate in shortened gut and associated malabsorption and malnutrition.

CD of the esophagus, stomach, and duodenum occurs in only 2% to 4% of patients and often is preceded by the presence of CD elsewhere in the gastrointestinal tract.[21] Gastric and duodenal CD tends to be structuring in nature and commonly includes multiple ulcers, nodularity, and irregular thickening, which may lead to gastric or duodenal obstruction. Standard treatment for primary duodenal disease is gastrojejunal bypass. Initial concerns of high marginal ulcer rates have been alleviated with the use of proton pump inhibitors. Duodenal strictureplasty has been proven safe, with low recurrence rates, but it may not be possible in lengthy strictures or when there are severely thickened duodenal walls. Gastroduodenal disease may also be the result of secondary involvement from fistulae after colon resections. Ileocolic resections often fistulize to the duodenal sweep, while gastric fistulae and fourth portion of the duodenum are likely to involve more distal colon.

Small bowel disease is a common manifestation of CD. Patients with stricturing often present with chronic, recurrent abdominal pain caused by luminal obstruction from narrowed segments of bowel. Unfortunately, stricturing disease rarely regresses with medical therapy, and surgery for the affected length of small bowel may be necessary. Traditionally, resection was used universally. For short solitary segments, resection remains effective and appropriate, but patients with multiple diffuse segments, long segments, or recurrent disease at the site of prior anastomosis may be at risk for loss of lengthy segments of bowel and associated complications. In these patients, bowel-sparing techniques provide the advantage of preserving intestinal length and may lead to regression of gross signs of CD following side-to-side and enterocolic strictureplasty (Figure 18-3).[22,23] It is believed that recurrence rates may be reduced up to 40% following strictureplasty, possibly with

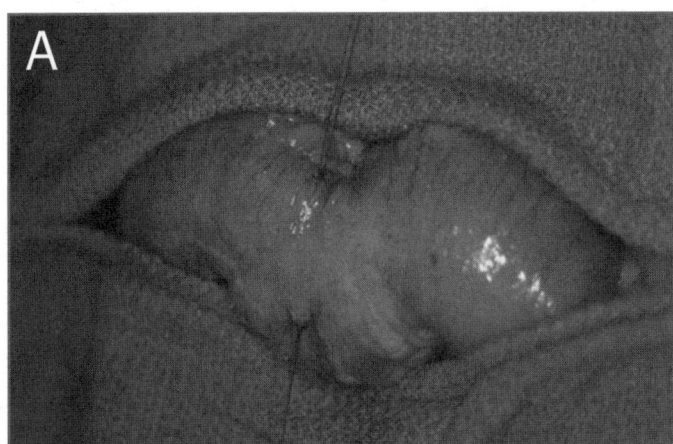

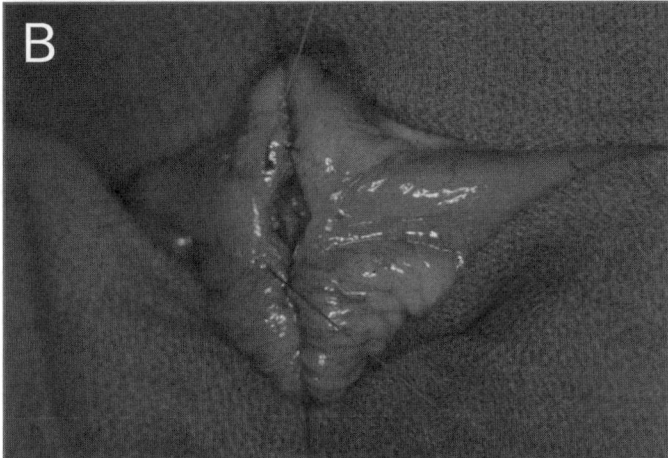

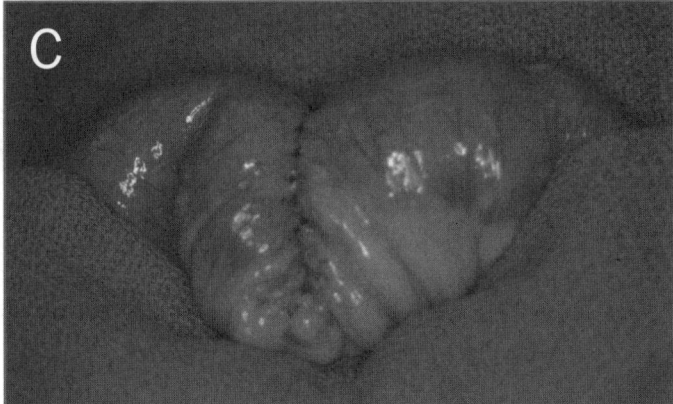

Figure 18-3. A Finney strictureplasty is performed on a narrowed segment of bowel. (A) Stitches are placed transversely across the bowel. (B) The bowel lumen is then entered longitudinally, through the area of stenosis. (C) Closure is performed transversely, increasing the internal lumen of the bowel throughout the strictured segment. (Reprinted with permission from Fabrizio Michelassi, MD.)

functional healing of the mucosa. Although initially strictureplasty was used conservatively, applications are now broader. Long-segment strictureplasty, ileocolic strictureplasty, and strictureplasty in active disease have all been successfully performed with good results.[24-26] Strictureplasty is an important tool in the armamentarium of surgeons, especially for young patients with anticipation of a long disease course.

The most common location for CD necessitating surgical intervention is disease of the terminal ileum.[27] Patients often present with recurrent right lower quadrant pain, weight loss, and intermittent obstruction. Operative rates are high for patients with terminal ileal involvement. A series from the Cleveland Clinic demonstrated that 90% of patients with ileocolitis and 70% of patients with isolated ileal disease required surgical intervention within 10 years of presentation. Obstruction, fistulae, and abscesses were the most common pathology necessitating surgical intervention.[28] Recurrent disease is common following ileocecal resection and may be treated with initial endoscopic dilation, resection, or increasingly with strictureplasty.

Concurrent right colon involvement is common with ileal disease and recommended treatment is a right hemicolectomy. Isolated right colon disease is treated similarly to avoid the morbidity associated with a colocolonic anastomosis. Because of the high rate of subsequent coloduodenal fistula, an omental flap is often used to cover the new anastomosis after exposure of the duodenum during right hemicolectomy.

Unlike UC, a subtotal or total colectomy does not cure patients with CD. Many patients with CD have involvement limited to a short segment, and several studies have demonstrated improved function with segmental resection over total abdominal colectomy, but there is an increased rate of disease recurrence. Patients undergoing segmental colectomy had fewer loose bowel movements and better stool control than patients undergoing total colectomy but were at increased risk of disease recurrence, even when adjustments were made for disease severity.[29,30] Patients with isolated, yet extensive involvement of the colon with relative rectal sparing are commonly treated with subtotal colectomy with ileorectal anastomosis. This provides a good functional result to patients with maintenance of normal capacitance and peristaltic functions, although colon resection may result in increased stool frequency. Ileorectal anastomosis is associated with a high rate of recurrent disease; between 40% and 60% of patients will have recurrence in the rectal stump and up to 50% of patients will ultimately require resection of the rectum at a later stage.[31-33] By comparison, proctocolectomy with end ileostomy has recurrence rates of 10% to 20%, and patients are often weaned off immunosuppressants and steroids more quickly following proctectomy.[33,34] However, patients are left with permanent ileostomy and the social and mental stigmata associated with a stoma.

If an anastomosis is not possible, a decision remains about whether to perform colostomy or ileostomy. With segmental resection of the colon, the patient remains at risk for subsequent recurrent disease, but fluid absorption is improved with increasing length of colon left in situ. Patients with end ileostomies may have difficulty with high ostomy output, leading to dehydration and electrolyte imbalance. For this reason, a colostomy is often considered in elderly patients and patients with concurrent renal disease.

Approximately 15% of patients with CD will have perianal symptoms, including anal skin tags, abscesses, fistulae, and fissures. Patients with CD may have trouble with continence secondary to the combination of bowel consistency and perianal disease. Paramount to treatment is preventing further loss of continence. For this reason, treatment is typically amelioration of symptoms with sphincter-sparing procedures, including abscess drainage, placement of setons, and advancement flaps (Figure 18-4). Combining surgical drainage of abscess and medical treatment of CD has been shown to induce response in up to 85% of patients although long-term recurrence rates are reported to be as low at 15%.[35]

Children with CD may require surgical intervention, often within 2 years of diagnosis. A recent population-based survey of patients with CD evaluated risk factors for surgery and noted 55% underwent an operative procedure within a 10-year study period and almost 20% required a second surgery in that period of time.[36] Children who were treated with immunomodulators or had extensive small bowel disease were less likely to undergo surgery. Pediatric patients with colitis may present a particular diagnostic dilemma. UC may be difficult to differentiate from CD in the pediatric population as both commonly present with skip lesions, periappendiceal inflammation, and ileitis. CD should be suspected in the setting of perianal disease, biopsies with granulomas (noncrypt), and presence of small intestinal disease. In a large study of pediatric patients who underwent IPAA, up to 15% of patients were eventually diagnosed with UC, and these patients

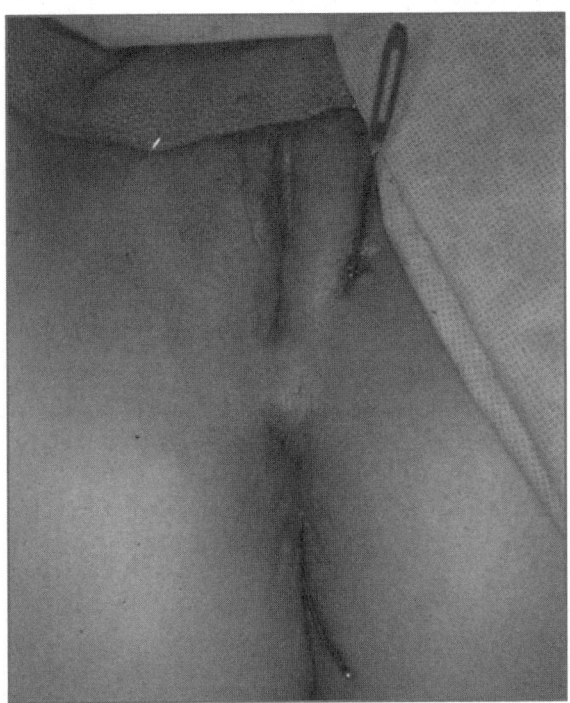

Figure 18-4. A patient with an anterior lateral fistula. A probe is placed from the external opening lateral to the vagina through the fistula tract into the rectum. (Reprinted with permission from Fabrizio Michelassi, MD.)

made up the vast majority of patients with chronic pouchitis, requiring pouch resection and ileostomy.[34] Female gender and perianal disease were associated with misdiagnosis. In indeterminate colitis, initial conservative resection may be warranted until a definitive diagnosis is established.

Pregnancy may also affect CD and surgical options. Studies demonstrate that symptoms of CD, particularly stricturing, may be ameliorated during and following pregnancy but other data demonstrate that there may be no decrease in rates of stenosis.[37,38] As in all pregnant patients, surgery should be minimized when possible, but emergency surgery may be necessary for the health and well-being of both the mother and child. Women with CD who underwent vaginal delivery demonstrated up to a 20% rate of perianal disease. In general, this was associated with episiotomy postdelivery.

Operative Options in Ulcerative Colitis

Approximately 20% of patients with UC will require colectomy. A review of a US insurance database determined that 44% of UC patients requiring surgery underwent TPC with IPAA, 22% underwent subtotal colectomy with Hartmann's procedure, 17% had TPC with end ileostomy, and the remainder underwent proctocolectomy or miscellaneous procedures.[39] In elective surgery, proctocolectomy is the definitive procedure recommended for patients with UC secondary to risk of recurrence and malignancy. TPC removes the entire colon and rectum. Options exist for either creation of a neorectum or ileostomy.

In the emergency setting, patients generally undergo a subtotal colectomy with end ileostomy. A subtotal colectomy is associated with less morbidity for an acutely ill patient. In addition to decreased operative time, risks of proctectomy include damage to nerves, ureter, bladder, and reproductive organs. In the acute setting, up to 30% of patients initially diagnosed with UC will be diagnosed with CD or indeterminate colitis by pathology, and one-third of UC patients decide to continue with ileostomy rather than undergo further surgery and reconstruction.[40] The first stage removes the abdominal colon and diverts the fecal stream to an ileostomy. A rectal stump of 20 to 35 cm is retained and may be sutured to the anterior abdominal wall or incision to allow for externalization in the case of ongoing inflammation. Patients generally have minimal symptoms from the retained rectum following subtotal colectomy. Passage of mucus and occasional bleeding may be present in some patients and can usually be treated with local pharmacologic agents such as topical 5-ASA derivatives or topical steroids. The second stage of the operation will include removal of the retained rectum. Most surgeons recommend an interval period prior to undergoing a completion proctectomy to allow the patient to recover from surgery, wean from medications (including steroids), and improve nutrition and anemia. Interval periods of 6 to 12 weeks are generally thought to reduce perirectal inflammation.

Options for reconstruction include Kock pouch, end ileostomy, or IPAA. Patients with poor anal sphincter tone, low rectal cancer, or who do not desire a IPAA may undergo creation of a Kock pouch or end ileostomy. A Kock pouch, or continent ileostomy, consists of the creation of an internal abdominal reservoir, with a valve mechanism allowing for cannulation and elective emptying of the pouch. Complications, such as fistula and leakage, occur in as many as 50% of patients and it is rarely performed. More commonly, patients undergo creation of an end ileostomy. The ostomy is generally created in a Brooke fashion, which elevates the end of the intestines above the abdominal wall, facilitating placement of an ostomy appliance. Complications such as prolapse of the intestines, parastomal hernias, and retraction can occur and may require surgical revision.

The IPAA is often referred to as a "J-pouch," but actual conformation of the pouch may vary and include S, W, or H pouch formation. The entire rectum is removed, and a neorectum is formed from the terminal ileum. Over time, storage function of the neorectum allows for decreased frequency of bowel movements, typically to 4 to 6 bowel movements per day. The distal end of the pouch is attached to the rectum or anus with either a stapled or hand-sewn technique. This varies by surgeon preference, but studies have demonstrated the hand-sewn technique with mucosectomy allows for more complete removal of rectal mucosa and reduced risk of cancer in the retained rectum, while the stapled technique provides improved sphincter function and decreased incontinence.[41] Patients with a history of colon or rectal cancer are generally offered a hand-sewn technique to reduce the risk of cancer.

Elective IPAA or pouch surgery can be done simultaneously with a colectomy. Often, a temporary loop ileostomy is performed at the time of pouch surgery. Internal reconstruction is completed, but a loop of ileum is raised on the anterior abdominal wall to divert stool while the pouch heals. Patients with suboptimal nutrition, multiple immunosuppressants, and poor general preoperative health generally have temporary diversion. A loop ileostomy provides temporary fecal diversion for the pouch and a period of healing prior to passage of stool through the new pouch. Some surgeons will perform a single-stage procedure, with removal of the colon and rectum and creation of pouch without diversion, but studies demonstrate early healing to be a crucial time in pouch healing and long-term effects may be marginalized should there be a problem with the pouch.[42]

Approximately 20% of patients will have some level of leakage, nighttime, stress incontinence, or actual accidents. Patients may develop pouchitis, or inflammation of the pouch, and require use of probiotics, antibiotics, or immunosuppressants. Incidence increases in patients who have perioperative complication such as a pelvic abscess, leak, or fistula. Problems are more significant in patients ultimately diagnosed with CD. Ten percent of patients may have long-term failure of their pouch.[43] In patients with J-pouch surgery, several studies have demonstrated only a mild increase in frequency of stools, mild incontinence, and need for protective garment over time; function was still deemed excellent even 20 years after the initial surgery.[44] Elderly patients with good preoperative continence and no contraindications may be candidates for IPAA even into their 60s and 70s. Patients over 65 do report more nighttime incontinence and less perfect continence than younger patients, but most elderly patients would undergo the procedure again and would recommend it to other patients. Current recommendations are to base decision to undergo IPAA on the patient characteristics and not age alone.[45]

Surgical treatment of children with UC raises some issues. While many adults are treated by colorectal surgeons, children are often treated by pediatric surgeons. Most pediatric surgeons may have only limited experience with complex surgical cases of inflammatory bowel disease. In a recent nationwide survey of British pediatric surgeons, the annual hospital caseload ranged from 0 to 23 laparotomies for IBD per year.[46] Surgeons who reported performing IPAA averaged only 1 case per year. Only 3 surgeons from this nationwide survey reported any experience with pouch revisions. Many pediatric surgeons are more comfortable with a traditionally straight ileoanal procedure as performed for Hirschsprung's, rather than ileorectal or IPAA and continue to perform straight coloanal anastomoses despite the benefits of IPAA, including decreased number of bowel movements and increased storage capacity.[47,48] Proctectomy in patients with UC differs from the same procedure in patients with Hirschsprung's, as patients are often treated preoperatively with immunosuppressants and may be malnourished and anemic.

Proctectomy and IPAA also have significant effects on patients' reproductive and sexual function. Women with UC have been shown to have decreased fertility rates even before surgery, but fecundity rates drop precipitously following restorative proctocolectomy.[49] Theories abound as to whether this is as a result of adhesive changes to the tubes or ovaries, inflammation, or other causes. Patients do well with in vitro fertilization, which tends to support a mechanical rather than endocrinologic cause for the decreased fertility; however, the risk is not increased in patients with postoperative abscess or leak.[50] In males, sexual dysfunction occurs in 0% to 25% of patients following pouch surgery. Proximity of the parasympathetic and sympathetic nerves in the pelvis may contribute to erectile dysfunction, including inability to maintain erection and retrograde ejaculation. Males planning to have a family following IPAA may be encouraged to cryobank sperm prior to surgery. Females also have an increased rate of dyspareunia, believed to be associated with the posterior displacement of the uterus following proctectomy.[51] Overall, most patients find that sexual activity improves following TPC/IPAA but this is certainly multifactorial in origin as acutely ill patients may be unlikely to participate in frequent sexual relations and improvement in overall health may contribute greatly to this outcome.[52]

Another area of concern following pouch surgery is vaginal delivery and its effects on pouch function. Traditionally, surgeons preferred caesarian section to avoid damage to the sphincter mechanism and rates of caesarian section for women after IPAA are close to 4 times the North American average.[53] Small trials have failed to demonstrate a change in pouch function or incontinence following vaginal delivery, and current recommendations are that vaginal delivery is safe and possible for patients following pouch surgery.

Minimally Invasive Surgery

Minimally invasive surgery is safe and possible for both patients with UC and CD. Numerous studies have demonstrated the feasibility of laparoscopic surgery in UC, including emergency resections.[54] In addition to potential cosmetic, narcotic use, and length-of-stay advantages, there are suggestions that patients incur additional benefits. A small study demonstrated a reduced number of adhesions both within the abdomen and enclosing the adnexa following IPAA.[55] The ability to improve sexual function following laparoscopic surgery is as of yet unproven.

CD appears ideally suited to laparoscopic surgery. Patients who may require multiple surgical resections may benefit from decreased adhesions, smaller incisions, and incisional hernias. Two randomized studies demonstrated decreased hospital stay for Crohn's patients who underwent laparoscopy, and differences were also noted in pulmonary function, length of postoperative ileus, and overall morbidity.[56,57] However, studies have demonstrated that laparoscopic resection in patients with CD may be more difficult than other laparoscopic procedures, leading to longer operative times, and higher conversion rates.[58] A relatively steep learning curve exists for surgeons performing laparoscopic Crohn's surgery, and recommendations include significant prior laparoscopic experience.[59]

The use of better monopolar and bipolar cautery instruments, ultrasonic dissection, and vascular sealants, as well as improvement in instrumentation and dissection tools, continue to advance the field of laparoscopic surgery. Magnification by the laparoscope can assist in visualization and preservation of vital structures, such as the hypogastric nerves. In the hands of trained laparoscopic surgeons, laparoscopic surgery is now possible to perform with precision equal to open surgical techniques and is a viable alternative for many patients.

Summary

Although medical therapy for inflammatory bowel disease has changed greatly in the past 20 years, surgical therapy has remained relatively stable. Indications including refractory disease, cancer, perforation, and bleeding continue to require surgical intervention. Advances in laparoscopic management and the ideologic move toward strictureplasty are the major changes that have occurred in surgical management.

References

1. Fazio VW, Wu JS. Surgical therapy for Crohn's disease of the colon and rectum. *Surg Clin North Am.* 1997;77:197-210.
2. Lee ECG, Papaioannou N. Minimal surgery for chronic obstruction in patients with extensive or universal Crohn's disease. *Ann R Coll Surg Eng.* 1982;64:229-233.
3. Hurst RD, Michelassi F. Strictureplasty for Crohn's disease: techniques and long-term results. *World J Surg.* 1998;22(4):359-363.
4. Hoie O, Wolters FL, Riis L, et al. European Collaborative Study Group of Inflammatory Bowel Disease: low colectomy rates in ulcerative colitis in an unselected European cohort followed for ten years. *Gastroenterology.* 2007;132:507-515.
5. Leijonmarck CE, Persson PG, Hellers G. Factors affecting colectomy rate in ulcerative colitis: an epidemiologic study. *Gut* 1990;31:329-333.
6. Newby E, Sawczenk A, Thomas AG, Wilson D. Interventions for growth failure in childhood Crohn's disease. *Cochrane Database Systematic Reviews.* 2005;4:CD003873.
7. Michelassi F, Stella M, Balestracci T, Giuliante F, Marogna P, Block GE. Incidence, diagnosis, and treatment of enteric and colorectal fistulae in patients with Crohn's disease. *Ann Surg.* 1993;218:660-666.
8. Gervais DA, Hahn PF, O'Neill MJ, Mueller PR. Percutaneous abscess drainage in Crohn's disease: technical success and short- and long-term outcomes during 14 years. *Radiology.* 2002;222(3):645-651.
9. Gutierrez A, Lee H, Sands BE. Outcome of surgical versus percutaneous drainage of abdominal and pelvic abscesses in Crohn's disease. *Am J Gastroenterol.* 2006;101:2283-2289.
10. Hordijk ML, Shivananda S. Risk of cancer in inflammatory bowel disease: why are the results in the reviewed literature so varied? *Scand J Gastroenterol Suppl.* 1989;170:70-74.
11. Ullman T. Preventing neoplastic progression in ulcerative colitis. *J Clin Gastroenterol.* 2005;39:S66-S69.
12. Hamilton SR. Colorectal carcinoma in patients with Crohn's disease. *Gastroenterology.* 1985;89(2):398-407.
13. Robert JR, Sachar DB, Greenstein AJ. Severe gastrointestinal hemorrhage in Crohn's disease. *Ann Surg.* 1991;213(3):207-211.
14. Campos AC, Meguid MM. A critical appraisal of the usefulness of perioperative nutritional support. *Am J Clin Nutr.* 1992;55:117-130.
15. Selvasekar CR, Cima RR, Larson DW, et al. Effect of infliximab on short-term complications in patients undergoing operation for chronic ulcerative colitis. *J Am Coll Surg.* 2007;205:956-962.
16. Appau KA, Fazio VW, Shen B, et al. Use of infliximab within 3 months of ileocolonic resection is associated with adverse postoperative outcomes in Crohn's patients. *J Gastrointest Surg.* 2008;12:1738-1744.
17. Page MJ, Poritz LS, Kunselman SJ. Factors affecting surgical risk in elderly patients with inflammatory bowel disease. *J Gastonintestin Surg.* 2002;6:606-613.
18. Ananthakrishnan AN, McGnley EL, Binion DG. Inflammatory bowel disease in the elderly is associated with worse outcomes: a national study of hospitalizations. *Inflamm Bowel Dis.* 2009;15:182-189.
19. Fazio VW. Regional enteritis (Crohn's disease): indications for surgery and operative strategy. *Surg Clin North Am.* 1983;63(1):27-48.

20. Fazio VW, Marchetti F, Church M, et al. Effect of resection margins on the recurrence of Crohn's disease in the small bowel: a randomized controlled trial. *Ann Surg.* 1996;224(4):563-571.

21. Yamamoto T, Allan RN, Keighley MR. An audit of gastroduodenal Crohn's disease: clinicopathologic features and management. *Scand J Gastroenterol.* 1999;34(10):1019-1024.

22. Michelassi F, Hurst RD, Melis M, et al. Side-to-side isoperistaltic strictureplasty in extensive CD. *Ann Surg.* 2000;232(3):401-408.

23. Fichera A, Lovadina S, Rubin M, Cimino F, Hurst RD, Michelassi F. Patterns and operative treatment of recurrent Crohn's disease: a prospective longitudinal study. *Surgery.* 2006;140(4):649-654.

24. Poggioli G, Stocchi L, Laureti S, et al. Conservative surgical management of terminal ileitis. *Dis Colon Rectum.* 1997;40:234-239.

25. Roy P, Kumar D. Strictureplasty for active Crohn's disease. *Int J Colorectal Dis.* 2006;21:427-432.

26. Michelassi F, Taschieri A, Tonelli F, et al. An international multicenter prospective observational study of the side-to-side isoperistaltic strictureplasty in Crohn's disease. *Dis Colon Rectum.* 2006;50:277-284.

27. Lapidius A, Bernell O, Hellers G, Lofberg R. Clinical course of colorectal Crohn's disease: a 35-year follow-up study of 507 patients. *Gastroenterology.* 1998;114(6):1151-1160.

28. Farmer RG, Hawk WA, Turnbull RB. Indications for surgery in Crohn's disease: analysis of 500 cases. *Gastroenterology.* 1976;71(2):245-250.

29. Andersson P, Olaison G, Hallbook O, Sjodahl R. Segmental resection or subtotal colectomy in Crohn's colitis? *Dis Colon Rectum.* 2002;45(1):47-53.

30. Fichera A, McCormack R, Rubin MA, Hurst RD, Michelassi F. Long-term outcome of surgically treated Crohn's colitis: a prospective study. *Dis Colon Rectum.* 2005;48(5):963-969.

31. Lefton HB, Fazio VW. Ileorectal anastomosis for Crohn's disease of the colon. *Gastroenterology.* 1975;69(3):612-617.

32. Lock MF, Fazio VW, Farmer RG, Jagelman DG, Lavery IC, Weakley FL. Proximal recurrence and the fate of the rectum following excisional surgery for Crohn's disease of the large bowel. *Ann Surg.* 1981;194(6):754-760.

33. Andrews, HA, Lewis P, Allan RN. Prognosis after surgery for colonic Crohn's disease. *Br J Surg.* 1989;76(11):1184-1190.

34. Alexander F, Sarigol S, DiFiore J, et al. Fate of the pouch in 151 pediatric patients after ileal pouch anal anastomosis. *J Ped Surg.* 2003;38:78-82.

35. Hyder SA, Travis SP, Jewell DP, et al. Fistulating anal Crohn's disease: results of combined surgical and infliximab treatment. *Dis Colon Rect.* 2006;49:1837-1841.

36. Vernier-Massouille G, Balde M, Salleron J, et al. Natural history of pediatric Crohn's disease: a population-based cohort study. *Gastroenterology.* 2008;135(4):1106-1113.

37. Nwokolo CU, Tan WC, Andrews HA. Surgical resection in parous patients with distal ileal and colonic Crohn's disease. *Gut.* 1994;35:220-223.

38. Castiglione F, Pignata S, Morace F, et al. Effect of pregnancy on the clinical course of a cohort of women with inflammatory bowel disease. *Ital J Gastroenterol.* 1996;4:199-204.

39. Loftus EV, Friedman HS, Delgado DJ, et al. Colectomy subtypes, follow up surgical procedures, postsurgical complications and medical charges among ulcerative colitis patients with private health insurance in the United States. *Inflamm Bowel Dis.* 2009;15(4):566-575.

40. Hyman NH, Cataldo P, Osler T. Urgent subtotal colectomy for severe inflammatory bowel disease. *Dis Colon Rectum.* 2005;48:70-73.

41. Chambers WM, Mortensen NJ. Should ileal pouch-anal anastomosis include mucosectomy? *Colorectal Dis.* 2007;9:384-392.

42. Davies M, Hawley PR. Ten years experience of end-stage restorative proctocolectomy for ulcerative colitis. *Int J Colorectal Dis.* 2007;22:1255-1260.

43. Wasmuth HH, Trano G, Endreseth B, et al. Long term surgical workload in patients with ileal pouch anal anastomosis. Available at www3.interscience.wiley.com.monstera.cc.columbia.ed:2048/journal/122301354/abstract. Accessed April 2, 2009.

44. Hahnloser D, Pemberton JH, Wolff BG, et al. Results at up to 20 years after ileal pouch–anal anastomosis for chronic ulcerative colitis. *Br J Surg.* 2007;94:333-340.

45. Delaney CP, Favio VW, Remzi FH, et al. Prospective, age-related analysis of surgical results, functional outcome and quality of life after ileal pouch anal anastomosis. *Ann Surg.* 2003;238:221.

46. Smith NP, Ba'ath ME, Perry D, et al. BAPS UK inflammatory bowel disease surgical practice survey. *J Pediatr Surg.* 2007;42:296-299.

47. Sako M, Kimura H, Arai K. Restorative proctocolectomy for pediatric patients with ulcerative colitis. *Surgery Today.* 2006;36:162.

48. Rintala RJ, Lindahl HG. Proctocolectomy and J-pouch ileo anal anastomosis in children. *J Ped Surg.* 2002;37:66-70.

49. Waljee A, Waljee J, Morris AM, Higgins PDR. Threefold increased risk of infertility: a meta-analysis of infertility after ileal pouch anal anastomosis in ulcerative colitis. *Gut.* 2006;55:1575-1580.

50. Gorgun E, Remzi FH, Goldberg JM, et al. Fertility is reduced after restorative proctocolectomy with ileal pouch anal anastomosis: a study of 300 patients. *Surgery.* 2004;136:795-803.

51. Oresland I, Palmblad S, Ellstrom M, Berndtsson I, Crona N, Hulten L. Gynaecological and sexual function related to anatomical changes in the female pelvis after restorative proctocolectomy. *International Journal of Colorectal Disease.* 1993;9:77-81.

52. Gorgun E, Remzi FH, Montague DK, et al. Male sexual function improves after ileal pouch anal anastomosis. *Colorectal Dis.* 2005;7:545-550.

53. McLeod RS. Ileal pouch anal anastomosis: pregnancy—before, during, and after. *J Gastrointest Surg.* 2008;12:2150-2152.

54. Ahmed AU, Keus F, Heikens JT, et al. Open versus laparoscopic (assisted) ileo pouch anal anastomosis for ulcerative colitis and familial adenomatous polyposis. *Cochrane Database Syst Rev.* 2009;1:CD006267

55. Indar AA, Efron JE, Young-Fadok TM. Laparoscopic ileal pouch-anal anastomosis reduced abdominal and pelvic adhesions. *Surg Endosc.* 2009;23:174-177.

56. Milsom JW, Hammerhofer KA, Bohm B, Marcello P, Elson P, Fazio VW. Prospective randomized trial comparing laparoscopy vs conventional surgery for refractory ileocolic CD. *Dis Colon Rectum.* 2001;44:1-9.

57. Maartense S, Dunker MS, Slors JFM, et al. Laparoscopic-assisted versus open ileocolic resection for Crohn's disease. *Ann Surg.* 2006;243:143-149.

58. Tan JJY, Tjandra JJ. Laparoscopic surgery for Crohn's disease: a meta-analysis. *Dis Colon Rectum.* 2007;50:576-585.

59. Evans J, Poritz L, MacRae H. Influence of experience on laparoscopic ileocolic resection for Crohn's disease. *Dis Colon Rectum.* 2002;45:1595-1600.

Financial disclosure: Dr. Stein is course instructor for a laparoscopic course receiving educational support from Olympus, Covidien, and Applied Medical.

CHAPTER 19

INFLAMMATORY BOWEL DISEASE IN THE CURRENT WORLD

CONTROVERSIES IN MANAGEMENT

Corey A. Siegel, MD

The field of inflammatory bowel disease (IBD) is evolving rapidly. In 2008, we had an armamentarium of treatment options that were unavailable just a few years ago, and there has been a rapid rise in the amount of research being performed in IBD. The number of annual IBD publications has more than doubled since 1998.[1] New and promising data from this work have generated new questions. Questions frequently lead to uncertainty, which ultimately breeds controversies in management (Table 19-1).

Clinicians take an oath to "prescribe regimens for the good of my patients according to my ability and my judgment and never do harm to anyone."[2] To guide us in this process, we look to evidence-based literature. However, when data are conflicting or still developing and controversy exists, treatment decisions become more challenging. For example, will 5-aminosalicylate (5-ASAs) drugs prevent the progression of Crohn's disease? Will biologic agents lead to serious side effects? Will low-grade dysplasia (LGD) of the colon progress to invasive cancer? The controversies of yesterday have led to the practice guidelines of today, and the controversies of today will lead to further research to develop the treatment strategies of tomorrow. This chapter reviews some of the most debated controversies of current IBD treatment and offers some insight into how they affect specific populations of patients.

5-ASAs for Crohn's Disease

Recently, the use of 5-ASA medications for the treatment of Crohn's disease has come under significant scrutiny. Used for years as a mainstay of Crohn's therapy, 5-ASA use is being abandoned based on more recent data. In 1993, Singleton et al published a randomized controlled trial showing efficacy of slow-release mesalamine capsules (Pentasa [Shire, Wayne, PA]) for the treatment of active Crohn's disease.[3] In this study of 310 Crohn's disease patients, 43% in the treatment group were in remission at 16 weeks as opposed to 18% in the placebo group. Based on these data, the presumed efficacy of this treatment went unchallenged for over 10 years.

Scherl EJ, Dubinsky MC.
*The Changing World of Inflammatory Bowel Disease:
Impact of Generation, Gender, and Global Trends (pp 231-244)*
© 2009 SLACK Incorporated.

Table 19-1

CURRENT CONTROVERSIES IN INFLAMMATORY BOWEL DISEASE

Controversies in Evaluation	Controversies in Treatment
Utility of capsule endoscopy	5-ASAs for Crohn's disease
Radiation exposure with CT scans	Risks of immunomodulators and biologics
Utility of MRI and ultrasound	Top-down therapy
Utility of serologic markers	Combination therapy versus monotherapy
Utility of genetic testing	Biologic therapy in pregnancy (see Chapter 13)
Utility of chromoendoscopy	Surveillance colonoscopy and the management of low-grade dysplasia

In 2004, Hanauer et al published a meta-analysis[4] to explore the utility of 5-ASAs for Crohn's disease that included the Singleton study, in addition to 2 previously unreported trials.[5,6] Although this analysis found a statistically significant improvement in the Crohn's Disease Activity Index in the treatment group, it was a negligible 18-point change and was felt by most to be clinically insignificant. Based on these results, experts have concluded that 5-ASAs are not useful in the treatment of Crohn's disease.[7] This has been corroborated by others, including a Cochrane analysis that found no data to support the use of 5-ASAs for the maintenance of remission of Crohn's disease. The authors added that further clinical trials are not warranted on this topic.[8]

Despite the Cochrane review's recommendations, many clinicians have anecdotal experience that 5-ASAs work for certain subgroups of patients (eg, colonic disease, mildly active disease) and that 5-ASAs may not all be alike (eg, sulfasalazine may be more effective if tolerated at higher doses). Published practice guidelines include 5-ASAs for the management of mild to moderately active Crohn's disease,[9] and 5-ASAs continue to be widely used in clinical practice. However, the concern is that using this weakly active medication will only delay the use of necessary, more active therapies. Of note, none of the 5-ASA drugs are Food and Drug Administration (FDA) approved for the treatment of Crohn's disease.

This controversy remains unanswered at the current time. It is unlikely that 5-ASAs will be significantly effective for Crohn's disease patients with more than mildly active disease. A reasonable approach is to exclude them from treatment algorithms in patients with moderate to severely active disease but allow a short trial in patients with mild colonic disease. Unless a convincing response is seen, there should be a low threshold to move to more effective medications.

HOW DOES THIS CONTROVERSY APPLY TO SPECIAL POPULATIONS?

5-ASA therapy is safe, so it is a particularly appealing treatment for children and the elderly. The biggest drawback is that it may not be effective, therefore delaying appropriate therapy in children who might be out of school and suffer from growth and pubertal delay and for the elderly who likely have other comorbidities. In addition, the large number of pills required for most formulations are inconvenient and can contribute to making children feel like "patients" and add to the pill burden in the elderly.

Risks of Immunomodulators and Biologics

A hot topic of debate involves the current understanding of risks of IBD therapies, specifically side effects associated with immunomodulators and biologics. Commonly used immunomodulator therapies include azathioprine (AZA), 6-mercaptopurine (6-MP), and methotrexate. Currently FDA-approved and available biologics are infliximab, adalimumab, certolizumab pegol, and natalizumab.

IMMUNOMODULATORS

AZA and 6-MP have been used for over 30 years for the treatment of IBD with established efficacy for the treatment of Crohn's disease[10-12] and ulcerative colitis (UC).[13] Side effects of these medications have been well-reported and relate to both direct and indirect toxicity. Direct toxicity refers to those events that come as a direct result from the medication and include pancreatitis, bone marrow suppression, and allergic reactions. In one report of nearly 400 patients, the rate of these events were 3%, 2%, and 2%, respectively.[14] Similar frequencies were seen in a Cochrane analysis with a number needed to harm (NNH) of 14 (for one patient to have an adverse event leading to withdrawal from the study).[15] Indirect toxicity refers to processes that result as sequelae from direct toxicity. These include infections (including rare deaths associated with sepsis) and an increased risk of malignancy (specifically for non-Hodgkin's lymphoma).

Significant infections have been reported in up to 7% of patients[14] and deaths attributable to leukopenia and sepsis as high as 0.3% (3/1000).[16,17] The rate of lymphoma associated with immunomodulators has been debated. Although the baseline risk of lymphoma in IBD patients not treated with immunomodulators has been uncertain, a large United Kingdom database did not show that IBD itself predisposes to lymphoma.[18] Based on population-based data[19] and a meta-analysis,[20] the risk of lymphoma (specifically non-Hodgkin's lymphoma) attributable to 6-MP/AZA in Crohn's disease appears to be about 2-fold higher than the general population. In absolute terms, the 1-year risk of lymphoma in the general population is approximately 2/10,000 patient-years.[21] Therefore, the 1-year risk of a patient with Crohn's disease developing lymphoma while on 6-MP/AZA is about 4/10,000 patient-years.

Methotrexate is used less often than 6-MP/AZA in most parts of the world, although it likely has similar efficacy for the treatment of Crohn's disease.[22] Although pulmonary and hepatic toxicity are well-reported in patients with rheumatoid arthritis (RA)[23] and psoriasis,[24] these events appear very rare in IBD patients.[25,26] Leukopenia is uncommon[22,27] but has been reported and can be life threatening.[28] There is a perception that lymphoma is more of a problem with 6-MP/AZA than methotrexate. However, lymphoma is well-reported in methotrexate-treated RA patients.[29-33] Methotrexate is teratogenic and a known abortifacient, so women need to use adequate birth control. In addition, methotrexate may be toxic to sperm, so men should stop taking it at least 3 months before trying to conceive.[25]

BIOLOGIC THERAPY

Currently available biologic therapies for IBD include the anti-tumor necrosis factor-alpha (anti-TNF) agents infliximab, adalimumab, certolizumab pegol as well as natalizumab (an anti-alpha-4 integrin molecule). The nature and rate of adverse events associated with these medications has generated significant controversy. Important limitations to accurately predicting the rate of serious side effects include the relatively short period of time that these agents have been on the market, the limited number of IBD patients who have been treated with these medications in clinical trials, and the lack of systematically collected data for all treated patients. Therefore, a broad range of incidence of events has been reported, contributing to considerable uncertainty.

Although a long list of adverse events has been reported with anti-TNF agents,[34,35] most of the attention has focused on the black box warnings that were added to the package labeling by the FDA during postmarketing surveillance. These include serious infections (including tuberculosis and life-threatening sepsis) and lymphoma. Most of the available data are related to infliximab (since it was FDA approved first), but adalimumab and certolizumab pegol likely have similar side effect profiles.

The rate of death as a result of severe life-threatening infections associated with anti-TNF therapy has been reported to be as high as 1% in the largest single-center experience.[36] On the other end of the spectrum, a large prospective registry of Crohn's disease patients (TREAT) found no increased risk of mortality independently associated with infliximab use.[37] A systematic analysis summarizing data from 6 different studies found a mortality rate due to sepsis of 0.4%.[38] Lymphoma estimates in the literature have the same problem of divergent results. The highest risk reported in Crohn's disease was from a Swedish population-based study of 1.6%[39] while there was no increased risk seen in the TREAT registry.[37] The same systematic analysis noted above found a 0.2% rate of lymphoma in Crohn's disease patients treated with infliximab.[38] A recent meta-analysis found a rate of non-Hodgkin's lymphoma of 0.6% (6/10,000 patient-years) in Crohn's disease patients taking combination immunomodulator and biologic therapy.[40]

A recently described type of lymphoma, hepatosplenic T-cell lymphoma (HSTCL), has generated significant concern.[41] To date, 16 cases of HSTCL have been reported in Crohn's disease patients taking infliximab in addition to an immunomodulator (6-MP/AZA) (data on file, Centocor, Horsham, PA). There were at least 9 cases in the literature of patients with Crohn's disease who were taking AZA without infliximab.[42-44] The average age of the 16 patients was 21 years of age, and the range of number of infliximab infusions was 1 to 24. Interestingly, 14 of these 16 reported patients were male. Unfortunately, this appears to be a nearly universally fatal disease. The incidence of HSTCL in IBD patients is unknown, as it is very difficult to estimate how many patients in this age group have been treated with infliximab worldwide.

Natalizumab has shown promise for the treatment of Crohn's disease in randomized controlled trials.[45] In 2005, significant concern was raised after 3 cases of progressive multifocal leukoencephalopathy (PML) associated with JC virus infection were reported. One case occurred in a patient with Crohn's disease.[46] PML is an opportunistic viral infection of the central nervous system that usually leads to death or severe disability. Natalizumab is not the only immune-suppressant medication with the potential to induce PML,[47] but these cases led to a temporary halting of all further clinical trials of natalizumab in Crohn's disease and withdrawal from the market for its other indication, multiple sclerosis (MS). In 2007, the FDA allowed natalizumab back on the market for the treatment of MS, and natalizumab is now approved for Crohn's disease in patients failing anti-TNFα therapies. To date, a total of 12 cases (11 in MS, 1 in Crohn's) of PML associated with the use of natalizumab have been reported. Its integration into the treatment algorithm of Crohn's disease will likely be a matter of significant attention in the coming years.

HOW DO THESE CONTROVERSIES APPLY TO SPECIAL POPULATIONS?

Risk is an emotional and complex topic, and how risk affects decision making will be influenced by the population in which the drug is prescribed. In the systematic analysis of the risks of infliximab,[38] the average age of patients with lymphoma was 52 and the average age of those who died of sepsis was 63. In contrast, HSTCL affects the younger population with an average age of 21 years.

Patients, parents of patients, and physicians have different thresholds of how much risk they are willing to accept of these adverse events. In a study to address this question, adult patients were willing to take higher risks for death related to sepsis, lymphoma, or PML than have been reported in the literature, with the highest thresholds for those with more severe disease who were promised a greater treatment benefit.[48] Parents of patients with Crohn's disease accepted even higher risks than the adult patients (up to a 1.05% risk of dying from lymphoma versus 0.81% for adults) when children were severely sick but were much more conservative when children were only mild-moderately sick.[49] When physicians were asked the same questions to ascertain their risk thresholds, they were generally more risk averse than adult patients when making choices for young patients, but they were more risk taking than adult patients when making choices for older patients.[50]

When addressing IBD medications risk with patients, physicians should be aware that patients' thresholds of acceptable treatment-related risk will vary based on their individual preferences and are highly dependent on the patient's age and level of disease activity. If early aggressive or "top-down" treatment becomes a proven means to improve the natural history of disease, the hesitance of using aggressive treatment in children who have recently been diagnosed will need to be addressed.

Top-Down Therapy

Recently, 2 important observations opened a dialogue regarding whether a more aggressive therapeutic approach early in the disease course of Crohn's disease, or "top-down" therapy, is a more effective strategy. The first was that our current algorithm of "step-up" treatment (safer, less effective drugs first, followed by more effective drugs after failure of the first-line agents) is not making a significant impact on the natural history of disease.[51,52] The second was that treatment with the strongest medications early in the disease course may lead to a better clinical response.[53-55] These latter data brought top-down therapy to the forefront of controversy in IBD. The basic premise is that treating patients during a window of opportunity before complications occur can change the natural history of the disease.

Natural history data have taught us that approximately 20% of patients with Crohn's disease undergo surgery within the first year of diagnosis, 50% within the first 5 years, and 80% after 20 years of disease.[56] The recent study by Cosnes et al showed that surgical rates have not changed over the past 25 years despite the increasing use of immunomodulators.[51] The authors stated that these results question the efficacy of current medical strategies. However, they raise the possibility that the reason immunomodulators did not make an impact on surgical rates was related to the timing of initiation. Specifically, a large majority of patients came to surgery while not on immunomodulators or were operated on within a few months of diagnosis (before immuno-modulators had a chance to take effect). In fact, only 16 patients (9%) who required surgery had been on immunomodulators for more than 3 months. Therefore, these data might imply that the failure to alter natural history is not due to a lack of effect of immunomodulators, but rather to a failure of not using them early enough in the disease course.

A study by Hommes et al presented in 1995 focused gastroenterologists' attention on top-down therapy,[54] but these ideas are not new. Rheumatologists had previously reported that the use of biologics (infliximab or adalimumab) along with methotrexate in patients with recently diagnosed RA provided better clinical, radiographic, and functional benefits than treatment with methotrexate alone.[57,58] Using similar reasoning, a randomized controlled trial was designed with 129 patients with recently diagnosed Crohn's disease.[54] They were randomized to either the top-down group, which received infliximab with AZA up front, or to the step-up group, which received corticosteroids at first with AZA added later to those patients requiring repeated corticosteroid courses. The proportion of patients in clinical remission and off of corticosteroids (the primary outcome) at week 26 was significantly higher in the top-down group (74.5% versus 48.1%, p = 0.006), and this significant statistical difference persisted at 52 weeks. Follow-up data were presented 1 year later on a subgroup of these patients who had colonoscopy 2 years after enrollment.[53] Complete ulcer disappearance was seen in 71% of patients in the top-down group as compared to 30% in the step-up group (p<0.001).

Post-hoc analyses of randomized controlled trials of other anti-TNF agents[59,60] provide a similar message that the use of biologic therapy earlier in the disease course increases efficacy. This is also supported by pediatric data. Children treated with infliximab show response and remission rates that are significantly higher than what has typically been seen with the adult Crohn's population.[55] Interestingly, the proportion of response in children (88% initial response rate and 49% overall remission rate) is very close to the proportion seen in the post-hoc analyses for adults who were treated within 1 to 2 years of diagnosis.

Although data supporting the concept of top-down therapy are compelling, larger prospective randomized controlled trials are necessary to confirm the benefit of this strategy. The keys to defining success of this strategy will focus on the risk-to-benefit ratio and the ability to predict which patients are at the most risk for disease progression. Until we are confident that we can separate out those destined to have complicated disease from those who will have a less complex disease course, it is difficult to adopt top-down therapy as a general approach.

HOW DOES THIS CONTROVERSY APPLY TO SPECIAL POPULATIONS?

Since the most common age of onset of Crohn's disease is in the late teens and early 20s, this age group has the most at stake. If in fact the early aggressive use of immunomodulators and/or biologics is proven to alter the natural history of disease, then a majority of newly diagnosed patients will be offered this aggressive treatment strategy. This has the potential to greatly improve the long-term quality of life of these patients, but it may be at the cost of side effects as noted previously. A decision to accept early aggressive or top-down therapy will need to ultimately be made together by a physician and his or her patient based on that patient's risk of disease progression and likelihood of adverse events.

Combination Versus Monotherapy

Once a decision has been made to use biologic therapy, the next important choice is whether or not to continue (or start) concomitant immunomodulators. The arguments to use combination therapy are 1) the combination of 2 effective drugs will increase clinical response, 2) immunomodulators will decrease the development of antibodies against the biologic agents (therefore increasing effectiveness and decreasing infusion reactions), and 3) the long-term results of biologic therapy are unknown, but there are over 30 years of data on immunomodulators in IBD. Arguments against the use of concomitant therapy primarily surround the issue of increased risk of side effects.

In RA, there are randomized controlled trial data showing that combination therapy is better than biologic monotherapy.[58,61] In fact, the infliximab package insert dosing instructions for RA state that infliximab should be given with methotrexate.[34] In the adalimumab package insert, dosing is recommended either every other week in combination with methotrexate or weekly if given without. This is based on the fact that 12% of RA patients using adalimumab monotherapy developed antibodies against adalimumab versus 1% who were taking combination therapy with methotrexate.[35] The development of anti-adalimumab antibodies has been associated with lower serum adalimumab levels and a diminished clinical response in RA. Anti-adalimumab antibodies formed less frequently in patients using concomitant methotrexate.[62]

In post-hoc analyses of Crohn's disease trials with infliximab,[63] adalimumab,[64] and certolizumab pegol,[65] there were no significant clinical differences between patients who were on biologic monotherapy versus those on concomitant immunomodulators. It should be noted, however, that the studies were not designed to examine this question, may be underpowered to detect a significant difference (Type II error), and long-term outcomes may differ from those based on 1 year of available data. Preliminary data regarding this topic are available for children as well, and they show similar results.[66]

Most recently, 2 randomized controlled trials addressed the question of anti-TNF monotherapy versus combination therapy with an immunomodulator. The Combination of Maintenance Methotrexate-Infliximab Trial (COMMIT)[67] studied patients who were induced into remission with corticosteroids along with infliximab with either methotrexate or placebo. Results did not show a difference in response or remission regardless of methotrexate use. A second study, Study of Biologic and Immunomodulator-Naive Patients in Crohn's Disease (SONIC), addressed a slightly different question.[68] These patients in general were earlier in their disease course and the majority were not taking corticosteroids. The investigators found that at 50 weeks, there was a statistically significantly increased rate of remission when using the combination of infliximab and AZA (versus either infliximab alone or AZA alone). Although at face value these 2 studies show discrepant results, the difference lies in the patient population. One can conceptualize these results as considering combination therapy in more recently diagnosed patients naive to both immunomodulators and anti-TNF agents and not receiving corticosteroids; however, in patients with a longer disease course who are being treated with corticosteroids, the addition of an immunomodulator may not be useful.

Other data focusing on serum infliximab levels suggest that combination therapy may be important to optimize response. Concomitant immunomodulators are associated with decreased production of antibodies to infliximab and higher infliximab levels.[69] As higher trough infliximab levels have been associated with improved clinical response,[70] it makes sense to prevent antibody formation. In addition, the timing of initiating immunomodulators appears to be important as we have seen that maintenance of a clinical response to infliximab is significantly improved in patients who started an immunomodulator greater than 3 months prior to initiating infliximab.[71]

The major concern about combination therapy is related to the risk of adverse events. This recently gained increased attention with the description of HSTCL as noted previously. Even before the report of HSTCL, many believed that immunomodulators with infliximab have a higher lymphoma rate than either agent alone, but there are no data to support this. In addition, opportunistic infections are more common in patients treated with more than one immunosuppressant drug.[72]

These data have led many physicians to stop immunomodulator use in their patients who are doing well on biologic therapy. Currently, there is no clear answer to whether biologic monotherapy or combination therapy is superior in efficacy or safety. Alternatives for patients starting biologics who are refractory to immunomodulators include stopping the immunomodulator completely, continuing 6-MP/AZA at the full weight-based dose, decreasing 6-MP/AZA dose, or switching to oral low-dose methotrexate.[73] For patients starting biologic therapy who are naïve to immunomodulators, the choice includes using biologic monotherapy, starting and maintaining combination therapy (with full- or low-dose 6-MP/AZA as above), or using biologic therapy as "bridge" therapy to immunomodulator monotherapy. Now that multiple anti-TNF agents are available (taking away some of the fear of starting and stopping biologics), the idea of using biologics to bridge immunomodulator-naïve patients for the 3 to 4 months until 6-MP/AZA takes effect is an appealing option. Early data on this strategy are promising,[54,74] but future studies will be needed before this can be a recommended approach.

HOW DOES THIS CONTROVERSY APPLY TO SPECIAL POPULATIONS?

This affects all patients with IBD, but particularly applies to children who seem to be at the most risk of HSTCL and their disease and to the elderly who are probably at the highest risk of drug-related adverse events.

Surveillance Colonoscopy and the Management of Low-Grade Dysplasia

Patients with long-standing UC and Crohn's colitis are at an increased risk of colorectal cancer.[75-77] The magnitude of this risk is uncertain. Long-accepted data that showed an approximately 20% cumulative risk of colon cancer after 30 years of disease[75] have recently come into question with population-based data reporting a much lower incidence.[78,79] The decreasing incidence of colon cancer noted in these recent publications might represent a true decrease in occurrence, but alternative explanations include bias in data acquisition, or a successful surveillance program.[80] Despite the uncertainty, clinicians agree that colorectal cancer surveillance is important in IBD patients. The current controversies on this topic relate to how to survey patients and what to do with the results.

HOW SHOULD PATIENTS BE SURVEYED?

Practice guidelines recommend surveillance colonoscopy with biopsies every 1 to 2 years in patients with colitis for longer than 8 years.[81] Based on a single publication, the recommended number of biopsies to detect dysplasia 90% of the time is 33, or 56 biopsies to increase confidence to 95%.[82] These biopsies are typically performed randomly of flat-appearing colonic mucosa with more directed biopsies taken of macroscopically visible lesions. The new technique of chromoendoscopy is threatening to change this standard protocol. Chromoendoscopy refers to the staining of the colonic mucosa with dye (indigo carmine or methylene blue) either with or without magnification colonoscopy. Early results are promising, but they raise new questions.

Kiesslich and colleagues performed the first large study of chromoendoscopy in Germany and found more neoplasia when using methylene blue dye as compared to standard endoscopy.[83] Rutter's group from Great Britain performed back-to-back colonoscopy in the same patients, first using conventional techniques and then performing directed biopsies based on abnormalities seen after indigo carmine staining.[84] In the Rutter study, no dysplasia was detected in the 2904 conventional nontargeted biopsies. In comparison, the targeted biopsy protocol with staining required fewer biopsies (157) yet detected 9 dysplastic lesions, 7 of which were only visible after indigo carmine application. It is not clear if this improved detection of dysplasia is simply due to looking harder or a true benefit of this new technique. There are some practical limitations to the widespread use of chromoendoscopy (time, cost, education), but a more important question is understanding the significance of finding "chromoendoscopy-detected dysplasia."[85]

WHAT SHOULD WE DO WITH LOW-GRADE DYSPLASIA?

There is little disagreement that a finding of high-grade dysplasia or cancer during colonoscopy in patients with long-standing UC or Crohn's disease warrants colectomy, but the management of flat LGD is more controversial. When flat LGD is identified, the reported rate of concomitant colorectal cancer in resected colon specimens is approximately 20%.[86,87] As many would agree that 20% is a high number, the general recommendation for a finding of flat LGD is for immediate colectomy. However, this may not be so straightforward. In the Ullman et al study that reported a nearly 20% risk of concomitant cancer with LGD, the average number of colon biopsies taken was 16.[86] The Thomas et al meta-analysis that showed a similar risk of cancer with LGD had an average of 18 biopsies per colonoscopy.[87] Therefore, the natural history data that we depend upon to make decisions are not based on the recommended 33 biopsies, but fewer biopsies. In fact, the recent publication by Rutter et al, which found a significantly lower incidence of dysplasia and cancer, had a median of only 8 biopsies,[79] and the only factor in Thomas' meta-analysis regression that was significantly associated with finding more advanced lesions was more biopsies.[87] These data suggest that looking harder finds more dysplasia. The question then is what is the natural history of LGD that is found using more sensitive sampling techniques (eg, more biopsies or chromoendoscopy)? If dysplasia found with 18 biopsies yields a concomitant cancer rate of 20%, what is the expected concomitant cancer rate when discovered with 33 biopsies or with chromoendoscopy? Currently, there are no data to guide us. As new methods for surveillance evolve, we need to consider the uncertainty of the clinical significance of the finding of dysplasia using these techniques.

HOW DOES THIS CONTROVERSY APPLY TO SPECIAL POPULATIONS?

The population at risk here is those who have long-standing, extensive UC or Crohn's colitis. For the elderly, at some point the risks of surveillance (and possible surgery) will outweigh the potential benefit. As patients get older, they (along with their physicians) need to carefully consider the utility of continued surveillance. Currently, there are no recommendations for the age at which to stop surveillance colonoscopy, so a decision needs to be made on an individual patient basis.

Summary

The issues discussed in this chapter are just some of the current controversies today in IBD. Other important debates include the risk of IBD medications during pregnancy; the effect of disease, treatment, and surgery on fertility; the efficacy of 5-ASAs (and other medications) for prophylaxis against colorectal cancer; the utility of "radiation sparing" imaging such as magnetic resonance imaging and ultrasound instead of standard computed tomography or fluoroscopy; the utility of capsule endoscopy; and the clinical applicability of serologic and genetic markers to diagnose and prognosticate IBD.

Future data will hopefully elucidate some of this uncertainty. It is likely that we will not have all of the answers and that we will have to make our best clinical judgment using the available data and experience. As we answer some questions, undoubtedly others will arise, leading to new controversies to be discussed and researched in the future.

References

1. Sands BE. How to read the inflammatory bowel disease literature. *Practical Gastroenterology.* 2005;XXIX:30-43.
2. Hippocrates. Circa 4th century BC.
3. Singleton JW, Hanauer SB, Gitnick GL, et al. Mesalamine capsules for the treatment of active Crohn's disease: results of a 16-week trial. Pentasa Crohn's Disease Study Group. *Gastroenterology.* 1993;104(5):1293-1301.
4. Hanauer SB, Stromberg U. Oral Pentasa in the treatment of active Crohn's disease: a meta-analysis of double-blind, placebo-controlled trials. *Clin Gastroenterol Hepatol.* 2004;2(5):379-388.
5. Hoechst. Marion Roussel Inc. Clinical study report: efficacy and safety of oral Pentasa in the treatment of active Crohn's disease. January 28, 1997.
6. Nordic. Research Inc. Clinical research report: efficacy and safety of oral Pentasa in the treatment of active Crohn's disease. October 23, 1991.
7. Feagan BG. 5-ASA therapy for active Crohn's disease: old friends, old data, and a new conclusion. *Clin Gastroenterol Hepatol.* 2004;2(5):376-378.
8. Akobeng AK, Gardener E. Oral 5-aminosalicylic acid for maintenance of medically-induced remission in Crohn's disease. *Cochrane Database Syst Rev.* 2005(1):CD003715.
9. Hanauer SB, Sandborn W. Management of Crohn's disease in adults. *Am J Gastroenterol.* 2001;96(3):635-643.
10. Candy S, Wright J, Gerber M, et al. A controlled double blind study of azathioprine in the management of Crohn's disease. *Gut.* 1995;37(5):674-678.
11. Present DH, Korelitz BI, Wisch N, et al. Treatment of Crohn's disease with 6-mercaptopurine: a long-term, randomized, double-blind study. *N Engl J Med.* 1980;302(18):981-987.
12. Sandborn W, Sutherland L, Pearson D, et al. Azathioprine or 6-mercaptopurine for inducing remission of Crohn's disease. *Cochrane Database Syst Rev.* 2000(2):CD000545.
13. Ardizzone S, Maconi G, Russo A, et al. Randomised controlled trial of azathioprine and 5-aminosalicylic acid for treatment of steroid-dependent ulcerative colitis. *Gut.* 2006;55(1):47-53.
14. Present DH, Meltzer SJ, Krumholz MP, et al. 6-mercaptopurine in the management of inflammatory bowel disease: short- and long-term toxicity. *Ann Intern Med.* 1989;111(8):641-649.
15. Pearson DC, May GR, Fick G, et al. Azathioprine for maintaining remission of Crohn's disease. *Cochrane Database Syst Rev.* 2000(2):CD000067.
16. Connell WR, Kamm MA, Ritchie JK, et al. Bone marrow toxicity caused by azathioprine in inflammatory bowel disease: 27 years of experience. *Gut.* 1993;34(8):1081-1085.
17. Pearson DC, May GR, Fick GH, et al. Azathioprine and 6-mercaptopurine in Crohn disease: a meta-analysis. *Ann Intern Med.* 1995;123(2):132-142.
18. Lewis JD, Bilker WB, Brensinger C, et al. Inflammatory bowel disease is not associated with an increased risk of lymphoma. *Gastroenterology.* 2001;121(5):1080-1087.
19. Lewis JD, Schwartz JS, Lichtenstein GR. Azathioprine for maintenance of remission in Crohn's disease: benefits outweigh the risk of lymphoma. *Gastroenterology.* 2000;118(6):1018-1024.

20. Kandiel A, Fraser AG, Korelitz BI, et al. Increased risk of lymphoma among inflammatory bowel disease patients treated with azathioprine and 6-mercaptopurine. *Gut.* 2005;54(8):1121-1125.
21. SEER. Surveillance, epidemiology, and end results database. Available at http://seer.cancer.gov. Accessed May 2, 2007.
22. Feagan BG, Rochon J, Fedorak RN, et al. Methotrexate for the treatment of Crohn's disease. The North American Crohn's Study Group Investigators. *N Engl J Med.* 1995;332(5):292-297.
23. Alarcon GS, Kremer JM, Macaluso M, et al. Risk factors for methotrexate-induced lung injury in patients with rheumatoid arthritis: a multicenter, case-control study. Methotrexate-Lung Study Group. *Ann Intern Med.* 1997;127(5):356-364.
24. Malatjalian DA, Ross JB, Williams CN, et al. Methotrexate hepatotoxicity in psoriatics: report of 104 patients from Nova Scotia, with analysis of risks from obesity, diabetes and alcohol consumption during long term follow-up. *Can J Gastroenterol.* 1996;10(6):369-375.
25. Siegel CA, Sands BE. Review article: practical management of inflammatory bowel disease patients taking immunomodulators. *Aliment Pharmacol Ther.* 2005;22(1):1-16.
26. Te HS, Schiano TD, Kuan SF, et al. Hepatic effects of long-term methotrexate use in the treatment of inflammatory bowel disease. *Am J Gastroenterol.* 2000;95(11):3150-3156.
27. Feagan BG, Fedorak RN, Irvine EJ, et al. A comparison of methotrexate with placebo for the maintenance of remission in Crohn's disease. North American Crohn's Study Group Investigators. *N Engl J Med.* 2000;342(22):1627-1632.
28. al-Awadhi A, Dale P, McKendry RJ. Pancytopenia associated with low dose methotrexate therapy: a regional survey. *J Rheumatol.* 1993;20(7):1121-1125.
29. Baird RD, van Zyl-Smit RN, Dilke T, et al. Spontaneous remission of low-grade B-cell non-Hodgkin's lymphoma following withdrawal of methotrexate in a patient with rheumatoid arthritis: case report and review of the literature. *Br J Haematol.* 2002;118(2):567-568.
30. Cleary AG, McDowell H, Sills JA. Polyarticular juvenile idiopathic arthritis treated with methotrexate complicated by the development of non-Hodgkin's lymphoma. *Arch Dis Child.* 2002;86(1):47-49.
31. Kennedy JW, Wong LK, Kalantarian B, et al. An unusual presentation of methotrexate-induced B-cell lymphoma of the metacarpophalangeal joint: a case report and literature review. *J Hand Surg [Am].* 2006;31(7):1193-1196.
32. Paul C, Le Tourneau A, Cayuela JM, et al. Epstein-Barr virus-associated lymphoproliferative disease during methotrexate therapy for psoriasis. *Arch Dermatol.* 1997;133(7):867-871.
33. Morris LF, Harrod MJ, Menter MA, et al. Methotrexate and reproduction in men: case report and recommendations. *J Am Acad Dermatol.* 1993;29(5 Pt 2):913-916.
34. Food and Drug Administration. Remicade (infliximab) for IV injection (prescribing information). Available at http://www.fda.gov/cder/foi/label/2002/inflcen022702LB.pdf. Accessed October 7, 2007.
35. Food and Drug Administration. Humira (adalimumab) [prescribing information]. Available at http://www.fda.gov/cder/foi/label/2002/adalabb123102LB.htm. Accessed April 30, 2007.
36. Colombel JF, Loftus EV Jr, Tremaine WJ, et al. The safety profile of infliximab in patients with Crohn's disease: the Mayo clinic experience in 500 patients. *Gastroenterology.* 2004;126(1):19-31.
37. Lichtenstein GR, Feagan BG, Cohen RD, et al. Serious infections and mortality in association with therapies for Crohn's disease: TREAT registry. *Clin Gastroenterol Hepatol.* 2006;4(5):621-630.
38. Siegel CA, Hur C, Korzenik JR, et al. Risks and benefits of infliximab for the treatment of Crohn's disease. *Clin Gastroenterol Hepatol.* 2006;4(8):1017-1024.
39. Ljung T, Karlen P, Schmidt D, et al. Infliximab in inflammatory bowel disease: clinical outcome in a population based cohort from Stockholm County. *Gut.* 2004;53(6):849-853.
40. Siegel CA, Marden SM, Persing SM, Larson RJ, Sands BE. Risk of lymphoma associated with combination anti-TNF and immunomodulator therapy for the treatment of Crohn's disease: a meta-analysis. *Clinical Gastroenterology and Hepatology.* In press.
41. Rosh JR, Gross T, Mamula P, et al. Hepatosplenic T-cell lymphoma in adolescents and young adults with Crohn's disease: a cautionary tale? *Inflamm Bowel Dis.* 2007;13(8):1024-1030.
42. Lemann M, Gerard de La Valussiere F, Bouhnik Y, et al. Intravenous cyclosporine for refractory attacks of Crohn's disease (CD): long-term follow-up of patients. *Gastroenterology.* 1998;114(4):A1020.
43. Mittal S, Milner BJ, Johnston PW, et al. A case of hepatosplenic gamma-delta T-cell lymphoma with a transient response to fludarabine and alemtuzumab. *Eur J Haematol.* 2006;76(6):531-534.
44. Navarro JT, Ribera JM, Mate JL, et al. Hepatosplenic T-gammadelta lymphoma in a patient with Crohn's disease treated with azathioprine. *Leuk Lymphoma.* 2003;44(3):531-533.
45. Targan SR, Feagan BG, Fedorak RN, et al. Natalizumab for the treatment of active Crohn's disease: results of the ENCORE Trial. *Gastroenterology.* 2007;132(5):1672-1683.
46. Van Assche G, Van Ranst M, Sciot R, et al. Progressive multifocal leukoencephalopathy after natalizumab therapy for Crohn's disease. *N Engl J Med.* 2005;353(4):362-368.
47. Warnatz K, Peter HH, Schumacher M, et al. Infectious CNS disease as a differential diagnosis in systemic rheumatic diseases: three case reports and a review of the literature. *Ann Rheum Dis.* 2003;62(1):50-57.

48. Johnson FR, Ozdemir S, Mansfield C, et al. Crohn's disease patients' risk-benefit preferences: serious adverse event risks versus treatment efficacy. *Gastroenterology.* 2007;133(3):769-779.

49. Johnson FR, Ozdemir S, Mansfield C, et al. Are adults more averse to treatment risks for their children than for themselves. Presented at the International Society of Pharmacoeconomics and Outcomes Research; Copenhagen, Denmark; October, 2006.

50. Sands BE, Siegel CA, Johnson FR, et al. Gastroenterologists' tolerance for Crohn's disease treatment risks. Presented at the United European Gastroenterology Week; Paris, France; October, 2007.

51. Cosnes J, Nion-Larmurier I, Beaugerie L, et al. Impact of the increasing use of immunosuppressants in Crohn's disease on the need for intestinal surgery. *Gut.* 2005;54(2):237-241.

52. Faubion WA Jr, Loftus EV Jr, Harmsen WS, et al. The natural history of corticosteroid therapy for inflammatory bowel disease: a population-based study. *Gastroenterology.* 2001;121(2):255-260.

53. D'Haens GR, Hommes D, Baert F, et al. A combined regimen of infliximab and azathioprine induces better endoscopic healing than classic step-up therapy in newly diagnosed Crohn's disease. *Gastroenterology.* 2006;130(4[Suppl. 2]):A110.

54. Hommes D, Baert F, Van Assche G, et al. A randomized controlled trial evaluating the ideal medical management for Crohn's disease (CD): top-down versus step-up strategies. *Gastroenterology.* 2005;128(4[Suppl. 2]):A577.

55. Hyams J, Crandall W, Kugathasan S, et al. Induction and maintenance infliximab therapy for the treatment of moderate-to-severe Crohn's disease in children. *Gastroenterology.* 2007;132(3):863-873; quiz 1165-6.

56. Munkholm P, Langholz E, Davidsen M, et al. Intestinal cancer risk and mortality in patients with Crohn's disease. *Gastroenterology.* 1993;105(6):1716-1723.

57. St Clair EW, van der Heijde DM, Smolen JS, et al. Combination of infliximab and methotrexate therapy for early rheumatoid arthritis: a randomized, controlled trial. *Arthritis Rheum.* 2004;50(11):3432-3443.

58. Breedveld FC, Weisman MH, Kavanaugh AF, et al. The PREMIER study: a multicenter, randomized, double-blind clinical trial of combination therapy with adalimumab plus methotrexate versus methotrexate alone or adalimumab alone in patients with early, aggressive rheumatoid arthritis who had not had previous methotrexate treatment. *Arthritis Rheum.* 2006;54(1):26-37.

59. Sandborn WJ, Columbel JF, Panes J, et al. Higher remission rate and maintenance of response rates with subcutaneous monthly certolizumab pegol in patients with recent-onset Crohn's disease: Data from PRECiSE 2. *Am J Gastroenterol.* 2006;101(9):S434.

60. Schreiber S, Reinisch W, Colombel JF, et al. Early Crohn's disease shows high levels of remission to therapy with adalimumab: sub-analysis of CHARM. *Gastroenterology.* 2007;132(4[Suppl. 2]):A147.

61. Klareskog L, van der Heijde D, de Jager JP, et al. Therapeutic effect of the combination of etanercept and methotrexate compared with each treatment alone in patients with rheumatoid arthritis: double-blind randomised controlled trial. *Lancet.* 2004;363(9410):675-681.

62. Bartelds GM, Wijbrandts CA, Nurmohamed MT, et al. Clinical response to adalimumab: relationship to anti-adalimumab antibodies and serum adalimumab concentrations in rheumatoid arthritis. *Ann Rheum Dis.* 2007;66(7):921-926.

63. Hanauer SB, Wagner CL, Bala M, et al. Incidence and importance of antibody responses to infliximab after maintenance or episodic treatment in Crohn's disease. *Clin Gastroenterol Hepatol.* 2004;2(7):542-553.

64. Colombel JF, Sandborn WJ, Rutgeerts P, et al. Adalimumab for maintenance of clinical response and remission in patients with Crohn's disease: the CHARM trial. *Gastroenterology.* 2007;132(1):52-65.

65. Sandborn WJ, Feagan BG, Stoinov S, et al. Certolizumab pegol for the treatment of Crohn's disease. *N Engl J Med.* 2007;357(3):228-238.

66. Kugathasan S, Ehlert R, Stephens MC, et al. Immunomodulators are not required to maintain efficacy with infliximab in pediatric inflammatory bowel disease (IBD). *Gastroenterology.* 2007;132(4[Suppl. 2]):A443.

67. Feagan BG, McDonald JWD, Panaccione R, et al. A randomized trial of methotrexate (MTX) in combination with infliximab (IFX) for the treatment of Crohn's disease (CD) [late-breaking abstract]. *Gastroenterology.* 2008;134:682c.

68. Sandborn WJ, Rutgeerts PJ, Reinisch W, et al. One year data from the SONIC study: A randomized, double-blind trial comparing infliximab and infliximab plus azathioprine to azathioprine in patients with Crohn's disease naive to immunomodulators and biologic therapy. Presented at Digestive Disease Week; Chicago, IL; June 2, 2009.

69. Vermeire S, Noman M, Van Assche G, et al. Effectiveness of concomitant immunosuppressive therapy in suppressing the formation of antibodies to infliximab in Crohn's disease. *Gut.* 2007;56(9):1226-1231.

70. Maser EA, Villela R, Silverberg MS, et al. Association of trough serum infliximab to clinical outcome after scheduled maintenance treatment for Crohn's disease. *Clin Gastroenterol Hepatol.* 2006;4(10):1248-1254.

71. Rudolph SJ, Weinberg DI, McCabe RP. Is infliximab a durable therapy for Crohn's disease? *Gastroenterology.* 2006;130(4 [Suppl 2]):A142.

72. Toruner M. Risk factors for opportunistic infections in IBD: a case-control study. *Gastroenterology.* 2006;130(4[Suppl 2]):A71.

73. Maini RN, Breedveld FC, Kalden JR, et al. Therapeutic efficacy of multiple intravenous infusions of anti-tumor necrosis factor alpha monoclonal antibody combined with low-dose weekly methotrexate in rheumatoid arthritis. *Arthritis Rheum.* 1998;41(9):1552-1563.

74. Lemann M, Mary JY, Duclos B, et al. Infliximab plus azathioprine for steroid-dependent Crohn's disease patients: a randomized placebo-controlled trial. *Gastroenterology.* 2006;130(4):1054-1061.

75. Eaden JA, Abrams KR, Mayberry JF. The risk of colorectal cancer in ulcerative colitis: a meta-analysis. *Gut.* 2001;48(4):526-535.

76. Ekbom A, Helmick C, Zack M, et al. Increased risk of large-bowel cancer in Crohn's disease with colonic involvement. *Lancet.* 1990;336(8711):357-359.

77. Siegel CA, Sands BE. Risk factors for colorectal cancer in Crohn's colitis: a case-control study. *Inflamm Bowel Dis.* 2006;12(6):491-496.

78. Jess T, Loftus EV Jr, Velayos FS, et al. Risk of intestinal cancer in inflammatory bowel disease: a population-based study from Olmsted County, Minnesota. *Gastroenterology.* 2006;130(4):1039-1046.

79. Rutter MD, Saunders BP, Wilkinson KH, et al. Thirty-year analysis of a colonoscopic surveillance program for neoplasia in ulcerative colitis. *Gastroenterology.* 2006;130(4):1030-1038.

80. Rubin DT. The changing face of colorectal cancer in inflammatory bowel disease: progress at last! *Gastroenterology.* 2006;130(4):1350-1352.

81. Kornbluth A, Sachar DB. Ulcerative colitis practice guidelines in adults (update): American College of Gastroenterology, Practice Parameters Committee. *Am J Gastroenterol.* 2004;99(7):1371-1385.

82. Rubin CE, Haggitt RC, Burmer GC, et al. DNA aneuploidy in colonic biopsies predicts future development of dysplasia in ulcerative colitis. *Gastroenterology.* 1992;103(5):1611-1620.

83. Kiesslich R, Fritsch J, Holtmann M, et al. Methylene blue-aided chromoendoscopy for the detection of intraepithelial neoplasia and colon cancer in ulcerative colitis. *Gastroenterology.* 2003;124(4):880-888.

84. Rutter MD, Saunders BP, Schofield G, et al. Pancolonic indigo carmine dye spraying for the detection of dysplasia in ulcerative colitis. *Gut.* 2004;53(2):256-260.

85. Ullman TA. Chromoendoscopy should be the standard method and more widely used for cancer surveillance colonoscopy in ulcerative colitis. *Inflamm Bowel Dis.* 2007;13(10):1273-1274.

86. Ullman T, Croog V, Harpaz N, et al. Progression of flat low-grade dysplasia to advanced neoplasia in patients with ulcerative colitis. *Gastroenterology.* 2003;125(5):1311-1319.

87. Thomas T, Abrams KA, Robinson RJ, et al. Meta-analysis: cancer risk of low-grade dysplasia in chronic ulcerative colitis. *Aliment Pharmacol Ther.* 2007;25(6):657-668.

Financial disclosure: Dr. Siegel receives grant support from Procter & Gamble; is on the advisory boards of Procter & Gamble, UCB, and Abbott; is a consultant for UCB, Abbott, and Elan; and performs CME activities for UCB and Abbott.

THE CHANGING WORLD OF INFLAMMATORY BOWEL DISEASE MANAGEMENT

THE IMPACT OF NEW THERAPIES ON OLD STRATEGIES

Ellen J. Scherl, MD, FACP, AGAF

> *These hormones (cortisone and adrenocorticotropic hormone) ... have demonstrated clearly
> the potential reversibility of many disease processes, which have been thought heretofore
> to be more or less relentlessly progressive.*[1]
> —Philip S. Hench, MD, Nobel Lecture, December 11, 1950

While defining the natural history of inflammatory bowel disease (IBD) has proven helpful in selecting treatment strategies for individual patients, it is less clear that individual therapies—specifically steroids—have altered the natural history of the disease. We have reviewed the impact of IBD on the life cycle of individuals and the evolution of the disease since it was first described. The purpose of this chapter is to contrast the life cycle of disease with the evolution of medical and surgical therapies. With the introduction of steroids in the mid-20th century, a dramatic decrease in mortality rates was noted, but the predicted reversal of disease progression has not been realized. With the recent advent of molecular-targeted therapies, the hope is that strategies will move away from treating symptoms and toward altering pathobiology of inflammation and clinical outcomes. As we enter a new millennium, we challenge the wisdom of relying on 1950s therapeutic strategies when we in fact have novel agents and approaches, namely earlier use of immunosuppression as well as personalized, targeted therapies in select patients with aggressive moderate-to-severe IBD.

It is too early to tell whether novel agents and approaches will alter the clinical outcomes or natural history of the disease. In order to understand the impact that the changing world of IBD holds for our patients, we need to step back and evaluate contextually what it means to be a patient living with IBD and a physician treating IBD in the 21st century.

Scherl EJ, Dubinsky MC.
*The Changing World of Inflammatory Bowel Disease:
Impact of Generation, Gender, and Global Trends (pp 245-260)*
© 2009 SLACK Incorporated.

History of Inflammatory Bowel Disease

The epidemiology of IBD is changing and the incidence is on the rise, raising the question as to whether it is a new disease or an old disease that is evolving.[2] In terms of first recognition, reports of IBD occurred as early as 1761, followed by other reports in the mid-1800s.[3] King Alfred the Great, who reigned as early as the 9th century, may be one of the earliest cases of IBD based on historical accounts that he experienced chronic remitting and recurring symptoms of abdominal pain and diarrhea.[4] In a retrospective study by Walker and Fielding, 29 cases of Crohn's disease were treated in Ireland in the second half of the 19th century.[5]

In 1901, tuberculosis (TB) infection of the intestines was reported in a patient, but TB tests were negative and inflammation of the intestines with nonspecific granuloma was observed.[6,7] It was the advent of the purified protein derivative (PPD) that later allowed Burrill Crohn to diagnose Crohn's disease by distinguishing it from TB and chronic appendicitis.[8-10] In 1909, researchers described 317 patients with ulcerative colitis at a symposium held at the World Society of London.[11] The earliest documented patient with Crohn's disease in Sweden was operated on in 1918 for suspected appendicitis.[12] The surgeons found a narrowing in the ileum and performed an ileobypass. It was not until 1969 that the same patient presented with perianal fistula, resection was performed, and histologic examination of the resected tissue (which included the bypassed segment of the ileum) confirmed the diagnosis of Crohn's disease.[12] This case suggests that there may be long periods before diagnosis and that the second peak incidence may actually represent missed or delayed diagnosis rather than late onset of Crohn's disease.

Dalziel, a Scottish surgeon, described IBD extensively.[13] However, it was not until 1932 that Crohn, Ginzburg, and Oppenheimer first described what is now known as Crohn's disease.[8] They described the disease as limited to the ileum and as sharply demarcated at the ileocecal valve with no colonic involvement. We now recognize that Crohn's disease can involve the colon, a combination of the ileum and colon, and in fact may involve the entire gastrointestinal tract as well as systemic extraintestinal manifestations.

A major question facing clinicians treating IBD is whether this is a single disease entity or a spectrum of multiple disorders. The nomenclature of IBD does not accurately reflect the diversity of clinical phenotypes. IBD involves a series of at least 3 diseases: ulcerative colitis, Crohn's disease, and indeterminate colitis. We often question whether there is an immunoinflammatory spectrum of diseases with mild ulcerative colitis at one end and aggressive fistulizing Crohn's disease at the other.

The life cycle of the various forms of IBD has not been extensively followed. Most randomized controlled trials are conducted over several years at best. Even clinical outcomes evaluate disease progression over a decade or a generation but not over a lifetime. One study examined biopsies from patients with long-standing ulcerative colitis who were receiving treatment and found diffuse involvement in 70% of biopsies.[14] The remaining 30% showed nondiffuse inflammation, rectal sparing, and a reversion to normal mucosa. This segmental inflammation does not necessarily reflect Crohn's disease and may accurately represent post-treatment alterations in ulcerative colitis.[14] A study of the role of serologic markers in indeterminate colitis predicted ulcerative colitis or Crohn's disease phenotype over time.[15]

The many forms of ulcerative colitis—proctitis, proctosigmoiditis, left-sided colitis, universal colitis, or proctosigmoiditis with a cecal patch—led Brooke to suggest that ulcerative colitis represents a pathologic state with various etiologies rather than a single disease entity.[16] Different bacteria and different antigens may result in diverse immunoinflammatory mucosal responses that translate into different clinical phenotypes.

Correlation of inflammatory molecular markers with different patterns of mucosal inflammation may offer a more accurate classification of Crohn's disease and ulcerative colitis, and ultimately may provide insight into heterogeneity of IBD behavior, genetic susceptibility, and stratifying therapeutic responses. The difference in types of IBD becomes important in determining appropriate treatment strategies. For example, the performance of ileal pouch-anal anastomosis in patients with indeterminate colitis is associated with a higher risk of complications compared with the same procedure performed in patients with ulcerative colitis.[17] Patients with perinuclear antineutrophil cytoplasmic antibody (pANCA)-positive titers also are more likely to fail infliximab therapy and follow a generally refractory course of the disease.[18,19] In addition, high levels of pANCA titers are consistently associated with chronic pouchitis after ileal pouch-anal anastomosis.[20,21] Serum pANCA expression in both ulcerative colitis and Crohn's disease provides evidence of a clinical, immunologic, and genetic heterogeneity among the 2 diseases and implies specific types of mucosal inflammation. Stratifying patients according to phenotypic behavior may be useful in determining more effective therapies from the outset.

In the Crohn's disease population, the presence of antibodies to *Saccharomyces cerevisiae* (ASCA) correlates with a younger age of disease onset. Patients who are double ASCA positive—express both immunoglobulin types IGA and IGG—are more likely to have stricturing, fistulizing disease and more like to require surgery.[22] Therefore, patients who are double ASCA positive may be candidates for more aggressive steroid-avoiding strategies such as earlier immunosuppression and/or targeted biologics.

Over time, Crohn's disease has changed and arguably has become more aggressive in select patients. It is debated whether steroid use is limited to more severe disease (see Chapter 6) or whether it is overused in mild-to-moderate disease, accelerating rather than ameliorating the natural history. Despite the increasing use of immunosuppression, surgical resection rates have remained stable, possibly reflecting the delayed introduction of immunosuppression after prolonged use of steroids.[23] Later use of immunologics in the context of long-term use of steroids and immunosuppression delays surgery and may negatively impact the natural history of the disease and increase the risk for infection, lymphoma in Crohn's disease, and colorectal cancer in ulcerative colitis.[24,25] Early initiation of anti-tumor necrosis factor (anti-TNF) therapy may decrease the risk for colitis-associated colorectal cancer.[26] Emerging data suggest that in select patients, early aggressive intervention with immunosuppression and/or immunologics may favorably impact the natural history of IBD.[27]

TNF-alpha is one of many proinflammatory cytokines, chemokines, and growth factors mediating intestinal inflammation. TNF-alpha mediates recruitment of leukocytes from blood vessels into intestinal mucosal through circulating cells interacting with adhesion molecules on the vascular endothelium.[28,29]

In evaluating the anti-TNF maintenance trials,[30-33] there is a trend toward more robust remission and response rates in the subgroup of patients treated early, within 2 years of onset of disease. Although the cumulative steroid dosing is difficult to quantify, many patients in these trials have been treated with steroids, immunomodulators, and in some cases previous anti-TNF therapies.[32-34] The role of regularly scheduled maintenance anti-TNF in combination with immunomodulators has not been clearly elucidated in many of the maintenance trials. In regularly scheduled combination, therapy with immunomodulators and anti-TNF agents or anti-TNF agents alone seems to make no difference on outcomes,)but these were subgroup post hoc analyses.

In contrast, the SONIC trial—a definitive large head-to-head prospective randomized controlled trial evaluating early intervention with 1 year of regularly scheduled infliximab and azathioprine in steroid-exposed moderate-to-severe Crohn's disease patients—showed that combination infliximab and azathioprine is superior in achieving steroid-free remission at 1 year in patients with moderate-to-severe disease and evidence of inflammation (elevated C-reactive protein [CRP] level and endoscopic lesions).[35] Post hoc subanalysis showed that in patients without evidence of inflammation (normal CRP and no endoscopic lesions), there was no statistical difference between azathioprine and infliximab monotherapy and marginal superiority with combination therapy in steroid-free remission rates (35%, 40%, and 50%, respectively) in patients with a CRP of less than 0.8 mg/dL.

Most gastroenterologists prescribe 6-mercaptopurine (6-MP) and azathioprine as a steroid-sparing therapy for patients with moderate Crohn's disease. However, fewer are using weight-based

6-MP orazathioprine at the time of steroid induction—6-MP/azathioprine top-down therapy. An examination of 6-MP/azathioprine maintenance of remission trials in the context of current prescribing patterns and the new SONIC data, which showed that azathioprine was consistently less effective than infliximab monotherapy or infliximab combination therapy, is instructive. A small head-to-head randomized controlled trial evaluating 6-MP in newly diagnosed Crohn's disease included 27 patients with moderate Crohn's disease who were treated with combination weight-based 6-MP 1.5 mg/kg and steroids versus 28 patients treated with steroids alone. At the end of 1.5 years, only 9% relapsed in the early intervention 6-MP combination group and more than 95% did not require repeat steroids.[36] In contrast, in the 28 patients treated with steroids alone, nearly two-thirds required repeat steroids and almost 50% relapsed. This trial is so small that the point estimates of efficacy have wide confidence intervals and the safety of the 2 regimens cannot be adequately assessed. In addition, the trial was conducted in children and does not provide strong evidence for the basis of clinical practice.

Alternatively, Candy et al found that when azathioprine weight-based 2.5 mg/kg was initiated in patients with long-standing disease, only 42% were in remission at 15 months, which compared favorably with only 7% in the placebo group (steroid taper without azathioprine maintenance).[37] However, this underscores the problem with maintenance azathioprine in steroid-exposed patients; 60% were not in remission at the end of 15 months. Furthermore, Costes et al found that long-term 4-year follow-up of steroid dependence (>6 months of steroid exposure) in moderate Crohn's disease patients showed that approximately 85% of patients treated with 6-MP or azathioprine alone or 6-MP/azathioprine in combination with 3-dose induction infliximab as a bridge strategy relapsed at 4 years.[38] Although the SONIC data are less robust in the Crohn's disease patients with less evidence of inflammation, maintenance studies[37,38] suggest that 6-MP/azathioprine does not maintain long-term clinical remission in the majority of moderate Crohn's disease patients previously treated with at least 6 months of steroids. This finding is also supported by the SONIC trial, which showed that azathioprine did not work in a large study. Furthermore, cost-benefit analyses of steroids in terms of pharmacoeconomic modeling show that patients who have had more than 3 months of steroids have increased costs to society in terms of time out of work and hospitalizations.[39] In contrast, 6-MP/azathioprine top-down therapy initiated in newly diagnosed Crohn's disease patients simultaneously with steroids was successful in achieving steroid-free remission in the majority of patients.[36] However, the study is too small to form the basis of clinical practice. In addition, in the context of SONIC, which showed less efficacy with azathioprine, it may not even be warranted to conduct a large prospective trial evaluating azathioprine/steroid top-down therapy.

SONIC data suggest that even in Crohn's disease without evidence of inflammation, combination therapy for 1 year initiated early in the disease course is more effective than azathioprine monotherapy in achieving steroid-free remission (50% versus 35%, respectively).[35] Likewise, the rates of steroid-free remission with azathioprine monotherapy were low in the Candy et al and Costes et al trials (42% at 15 months and 15% at 4 years, respectively).[37,38]

SONIC is the first definitive randomized controlled trial evaluating 1-year regularly scheduled infliximab and azathioprine as early intervention in steroid-exposed moderate-to-severe Crohn's disease patients. The SONIC trial also included patients who failed to respond to mesalamine. While infliximab and azathioprine combination therapy was superior to monotherapy in moderate-to-severe Crohn's disease of short-duration, patients with severe disease and evidence of inflammation (elevated CRP and endoscopic lesions) had the most significant improvement with combination treatment. In patients with moderate-to-severe disease and evidence of inflammation (elevated CRP and endoscopic lesions), infliximab monotherapy was superior to azathioprine monotherapy and combination therapy was more effective than either forms of monotherapy. In conclusion, SONIC is important because it is the first large prospective head-to-head trial supporting the tectonic shift toward early intervention with anti-TNF therapy and away from unlimited steroid use in moderate-to-severe Crohn's disease. The superiority of combination therapy may reflect the synergistic effect of 2 effective drugs rather than reduced immunogenicity. Serious adverse events were similar in each of the 3 arms of the SONIC trial. Although the study is not designed to evaluate combination therapy beyond 1-year duration and did not evaluate combination therapy in patients with long-standing Crohn's disease treated with long-standing sequential or simultaneous steroids, immunomodulators, or anti-TNF and biologic agents or in male adolescents and young adults, it is still the best large randomized controlled prospective head-to-head trial evaluating infliximab and azathioprine. It clearly demonstrates the superiority of infliximab monotherapy and combination therapy in the treatment of moderate-to-severe Crohn's disease with evidence of inflammation (elevated CRP and endoscopic lesions). The study also underscores the importance in determining the extent and severity of inflammation in patients with Crohn's disease prior to embarking on biologic therapy. The SONIC trial provides strong evidence for early infliximab therapy and challenges not only ending the steroid era, but also ending the immunomodulator era.

History of Therapies

Medications used to treat IBD have evolved from sulphas in the 1930s, to antibiotics in the 1940s, to steroids in the 1950s. While steroids remain the mainstay of treatment for moderate-to-severe IBD, controversy exists over whether the benefits of steroids outweigh the risks and, when used as long-term treatment, whether these agents may mask the underlying disease process, allowing for progression. In contrast, immunosuppressive agents introduced in the 1960s and immunologics introduced in the 1990s may prove to be steroid sparing, steroid avoiding, as well as disease modifying.

STEROID ERA

In 1950, with the introduction of adrenocorticotropic hormone and prednisone, it was felt that disease progression would be reversed in both IBD and rheumatoid arthritis. That same year, Hench et al described steroids as clearly demonstrating the potential reversibility of disease processes, which had been thought to be relentlessly progressive.[40] In the presteroid era, the mortality rate for ulcerative colitis was as high as 35%.[41] With the advent of steroids, this mortality rate decreased dramatically to less than 1%.[41]

In 1955, Truelove and Witts noted that steroid-treated patients showed improved clinical outcomes compared with placebo-treated patients but at the expense of increased infectious complications and with no prevention of recurrence.[42] In 1959, they went on to recognize a higher relapse rate in patients treated with adrenocorticotropic hormone.[43] This paper ushered subsequent observations that repeated steroid use resulted in shorter duration of response. In 1965, Lennard-Jones et al concluded that prednisone was ineffective in preventing relapse of ulcerative colitis.[44]

In a more recent population-based study by Faubion et al, steroids were effective in 84% of patients with Crohn's disease and induced either complete or partial remission within 1 month.[45] However, the 1-year outcomes were less encouraging, with 38% of patients requiring surgery and 28% developing steroid dependence. Patients with ulcerative colitis also showed dramatic results initially with 84% showing complete or partial remission at 1 month, but at the end of 1 year more than 50% of patients were either steroid dependent (22%) or steroid refractory (29%), requiring total proctocolectomy. A prospective cohort study by Munkholm et al showed similar findings for patients with Crohn's disease.[46] Furthermore, while the acute natural history of ulcerative colitis changed favorably with the advent of steroids, the longstanding natural history in terms of surgical therapies for both ulcerative colitis and Crohn's disease has not been reversed and remains at 30% and 70%, respectively. Thus, steroids appear to be effective in induction of remission for IBD, but not in maintaining remission. Pharmacoeconomic modeling has demonstrated that continuous steroid use for greater than 3 months results in significant costs to society and third-party payers.[39]

In patients with Crohn's disease who are steroid dependent (defined as greater than 6 months of steroid use), short-term infliximab was ineffective as a bridge to azathioprine maintenance therapy in both azathioprine-naïve and azathioprine-experienced patients over a 4-year follow-up period.[38] Furthermore, the risks of prolonged use of steroids include metabolic disturbances, infections, glaucoma, emotional and psychiatric disturbances, impaired wound healing, and metabolic bone disease.[47]

While our use of steroids has remained unchanged since the 1950s, much has changed in our understanding of the science of IBD. We now understand that IBD is in part due to an overactive immune response requiring suppressive therapy but also to an underactive innate immune response requiring immunostimulation with agents such as granulocyte-macrophage colony stimulating factors.[48] There has been a movement at a cellular level toward understanding that TNF as well as TH1- and TH2-type immune responses may be observed in both Crohn's disease and ulcerative colitis.[49,50] Research also has focused on identifying serologic immunomarkers and genotyping in IBD. Despite this progress and the introduction of immunomodulators, novel biologics, and the promise of small molecules, we continue to use steroids much the way we did in mid-century.[51,52]

The American College of Gastroenterology (ACG) guidelines underscore the recommendations for steroids for induction of remission in both moderate and severe ulcerative colitis and Crohn's disease, much as they were used in the 1950s.[47,53] The guidelines on Crohn's disease highlight that "corticosteroids should not be used as long-term agents to prevent relapse of Crohn's disease. Azathioprine/mercaptopurine have demonstrable maintenance benefits after inductive therapy with corticosteroids. Mesalamine or azathioprine/mercaptopurine should be considered after ileocolonic resections to reduce the likelihood of symptomatic recurrence."[47] A recent American Gastroenterological Association position paper echoes the ACG guideline recommendations to use steroids as initial treatment in moderate-to-severe Crohn's disease and ulcerative colitis but not as maintenance therapy.[54] Developing an exit strategy seems prudent in the management of patients receiving steroids for treatment of ulcerative colitis or Crohn's disease. However, no guidelines for limiting steroid duration or tapering strategies exist.

The real issue is to understand the impact of steroids on the natural history of both ulcerative colitis and Crohn's disease and to determine whether steroids mask the underlying disease process, confounding the underlying natural history of Crohn's disease and ultimately revealing a gaping wound whereby steroids become nothing but a superimposed salve. Do steroids disarm the immune balance and mask the dreaded signals of a disease gone unchecked? Are we missing signals that are muted by steroids, which are used to treat flare-to-flare, day-to-day manifestations of the disease rather than addressing the underlying causes of the disease?

If IBD is in part the result of inappropriately activated T cells and a failure of T regulatory cells, and if steroids are thought in part to propagate-activated, IBD-associated T cells, then in the long run it is conceivable that steroids perpetuate activated IBD-associated T cells and will be unable to reverse the natural history of progressive IBD.[55] These newly gained perspectives of the mechanism of disease may allow research to move in a more proactive direction toward targeting molecules instead of treating symptoms. The hope is that long-term outcomes will be altered favorably with a decrease in colectomy rates and fistulizing structural damage in Crohn's disease.

Is This the End of the Steroid Era?

The goal of therapy is to reverse progression of disease and favorably affect the natural history of disease. An assumption is made to identify more aggressive disease at an earlier onset and to treat select patients more aggressively with immunomodulators or biologics and eventually small molecules and stem cells. Defining the natural history of IBD in identifying more aggressive disease has proven helpful in selecting treatment for patients with Crohn's disease/IBD and also rheumatoid arthritis. Generally, Crohn's disease and rheumatoid arthritis are regarded as chronic, lifelong diseases that may be aggressive and unpredictable with systemic manifestations resulting in tissue and structural damage—either fistulizing and stricturing disease in IBD or joint destruction in rheumatoid arthritis.

In the 1950s, steroids were the basis for treatment of rheumatoid arthritis. There was a paradigm shift in the 1990s with the introduction of infliximab, which has resulted in a 5-fold decrease in joint replacement (25% to 5%).[56] The therapeutic approach in rheumatoid arthritis has shifted toward aggressive, early intervention with methotrexate and biologics (namely anti-TNF therapy) with lifelong maintenance strategies aimed at reversal of joint destruction.[57] In contrast, earlier top-down intervention with azathioprine and infliximab results in durable mucosal healing and clinical remission in Crohn's disease.[27]

Certainly, there has been increasing concern among patients with IBD regarding adverse events in relation to combination treatment, resulting largely from layering immunomodulators and biologics in the context of steroids.[24] Studies have shown complications of progressive multifocal leukoencephalopathy related to combination therapy with nataluzimab and azathioprine[58] and hepatosplenic T-cell lymphomas largely in patients with Crohn's disease related to combination therapy with steroids, azathioprine, and infliximab. These increasing reports of adverse events have prompted a movement toward monotherapy. Re-evaluation of more aggressive, early intervention is challenging our prolonged use of steroids.

A recent study by D'Haens et al showed that early use of combined immunosuppression in steroid-naïve moderate-to-severe Crohn's disease avoided the need for steroids and resulted in early onset of remission and sustained mucosal healing over 2 years.[27] A new therapeutic goal is steroid-free remission with durable mucosal and histologic healing.[35]

The evolution of IBD has occurred in the context of unlimited steroid use. Since the first description of IBD in the early 20th century, the disease has evolved from limited ileal inflammation to more extensive and more aggressive intestinal as well as extraintestinal manifestations in select patients. Whether steroids are an epiphenomenon or are associated with acceleration of the disease is yet unknown. IBD was recognized as a rarity at the turn of the 20th century and is increasingly recognized in epidemic proportions at the beginning of the 21st century, suggesting that alterations in enteric bacteria should be strongly considered as a cause, raising the question of industrialization as a contributing factor and challenging the unlimited dosing and duration of steroids.

Evidence for Infection

At the beginning of the 20th century, the challenge was to unmask IBD masquerading as TB. The goal in the new millennium is to unmask TB masquerading as IBD in immunosuppressed individuals and to understand the interaction of luminal bacteria and intestinal immunoregulation in genetically susceptible hosts.

At the turn of the last century, Lartigau—a pathologist at Columbia—first described differences in classic TB and a new entity of a thickening of the distal two-thirds of the ileum associated with a rigid ileocecal valve.[6] He described nonepithelial granuloma, which were aggregates of lymphoid cells with occasional giant cells with little or no necrotic changes. He recognized that this process—later to be called Crohn's disease—was different than pulmonary or intestinal TB.

Research has studied the phagocytosis of TB bacilli and granuloma formation with the associated corralling of TNF and interferon gamma. There is secondary cytokine and chemokine release and recruitment of lymphocytes with a multiplying cascade of activated T cells and macrophages, leading to intracellular phagocytosis, bacilli death, and granuloma formation.

Granulomas (TB positive and negative) are active immune processes that corral TNF. The risk of TB in association with anti-TNF agents is increasingly recognized; however, the risk of TB in patients on steroids and/or immunosuppressive agents (methotrexate, 6-MP, azathioprine) historically has not been addressed.

Although steroids are increasingly recognized as risk factors for infection and increased mortality,[24,59,60] consensus recommendations for evaluating the risk of TB in negative chest x-ray, PPD-positive IBD patients are warranted. It is prudent to perform computed tomography scan of the chest, TB polymerase chain reaction (PCR) analysis, intestinal biopsies with cultures for acid-fast bacillus smear, as well as stool TB PCR and acid-fast bacilli testing in patients who are PPD positive and have negative findings on chest x-ray prior to initiating isoniazid therapy. Quantiferon-TB gold test for interferon-gamma release is another method for detecting TB, especially in immunosuppressed patients with IBD.[61] There are no guidelines for TB screening in IBD patients taking steroid and/or immunosuppressive agents (methotrexate, 6-MP, azathioprine). The focus has been on patients treated with biologics.

Molecular genotyping or fingerprinting of bacterial TB has enhanced our understanding of the pathogenesis and transmission of TB[62] and reflects huge strides from 1890 when Koch first announced the discovery of tuberculin, a substance derived from the tubercle bacilli.[63] The initial diagnosis of TB occurred with the description of acid-fast bacteria by Ehrlich in 1882, the development of x-rays by Roentgen in 1895, tuberculin skin test by Mantoux and Von Pirquet in 1907, and finally the PPD of tuberculin by Florence Siebert in 1930.[63]

Koch's studies on TB, known as Koch's postulates, required that one observe the tubercle bacilli in association with all diagnosed TB cases, grow the bacteria in culture, and that the disease be reproduced in a susceptible host into whom the bacterium is inoculated.[63] The role of bacteria in IBD has been documented, but no isolated bacteria or cluster of bacteria have fulfilled Koch's postulates in reproducing IBD.

The best evidence for the role of bacteria in IBD is from numerous genetically engineered animal models that are susceptible to developing IBD only in the presence of luminal bacteria and fail to develop the disease in a germ-free environment.[64] D'Haens et al have demonstrated that resection of Crohn's ileocolitis with proximal ileal diversion (ileostomy) results in no recurrent disease.[65] Reanastomosis results in clinical recurrence in less than a month and reinfusion of the luminal contents results in inflammation in 1 week. Increased mucosa-associated bacteria has been identified on ileal biopsies.[66] Adherent-invasive *Escherichia coli* strains have been associated with ileal Crohn's disease.[67] Recently, a selective increase in a novel group of invasive *E. coli* using library array and other culture-independent analysis of bacterial diversity (16S rDNA library analysis, quantitative PCR and fluorescence in situ hybridization, and molecular characterization of cultured bacteria) has been observed in patients with ileal Crohn's disease and may be involved in the disease pathogenesis.[68]

The path of IBD immunology has run parallel to our criminal justice system in that both are moving away from a reliance on biological phenotyping, clinical diagnosis, and fingerprinting in favor of more reliable and quantifiable markers, such as variations in DNA sequencing.[69] Mutations in a variety of genes have been associated with IBD and specific IBD phenotypes. The NOD2 gene (encoding nucleotide-binding oligomerization domain protein 2) is associated with the sensing of and tolerance to intraluminal bacteria and underscores the importance of regulating responses to bacteria while maintaining intestinal immune tolerance and homeostasis. NOD2 mutations may be associated with fibrostenosing ileal Crohn's disease phenotypes. Both NOD2 and autophagy-related genes ATG16L1 (encoding autophagy related 16-like 1 protein) and IRGM (encoding immunity-related GTPase family M) are associated with innate immune responses in Crohn's disease and emphasize that this disease may result from dysregulated immune responses to luminal bacteria in genetically vulnerable individuals. The gene encoding interleukin 23 (IL-23) receptor is associated with the acquired immune response mediating T helper 17 (TH17) regulatory cells in both ulcerative colitis and Crohn's disease.[70] Recently published genome-wide association studies have confirmed findings related to the NOD2 gene and the IBD5 locus. The studies have also identified more than 30 novel loci and several promising associations between

Crohn's disease and gene variants, the two most widely replicated being variants in the IL23R and ATG16L1 genes. These findings further support the importance of the immune system and its interactions with the intestinal flora in the pathogenesis of inflammatory bowel disease.[71]

Much has changed in our understanding of microbiology and immunogenetics since the 1950s. There has been a shift in focus from acquired immune responses occurring in the deeper layers of the lamina propria to include the superficial epithelial layers of the innate immune response. Our bacterial microflora/microbiome along with dendritic cells form part of our first-line defense.[72] We have redefined mucosal barriers to include dendritic cells sampling luminal bacteria and learned that bacteria microflora compose a protective biofilm, allowing for colonization resistance as well as local gene regulation in the intestinal epithelial. This continuous crosstalk between bacteria and gut immune responses lead to activation of T and B cells. T cells may be inhibited by anti-inflammatory immunosuppressive cytokine and regulatory cells.[73,74]

Cytokines are a diverse family of soluble immunomodulatory proteins and peptides that act as hormone regulators under both normal and pathologic conditions. Cytokines modulate the functional activities of individual cells and tissues and enable communication between cells, controlling cellular proliferation. They are involved in activating many cell types and are pleiotropic, playing pivotal roles in a variety of functions such as immune regulation, tumor surveillance, tissue repair, hemangiogenesis, and T-cell subset differentiation.

With this enlarging view of gut immune response to include not only acquired immune response but also innate immune response, there is a shift from immunosuppression of an overactive acquired immune system to include elements of immunostimulation of an underactive innate immune system with granulocyte-macrophage colony stimulating factors targeting the granulocyte, the common effector cell of the innate immune system. Another change is the introduction of serologic markers and antibody profiling as a window into observing and characterizing the disregulated immune response.

Evidence Versus Experience: How to Address Issues of the Life Cycle in Patients With Inflammatory Bowel Disease?

Since the first descriptions of IBD, the evidence and the experience of managing the disease is changing as the disease itself is evolving into a more aggressive, extensive, and systemic disease. A nuanced view presents IBD as an immunoinflammatory spectrum of chronic recurring inflammation beginning with mild ulcerative colitis at one end and severe ulcerative colitis and stricturing, fistulizing Crohn's disease with extraintestinal manifestations at the other.

IBD affects younger, older, and more diverse populations than initially appreciated. The changing world of IBD underscores the difference between IBD populations and the general population, with the highest prevalence occurring in industrialized countries and intermediate prevalence occurring in post-World War II developing countries: Japan, Korea, the Middle East, Hong Kong, Israel, and South Africa. Areas with the lowest prevalence have the highest frequency of intestinal infections, specifically helminthic infections. IBD is increasingly recognized globally in epidemic proportions, suggesting alterations in enteric bacterial flora as a cause, with different antigens possibly related to diverse mucosal immune responses. The role of probiotics and antibiotics in IBD is being elucidated. Historically treatment has been started with 5-aminosalicylic acid anti-inflammatory mesalamines and stepped up to steroids. With the advent of immunosuppressants and the novel array of biologics (anti-TNF agents, anti-integrins), small molecules, stem cells, and the failure of steroids to alter the long-term natural history of these disabling diseases, the pyramidal approach to treatment is being challenged.

STEROIDS

While evidence from randomized controlled trials still supports the role of steroids in treating IBD, clinicians' experience and observations question the long-term impact steroids have on disease progression. Within the first decade of steroid introduction, it was noted that they were ineffective in preventing relapse. Furthermore, repeated use of steroids was associated with shorter duration of response and increased pyogenic complications.[42-44]

Yet, clinicians currently prescribe steroids much the way they did half a century ago. We persist in using 1950s strategies when we have novel targeted molecular and cellular therapies. Although we are concerned about long-term steroid toxicity, there is a discrepancy between our clinical experience and evidence-based trials.[75]

Evidence shows 80% response rates to steroids in the first month of use. However, at the end of a year, approximately two-thirds of patients are either steroid dependent or steroid refractory. Steroids have not altered the natural history of ulcerative colitis, colectomy rates, or stricturing, fistulizing damage in Crohn's disease.[23,76,77]

Despite the 80% response rate with infliximab within 2 weeks in medically refractory Crohn's disease, the medical community has been slow to embrace early anti-TNF therapy in moderate-to-severe Crohn's disease.[49] In randomized controlled trials evaluating infliximab in ulcerative colitis and Crohn's disease, between 50% to 60% of patients entering those trials were on steroids, arguably blunting the full impact of anti-TNF therapy on reversing progression of disease and blunting the steroid-sparing effect of anti-TNF therapy.[30,78,79] A trial evaluating early infliximab and immunosuppression (azathioprine) suggested that this combination was steroid avoiding and was associated with mucosal healing and sustained remission rates at 2 years in patients with Crohn's disease.[27]

Steroids and Crohn's Disease

Emerging evidence suggests that mucosal healing in Crohn's disease is associated with durable clinical remission[80] and is more likely to occur with scheduled infliximab therapy rather than episodic therapy.[81] Scheduled maintenance infliximab therapy has been associated with decreased hospitalization and surgery rates.[82,83]

A study by Costes et al showed that short-term use of infliximab combined with azathioprine maintenance was ineffective in patients with steroid-dependent Crohn's disease (greater than 6 months of steroid use), regardless of whether the patients were azathioprine experienced or naïve. The findings suggest that if immunologics or azathioprine are introduced late in the course of Crohn's disease, the full therapeutic effects of these agents may be diluted by background use of steroids.[38] That being said, infliximab maintenance monotherapy may prove more effective than azathioprine (with or without infliximab) in steroid-dependent Crohn's disease.

A study examining the efficacy of azathioprine in maintaining remission in conjunction with prednisone taper over 12 weeks showed that only 42% of patients were in remission at the end of 15 months.[37] Among the predictors of a disabling course in Crohn's disease is a requirement for corticosteroids during the first flare.[84] A large definitive head-to-head randomized controlled study demonstrated that 1-year combination therapy with infliximab and azathioprine is superior to infliximab or azathioprine monotherapy in achieving steroid-free remission.[35]

Steroids and Ulcerative Colitis

Similarly, steroids are ineffective in altering colectomy rates over time, and even when used in newly diagnosed ulcerative colitis within the first year of diagnosis, nearly three-quarters of patients relapse within 1 year of the first steroid course.[75] Infliximab is effective for inducing mucosal healing and remission in steroid-dependent ulcerative colitis and may prove more effective if used earlier in steroid-naïve patients with colitis.[50,85,86]

EARLY IMMUNOSUPPRESSION AND BIOLOGICS

In contrast, early introduction of immunosuppression in newly diagnosed Crohn's disease is steroid sparing in 96% of patients over a 1.5-year period[36] and steroid avoiding over a 2-year period.[27] Earlier introduction of biologics also is associated with prolonged steroid-free remission rates.[32-35,77,81] When scheduled maintenance therapy with infliximab is introduced within 2 years of disease onset, 50% of children remain off steroids and in clinical remission at the end of the first year of treatment.[80] In contrast, later introduction of anti-TNF therapy (after 5 to 7 years of disease) results in less robust steroid-free remission rates.[30,79,87] Similarly, in a study involving patients with Crohn's disease of less than 2 years duration, 50% were in remission at 1 year after receiving 40 mg adalimumab subcutaneously once a week or every other week.[33] Early intervention with induction and maintenance therapy for 1 year consisting of infliximab combination therapy or monotherapy is superior to azathioprine monotherapy in achieving steroid-free remission in moderate-to-severe Crohn's disease. Natalizumab induction and maintenance of remission occurs in consistently higher rates with nearly 25% of patients with Crohn's disease of less than 3 years showing sustained remission.[58,88] Of the 10-week natalizumab responders, 55% of patients receiving natalizumab 300 mg every 4 weeks were in steroid-free remission at week 36.[89]

CLINICAL OUTCOMES AND ADVERSE EVENTS

Although the long-term clinical outcomes of early immunosuppression and biologics on IBD are largely unknown, pharmacoeconomic studies reveal beneficial effects of early intervention on hospitalization and surgical rates as well as cost to society and third-party payers.[39] Early intervention may minimize the adverse events related to sequential and/or simultaneous combination therapy and delayed surgery seen with prolonged steroid use and by definition delayed immunosuppression and biologic use. The TREAT registry echoes the pyogenic complications recognized shortly after steroids were initially introduced.[24,44] Long-term follow-up of approximately 2000 Crohn's disease patients in the ENCORE registry underscores the TREAT registry findings that steroids, not infliximab, pose increased risk for serious infections.[60,90] Earlier introduction of more aggressive therapies may be chemopreventive.[26]

Combined cyclosporine and infliximab as acute salvage therapies for each other in severe steroid-refractory ulcerative colitis resulted in a 15% rate of serious adverse events including a single death due to *E. coli* sepsis.[91] Patients with IBD who receive more than 3 immunosuppressants and/or biologic therapies may react like post-transplant patients and are at increased risk for developing Epstein-Barr virus-positive lymphoma.[92] As we use combinations of immunosuppressives and/or biologics—in steroid-naïve, steroid-dependent, or steroid-refractory patients—clear guidelines for preventing opportunistic infections and registries for correlating early versus late introduction of immunosuppressants or biologics and for documenting lymphomas and cancer risks need to be implemented.[59] Hepatosplenic T-cell lymphoma has been associated with azathioprine monotherapy or in combination with infliximab or adalimumab in male adolescents and young adults.[93]

SURGICAL OUTCOMES

Surgical complication rates remain low. In a study by Rutgeerts et al involving a cohort of 743 patients treated with infliximab for Crohn's disease and ulcerative colitis, only one complication occurred following surgery.[50] Just as earlier intervention with immunosuppression and targeted molecular and cellular therapies may prove beneficial, earlier surgical intervention also may be of benefit with minimally invasive laparoscopic techniques and novel bowel-sparing strictureplasty.[94,95] Optimally timed surgery should be viewed as a treatment not as a failure of therapy. Delayed introduction of immunologics and/or immunosuppression in the context of long-term steroid use (ie, greater than 3 to 6 months) may delay surgery thereby increasing infectious complications as well as the risk for cancer and lymphoma.[24,25]

Summary

With increasing and ever changing medical and surgical options for patients living with IBD and for physicians managing IBD, the best approach is a multidisciplinary and interactive collaboration. In select patients with moderate-to-severe disease, an earlier aggressive approach will be indicated; in other patients with mild-to-moderate disease, stepping back and challenging the diagnosis, de-escalating medication dose, and stressing adherence to therapeutic regimens are in order. Identifying immunologically vulnerable subsets of patients with emerging serologic markers, biomarkers, and ultimately genotyping may allow for stratification of therapeutic responses and personalized medicine.

Decoding the human genome is redefining the science of individuality, reminding us that less than 0.1% of our DNA is responsible for disease susceptibility and therapeutic response.[96-98] While we are poised to recognize the potential for genotyping informing our therapeutic options, we are not yet using genotyping as routine in selection of optimal therapies. We are at a threshold for genotyping both individual patients and bacteria, which will lead to a greater understanding of the pathobiology of IBD and improving clinical outcomes.[99]

Until the science of the human genome and microbiome translates into personalized medicine, predicting the outcome of disease progression may best be achieved by looking back at our past therapies, specifically steroids. There has been a tectonic shift toward early biologic or immunosuppressive therapy aimed at steroid-free remission with mucosal and histologic healing. Identifying select patients with evidence of moderate-to-severe disease for early intervention with immunosuppression and/or biologic therapies—and limited steroids—will make current therapies safer and may favorably affect the natural history of IBD.

References

1. Hench PS. The reversibility of certain rheumatic and non-rheumatic conditions by the use of cortisone or of the pituitary adrenocorticotropic hormone. Nobel Lecture, December 11, 1950.
2. Diamond J. *Guns, Germs and Steel. The Fates of Human Societies.* New York, NY: W. W. Norton & Company, 1997.
3. Kirsner JB. Historical aspects of inflammatory bowel disease. *J Clin Gastroenterol.* 1988;10(3):286-297.
4. Craig, G. Alfred the Great: a Diagnosis. *J R Soc Med.* 1991;84:303-305.
5. Walker JF, Fielding JF. Crohn's disease in Dublin in the latter half of the nineteenth century. *Ir J Med Sci.* 1988;157(7):235-237.
6. Lartigau AJ. A study of chronic hyperplastic tuberculosis of the intestine with report of a case. *J Exp Med.* 1901;6:23-51. Cited by Kyle J. *Crohn's Disease.* New York, NY: Appleton-Century-Crofts.;1972.
7. Braun H. Uber entzundliche geschwulste es netz. *Arch Klin Chir.* 1901;63:378-381.
8. Crohn BB, Ginzburg L, Oppenheimer GD. Regional ileitis: a pathological and clinical entity. *JAMA.* 1932;99:1323-1328.
9. Seibert FB. Precipitin tests and differentiation of various tuberculin and timothy-bacillus proteins. *Amer Rev Tuberc.* 1930;21:370-382.
10. McCarter J, Kanne EM, Hastings EM. Precipitins for the tuberculin proteins of acid-fast bacteria. *J Bacteriol.* 1939;37:461-469.
11. Hawkins HP. An address on the natural history of ulcerative colitis and its bearing on treatment. *BMJ.* 1909;1:765-770
12. Ekbom A. The changing faces of Crohn's disease and ulcerative colitis. In: Targan S, Shanahan F, Karp LC, eds. *Inflammatory Bowel Disease: From Bench to Bedside.* 2nd ed. New York, NY: Kluewer Academic Publishers; 2003:5-20.
13. Dalziel TK. Chronic interstitial enteritis. *BMJ.* 1913;2:1068-1070.
14. Kleer CG, Appelman HD. Ulcerative colitis: patterns of involvement in colorectal biopsies and changes with time. *Am J Surg Pathol.* 1998;22(8):983-989.
15. Joossens S, Reinisch W, Vermeire S, et al. The value of serologic markers in indeterminate colitis: a prospective follow-up study. *Gastroenterology.* 2002;122(5):1242-1247.
16. Brooke BN. *Ulcerative Colitis and Its Surgical Treatment.* Edinburgh, Scotland: E&S Livingston; 1954.
17. Koltun, Schoetz DJ, Roberts PL, Murray JJ, Coller JA, Veidenheimer MC. Indeterminate colitis predisposes to perineal complications after ileal pouch-anal anastomosis. *Dis Colon Rectum.* 1991;34(10):857-860.

18. Vasiliauskas EA, Plevy SE, Landers CJ, et al. Perinuclear antineutrophil cytoplasmic antibodies in patients with Crohn's disease define a clinical subgroup. *Gastroenterology.* 1996;110(6):1810-1819.

19. Esters N, Vermeire S, Joossens S, et al. Serological markers for prediction of response to anti-tumor necrosis factor treatment in Crohn's disease. *Am J Gastroenterol.* 2002;97:1458-1462.

20. Fleshner PR, Vasiliauskas EA, Kam LY, et al. High level perinuclear antineutrophil cytoplasmic antibody (pANCA) in ulcerative colitis patients before colectomy predicts the development of chronic pouchitis after ileal pouch-anal anastomosis. *Gut.* 2001;49(5):671-677.

21. Fleshner P, Ippoliti A, Dubinsky M, et al. Both preoperative perinuclear antineutrophil cytoplasmic antibody and anti-CBir1 expression in ulcerative colitis patients influence pouchitis development after ileal pouch-anal anastomosis. *Clin Gastroenterol Hepatol.* 2008;6(5):561-568.

22. Vasiliauskas EA, Kam LY, Karp LC, Gaiennie J, Yang H, Targan SR. Marker antibody expression stratifies Crohn's disease into immunologically homogeneous subgroups with distinct clinical characteristics. *Gut.* 2000;47(4):487-496.

23. Cosnes J, Nion-Larmurier I, Beaugerie L, Afchain P, Tiret E, Gendre JP. Impact of the increasing use of immunosuppressants in Crohn's disease on the need for intestinal surgery. *Gut.* 2005;54(2):237-241.

24. Lichtenstein GR, Feagan BG, Cohen RD, et al. Serious infections and mortality in association with therapies for Crohn's disease: TREAT registry. *Clin Gastroenterol Hepatol.* 2006;4(5):621-630.

25. Beaugerie L, Carrat F, Bouvier A-M, et al. Excess risk of lymphoproliferative disorders in inflammatory bowel disease: interim results of the Cesame cohort. *Gastroenterology.* 2008;134:A-116[abstract 818].

26. Wilson JA. Tumor necrosis factor alpha and colitis-associated colon cancer. *N Engl J Med.* 2008;358:2733-2734.

27. D'Haens G, Baert F, van Assche G, et al. Early combined immunosuppression or conventional management in patients with newly diagnosed Crohn's disease: an open randomised trial. *Lancet.* 2008;371(9613):660-667.

28. Podolsky DK. Inflammatory bowel disease. *N Engl J Med.* 2002;347(6):417-429.

29. Brown SJ, Mayer L. The immune response in inflammatory bowel disease. *Am J Gastroenterol.* 2007;102(9):2058-2069.

30. Hanauer SB, Feagan BG, Lichtenstein GR, et al. Maintenance infliximab for Crohn's disease: the ACCENT I randomised trial. *Lancet.* 2002;359(9317):1541-1549.

31. Sands BE, Blank MA, Patel K, van Deventer SJ; ACCENT II Study. Long-term treatment of rectovaginal fistulas in Crohn's disease: response to infliximab in the ACCENT II Study. *Clin Gastroenterol Hepatol.* 2004;2(10):912-920.

32. Sandborn WJ, Feagan BG, Stoinov S, et al, and the PRECiSE 1 Study Investigators. Certolizumab pegol for the treatment of Crohn's disease. *N Engl J Med.* 2007;357(3):228-238.

33. Colombel JF, Sandborn WJ, Rutgeerts P, et al. Adalimumab for maintenance of clinical response and remission in patients with Crohn's disease: The CHARM trial. *Gastroenterology.* 2007;132(1):52-65.

34. Schreiber S, Khaliq-Kareemi M, Lawrance IC, et al, and the PRECiSE 2 Study Investigators. Maintenance therapy with certolizumab pegol for Crohn's disease. *N Engl J Med.* 2007;357(3):239-250.

35. Sandborn WJ, Rutgeerts PJ, Reinisch W, et al. One year data from the SONIC Study: a randomized, double-blind trial comparing infliximab and infliximab plus azathioprine to azathioprine in patients with Crohn's disease naive to immunomodulators and biologic therapy. Presented at: Digestive Diseases Week 2009; June 2, 2009; Chicago, Illinois. Abstract 751F.

36. Markowitz J, Grancher K, Kohn N, Lesser M, Daum F. A multicenter trial of 6-mercaptopurine and prednisone in children with newly diagnosed Crohn's disease. *Gastroenterology.* 2000;119(4):895-902.

37. Candy S, Wright J, Gerber M, Adams G, Gerig M, Goodman R. A controlled double blind study of azathioprine in the management of Crohn's disease. *Gut.* 1995;37(5):674-678.

38. Costes L, Colombel J-F, Mary J-Y, et al. Long term follow-up of a cohort of steroid-dependent Crohn's disease patients included in a randomized trial evaluating short term infliximab combined with azathioprine. *Gastroenterology.* 2008;134;A-134[abstract 921].

39. Feagan BG, Loftus EV, Kamm MA, et al. Impact of steroid discontinuation on healthcare resource utilization in Crohn's disease. *Am J Gastroenterol.* 2007;102(suppl 2):S445-S446.

40. Hench PS, Slocumb CH, Polley HF, Kendal EC. Effect of cortisone and pituitary adrenocorticotropic hormone (ACTH) on rheumatic diseases. *JAMA.* 1950;144(16):1327-1335.

41. Truelove SC, Jewell DP. Intensive intravenous regimen for severe attacks of ulcerative colitis. *Lancet.* 1974;1:1067-1070.

42. Truelove SC, Witts LJ. Cortisone in ulcerative colitis; final report on a therapeutic trial. *Br Med J.* 1955;2(4947):1041-1048.

43. Truelove SC, Witts LJ. Cortisone and corticotrophin in ulcerative colitis. *Br Med J.* 1959;1(5119):387-394.

44. Lennard-Jones JE, Misiewicz JJ, Connell AM, Baron JH, Jones FA. Prednisone as maintenance treatment for ulcerative colitis in remission. *Lancet.* 1965;1(7378):188-189.

45. Faubion WA Jr, Loftus EV Jr, Harmsen WS, Zinsmeister AR, Sandborn WJ. The natural history of corticosteroid therapy for inflammatory bowel disease: a population-based study. *Gastroenterology.* 2001;121:255-260.

46. Munkholm P, Langholz E, Davidsen M, Binder V. Frequency of glucocorticoid resistance and dependency in Crohn's disease. *Gut.* 1994;35(3):360-362.

47. Kornbluth A, Sachar DB. Ulcerative colitis practice guidelines in adults (update): American College of Gastroenterology, Practice Parameters Committee. *Am J Gastroenterol.* 2004;99:1371-1385.

48. Dieckgraefe BK, Korzenik JR. Treatment of active Crohn's disease with recombinant human granulocyte-macrophage colony-stimulating factor. *Lancet.* 2002;360(9344):1478-1480.

49. Targan SR, Hanauer SB, van Deventer SJ, et al. A short-term study of chimeric monoclonal antibody cA2 to tumor necrosis factor alpha for Crohn's disease. Crohn's Disease cA2 Study Group. *N Engl J Med.* 1997;337(15):1029-1035.

50. Rutgeerts P, Sandborn WJ, Feagan BG, et al. Infliximab for induction and maintenance therapy for ulcerative colitis. *N Engl J Med.* 2005;353:2462-2476.

51. Summers RW, Switz DM, Sessions JT Jr, et al. National Cooperative Crohn's Disease Study: results of drug treatment. *Gastroenterology.* 1979;77(4 Pt 2):847-869.

52. Malchow H, Ewe K, Brandes JW, et al. European Cooperative Crohn's Disease Study (ECCDS): results of drug treatment. *Gastroenterology.* 1984;86(2):249-266.

53. Lichtenstein GR, Hanauer SB, Sandborn WJ; Practice Parameters Committee of American College of Gastroenterology. Management of Crohn's disease in adults. *Am J Gastroenterol.* 2009;104(2):465-483.

54. Lichtenstein GR, Abreu MT, Cohen R, Tremaine W; American Gastroenterological Association. American Gastroenterological Association Institute medical position statement on corticosteroids, immunomodulators, and infliximab in inflammatory bowel disease. *Gastroenterology.* 2006;130(3):935-939.

55. Williams AM, Whiting CV, Bonhagen K, et al. Tumour necrosis factor-alpha (TNF-alpha) transcription and translation in the CD4+ T cell-transplanted scid mouse model of colitis. *Clin Exp Immunol.* 1999;116(3):415-424.

56. Maini R, St Clair EW, Breedveld F, et al. Infliximab (chimeric anti-tumor necrosis factor alpha monoclonal antibody) versus placebo in rheumatoid arthritis patients receiving concomitant methotrexate: a randomised phase III trial. ATTRACT Study Group. *Lancet.* 1999;354(9194):1932-1939.

57. Van der Bijl AE, Goekoop-Ruiterman YP, de Vries-Bouwstra JK, et al. Infliximab and methotrexate as induction therapy in patients with early rheumatoid arthritis. *Arthritis Rheum.* 2007;56(7):2129-2134.

58. Sandborn WJ, Colombel JF, Enns R, et al. Natalizumab induction and maintenance therapy for Crohn's disease. *N Engl J Med.* 2005;353(18):1912-1925.

59. Poppers DM, Scherl EJ. Prophylaxis against *Pneumocystis pneumonia* in patients with inflammatory bowel disease: toward a standard of care. *Inflamm Bowel Dis.* 2008;14(1):106-113.

60. D'Haens G, Colombel J-F, Hommes D, et al. Corticosteroids pose an increased risk for serious infection: an interim safety analysis of the ENCORE registry. *Gastroenterology.* 2008;134:A-140[abstract 946].

61. Mazurek GH, Jereb J, Lobue P, Iademarco MF, Metchock B, Vernon A; Division of Tuberculosis Elimination, National Center for HIV, STD, and TB Prevention, Centers for Disease Control and Prevention (CDC). Guidelines for using the QuantiFERON-TB Gold test for detecting *Mycobacterium tuberculosis* infection, United States. *MMWR Recomm Rep.* 2005;54(RR-15):49-55.

62. Barnes PF, Cave MD. Molecular epidemiology of tuberculosis. *N Engl J Med.* 2003;349(12):1149-1156.

63. Centers for Disease Control and Prevention. Historical perspectives centennial: Koch's discovery of the tubercle bacillus. *MMWR.* 1982;31(10):121-123.

64. Sartor RB. Intestinal microflora in human and experimental inflammatory bowel disease. *Curr Opin Gastroenterol.* 2001;17(4):324-330.

65. D'Haens GR, Geboes K, Peeters M, Baert F, Penninckx F, Rutgeerts P. Early lesions of recurrent Crohn's disease caused by infusion of intestinal contents in excluded ileum. *Gastroenterology.* 1998;114(2):262-267.

66. Swidsinski A, Ladhoff A, Pernthaler A, et al. Mucosal flora in inflammatory bowel disease. *Gastroenterology.* 2002;122(1):44-54.

67. Darfeuille-Michaud A, Boudeau J, Bulois P, et al. High prevalence of adherent-invasive *Escherichia coli* associated with ileal mucosa in Crohn's disease. *Gastroenterology.* 2004;127(2):412-421.

68. Baumgart M, Dogan B, Rishniw M, et al. Culture independent analysis of ileal mucosa reveals a selective increase in invasive Escherichia coli of novel phylogeny relative to depletion of *Clostridiales* in Crohn's disease involving the ileum. *ISME J.* 2007;1(5):403-418.

69. Cummings CA, Relman DA. Genomics and microbiology: microbial forensics—'cross-examining pathogens'. *Science.* 2002;296:1976-1979.

70. Cho JH. The genetics and immunopathogenesis of inflammatory bowel disease. *Nature.* 2008;8:458-466.

71. Noomen CG, Hommes DW, Fidder HH. Update on genetics in inflammatory disease. *Best Pract Res Clin Gastroenterol.* 2009;23(2):233-243.

72. Banchereau J, Steinman RM. Dendritic cells and the control of immunity. *Nature.* 1998;392(6673):245-252.

73. Rescigno M, Urbano M, Valzasina B, et al. Dendritic cells express tight junction proteins and penetrate gut epithelial monolayers to sample bacteria. *Nat Immunol.* 2001;2(4):361-367.

74. Seksik P, Sokol H, Lepage P, et al. The role of bacteria in onset and perpetuation of inflammatory bowel disease. *Aliment Pharmacol Ther.* 2006;24(Suppl 3):11-18.

75. Ayres I. *Super Crunchers: Why Thinking-by-Numbers Is the New Way to Be Smart.* New York, NY: Bantam Dell; 2007:81.

76. Ardizzone S, Cassinotti A, Penati CM, et al. Clinical and endoscopic outcomes after the first corticosteroid course in newly diagnosed ulcerative colitis: a 5-year follow-up inception cohort study. *Gastroenterology.* 2007;132: A-16[abstract 78].

77. Langholz E, Munkholm P, Davidsen M, Binder V. Course of ulcerative colitis: analysis of changes in disease activity over years. *Gastroenterology.* 1994;107(1):3-11.

78. Rutgeerts P, Sandborn WJ, Feagan BG, et al. Infliximab for induction and maintenance therapy for ulcerative colitis. *N Engl J Med.* 2005;353(23):2462-2476.

79. Sands BE, Anderson FH, Bernstein CN, et al. Infliximab maintenance therapy for fistulizing Crohn's disease. *N Engl J Med.* 2004;350(9):876-885.

80. Schnitzler F, Fidder H, Ferrante M, et al. Maintenance Q8 therapy of Crohn's disease with infliximab is associated with endoscopic mucosal healing in the long-term. *Gastroenterology.* 2008;134:A-133[abstract919].

81. Hyams J, Crandall W, Kugathasan S. Induction and maintenance infliximab therapy for the treatment of moderate-to-severe Crohn's disease in children. *Gastroenterology.* 2007;132(3):863-873.

82. Taxonera C, Rodrigo L, Casellas, et al. Infliximab maintenance therapy decreases the use of non-pharmacological resources in patients with Crohn's disease. *Gastroenterology.* 2008;134:A-347[abstract M1141].

83. Yoshimura N, Kawaguchi T, Sako M, Takazoe M. Clinical efficacy of infliximab in the management of postsurgical recurring Crohn's disease. *Gastroenterology.* 2008;134:abstract T1051.

84. Beaugerie L, Seksik P, Nion-Larmurier I, Gendre JP, Cosnes J. Predictors of Crohn's disease. *Gastroenterology.* 2006;130(3):650-656.

85. Barreiro M, Aurelio L, Mera J. Prospective, open pilot study for evaluating the clinical efficacy and mucosal healing rate of infliximab in steroid-dependent ulcerative colitis. *Gastroenterology.* 2008;134:A-667[abstract W1262].

86. Present DH, Sandborn WJ, Rutgeerts PJ, et al. Infliximab treatment for ulcerative colitis: Clinical response, clinical remission, and mucosal healing in patients with moderate or severe disease in the active ulcerative colitis trials (ACT1 & ACT2). *Gastroenterology.* 2008;134:A-493[abstract T1142].

87. Sandborn WJ, Rutgeerts P, Feagan BG, et al. Infliximab reduces colectomy in patients with moderate-to-severe ulcerative colitis: colectomy analysis from ACT 1 and ACT 2. *Gut.* 2007;56(Suppl 3):A26.

88. Targan SR, Feagan BG, Fedorak RN, est al. Natalizumab for the treatment of active Crohn's disease: results of the ENCORE Trial. *Gastroenterology.* 2007;132(5):1672-1683.

89. Sandborn WJ, Colombel JF, Enns R, et al, and the International Efficacy of Natalizumab as Active Crohn's Therapy (ENACT-1) Trial Group and Evaluation of Natalizumab as Continuous Therapy (ENACT-2) Trial Group. Natalizumab induction and maintenance therapy for Crohn's disease. *N Engl J Med.* 2005;353(18):1912-1925.

90. Colombel JF, Prantera C, Rutgeerts PJ, et al. No new safety signals identified in Crohn's disease patients treated with infliximab in an interim review of the ENCORE registry. *Gastroenterology.* 2008;134:A-472[abstract T1048].

91. Maser EA, Deconda D, Lichtiger S, et al. Cyclosporine (CSA) and infliximab (INF) as acute salvage therapies for each other, in severe steroid refractory ulcerative colitis. *Gastroenterology.* 2007;132 (Suppl 2):S1132[abstract 180].

92. Schwartz LK, Kim MK, Coleman M, Lichtiger S, Chadburn A, Scherl E. Case report: lymphoma arising in an ileal pouch anal anastomosis after immunomodulatory therapy for inflammatory bowel disease. *Clin Gastroenterol Hepatol.* 2006;4(8):1030-1034.

93. Rosh JR, Gross T, Mamula P, Griffiths A, Hyams J. Hepatosplenic T-cell lymphoma in adolescents and young adults with Crohn's disease: a cautionary tale? *Inflamm Bowel Dis.* 2007;13(8):1024-1030.

94. Michelassi F, Taschieri A, Tonelli F, et al. An international, multicenter, prospective, observational study of the side-to-side isoperistaltic strictureplasty in Crohn's disease. *Dis Colon Rectum.* 2007;50(3):277-284.

95. Michelassi F, Milsom JW (eds). *Operative Strategies in Inflammatory Bowel Disease.* New York, NY: Springer-Verlag; 1999.

96. Lander ES, Linton LM, Birren B, et al. Initial sequencing and analysis of the human genome. *Nature.* 2001;409(6822):860-921.

97. Venter JC, Adams MD, Myers EW, et al. The sequence of the human genome. *Science.* 2001;291(5507):1304-1351.

98. Jasny BR, Roberts L. Building on the DNA revolution. *Science.* 2003;300:277-296.

99. Kevles D, Hood L, eds. *The Code of Codes: Scientific and Social Issues in the Human Genome Project.* Cambridge, Mass: Harvard University Press; 1992:3-363.

INDEX

abscesses
    in Crohn's disease, 216–217, 218
    surgical drainage of, 222
adalimumab
    for Crohn's disease in elderly patients, 197
    in erectile dysfunction, 187
    during pregnancy, 166, 169
    risks of, 233–234, 255
adenocarcinoma, bowel, 207
adolescents
    IBD hallmark in, 119
    inflammatory bowel disease in, 119–123
        management of, 120–121
    long-term care in, 210–211
adult medical setting, 128
Africa
    dietary changes and IBD incidence in, 25–26
    IBD incidence and prevalence in, 22, 23
aging, effects of, 193–198
Americans with Disabilities Act of 1990, 122
aminosalicylates
    in combination versus monotherapy, 237
    in developing world, 26
    in elderly patients, 196
    risks of, 233
anastomosis, 222, 252. *See also* ileal pouch anal anastomosis (IPAA)
anti-TNF agents, 251–252, 254
    for Crohn's disease in elderly patients, 197
    male infertility and, 155–156
    during pregnancy and nursing, 166
    risks of, 233–234
    trials of, 235, 247
antibiotics, 253
    during pregnancy, 170
anticytokine monoclonal antibodies, 45
anxiety, in adolescents, 121
appendectomy, protective effect of, 25
arthritis, 8
Asia, IBD incidence and prevalence in, 21–23
at-risk patients, colorectal cancer prevention in, 209–210
ATG16L1 gene, 74, 253
autoimmune disease, 25, 57–58
autophagy, 74–75
azathioprine, 247–248
    adverse effects of, 255
    long-term use of, 208
    during pregnancy, 166, 168

    sperm and, 155

bacterial colonization, 33, 38–40
bacterial infection, 252–253
balsalazide, 167
Bifidobacterium, 25–26
biologics
    complications of, 206
    in early therapy, 255
    for IBD in developing world, 26
    outcomes and adverse effects of, 255
    risks of, 232–235
bisphosphonates, 109–110
body composition, in medication responsiveness, 93–95
bone
    biopsy of, 105
    density of, 209
    metabolic disease of in elderly patients, 198
    normal physiology of, 101–103
bone cells, 101–102
bone loss. *See also* osteoporosis
    age-related, 102
    mechanisms of, 107–110
bone mass
    deficits in, 106
    deficits of, 103–104
    evaluation of, 102–103
    peak, 102
    therapies to increase, 109–110
bone mass density (BMD), 103
bone modeling/remodeling, 102
bone turnover markers, 104–105
bowel habits, in adolescents, 122
breastfeeding
    IBD medications and, 171
    in pediatric IBD, 60
budesonide
    in elderly patients, 197
    during pregnancy, 166, 167–168

calcium
    bone loss and, 107
    bone mass and, 109–110
    for metabolic bone disease, 198
cancer, IBD related, 207
carbohydrates
    in IBD, 25–26
    in pediatric IBD, 59–60

Scherl EJ, Dubinsky MC.
*The Changing World of Inflammatory Bowel Disease:
Impact of Generation, Gender, and Global Trends (pp 261-270)*
© 2009 SLACK Incorporated.

WAIT
...There's More!

SLACK Incorporated's Health Care Books and Journals offers a wide selection of products in the field of Gastroenterology. We are dedicated to providing important works that educate, inform and improve the knowledge of our customers. Don't miss out on our other informative titles that will enhance your collection.

The exciting and unique *Curbside Consultation Series* is designed to effectively provide gastroenterologists with practical, to the point, evidence based answers to the questions most frequently asked during informal consultations between colleagues.

Each specialized book included in the *Curbside Consultation Series* offers quick access to current medical information with the ease and convenience of a conversation. Expert consultants who are recognized leaders in their fields provide their advice, preferences, and solutions to 49 of the most frequent clinical dilemmas in gastroenterology.

Written with a similar reader-friendly Q and A format and including images, diagrams, and references, each book in the *Curbside Consultation Series* will serve as a solid, go-to reference for practicing gastroenterologists and residents alike.

Series Editor: Francis A. Farraye, MD, MSc, FACP, FACG

Curbside Consultation of the Colon: 49 Clinical Questions
Brooks D. Cash MD, FACP, CDR, MC, USN
208 pp., Soft Cover, 2009, ISBN 13 978-1-55642-831-9, Order #78316, **$79.95**

Curbside Consultation in Endoscopy: 49 Clinical Questions
Joseph Leung MD; Simon Lo MD
250 pp., Soft Cover, 2009, ISBN 13 978-1-55642-817-3, Order #78170, **$79.95**

Curbside Consultation in GERD: 49 Clinical Questions
Philip Katz MD
192 pp., Soft Cover, 2008, ISBN 13 978-1-55642-818-0, Order #78189, **$79.95**

Curbside Consultation in IBD: 49 Clinical Questions
David Rubin MD; Sonia Friedman MD; Francis A. Farraye MD
240 pp., Soft Cover, 2009, ISBN 13 978-1-55642-856-2, Order #78562, **$79.95**

Curbside Consultation of the Liver: 49 Clinical Questions
Mitchell Shiffman MD
272 pp., Soft Cover, 2008, ISBN 13 978-1-55642-815-9, Order #78154, **$79.95**

Curbside Consultation of the Pancreas: 49 Clinical Questions
Scott Tenner MD, MPH; Alphonso Brown MD, MS Clin Epi; Frank Gress MD
272 pp., Soft Cover, 2009, ISBN 13 978-1-55642-814-2, Order #78146, **$79.95**

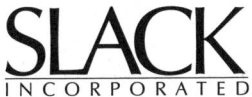